Panic and Phobias 2

Treatments and Variables Affecting Course and Outcome

Edited by
Iver Hand and Hans-Ulrich Wittchen

Foreword by G.L. Klerman

Epilogue by I.M. Marks

Springer-Verlag
Berlin Heidelberg New York
London Paris Tokyo

Iver Hand, Prof. Dr. med
Psychiatrische Universitätsklinik
Verhaltenstherapie - Ambulanz
Martinistraße 52
D-2000 Hamburg 20

Hans-Ulrich Wittchen, Prof. Dr. phil., Dipl.-Psych.
Universität Mannheim
Klinische Psychologie and
Max Planck Institut für Psychiatrie
Unit for Evaluation Research
Kraepelinstraße 10
D-8000 München 40

ISBN-13:978-3-642-73545-5 e-ISBN-13:978-3-642-73543-1
DOI: 10.1007/978-3-642-73543-1

Softcover reprint of the hardcover 1st edition 1988

2125/3140/543210

Preface

Behavioral and biological research in recent years have produced partially contradictory treatment results and recommendations for phobias with and without panic attacks, for panic disorder, and for anxiety disorders in a broader sense.

The new classification of anxiety disorders in both DSM-III (1980) and its revision DSM-IIIR (1987), which gives panic attacks a key role with regard to etiology, differential diagnoses, and treatment has not only stimulated research in this field but has also provoked growing controversy among clinicians and researchers. Biologically oriented authors have interpreted anxiety disorders with panic attacks as "endogenous" disorders linked to depression, claiming pharmacological treatments to be the essential interventions. The concept of panic attacks has recently been expanded even further by its new operationalization in DSM-IIIR. In the future, it will be applied to almost all kinds of anxiety disorders, as long as they involve at least one attack-like event followed by a persistent anticipatory fear of further such attacks.

On the other hand, over the past two decades a vast number of carefully controlled, clinical studies have accumulated evidence that phobias, including agoraphobia with and without panic attacks, can in the majority of cases be successfully treated with behavioral methods, such as exposure in vivo (most recent review by Marks 1987). For acute panic states in the context of phobic responses, effective behavioral techniques were developed already in the early 1970s (Hand et al. 1974) and have proved extremely successful in long-term follow-ups (Hand et al. 1986). The occurrence of panic attacks independent of phobic trigger situations is almost never mentioned as an obstacle to the effective behavioral therapy of phobias.

Until very recently, professional interaction and mutual evaluation regarding these contradictory views and results have been almost non-existent. Together with European and American colleagues, we addressed these questions in a previous volume, examining in more detail the epidemiological, psychopathological, and experimental evidence for each of these positions (Hand and Wittchen 1986).

This new volume has a more intervention-oriented perspective. The time appears to have come for an attempt to resolve some of the treatment controversies: pharmacological research now investigates the effects of both long-term medication and of its discontinuation, while behavioral research has begun to focus on patients who have either failed or dropped out of exposure treatments.

Thus, both the behavioral-cognitive and the biological researchers and clinicans are now ready to face inconsistencies in their theoretical models and failures in their treatment methods. There is now evidence of a growing willingness to engage in joint efforts not only to improve treatments, but also to advance know-

ledge of why a considerable proportion of anxiety patients still refuse, drop out or fail from and relapse after either of these treatment approaches.
The authors of this book met at an international Symposium at the Ringberg Castle in Bavaria (sponsored by the Max Planck Society) to engage in intensive discussions of behavioral, cognitive, and biological treatments of anxiety disorders. This joint venture definitely broadened views and modified initial cautious interactions into an open-minded and productive exchange of knowledge and opinions.
Panic and Phobias II is the outcome of this exciting conference and evaluates in detail not only those behavioral, cognitive, and pharmacological treatments that are currently best elaborated, but also the most promising new research in this field. This book does not however provide final answers to the question "What is the best treatment?," but it does give the most current and comprehensive description of results in the three major areas of research relevant to the treatment of anxiety disorders.
We hope that the very fact that the many authors in this book partly use the same data to draw conclusions that differ in part from one another will also stimulate the reader to join the discussion for the welfare of the patients.

References

Hand I, Lamontagne Y, Marks IM (1974) Group exposure (flooding) in vivo for agoraphobics. Br J Psychiatry 124:588–602

Hand I, Wittchen HU (eds) (1986) Panic and phobias. Empirical evidence of theoretical models and longterm effects of behavorial treatments. Springer, Berlin Heidelberg New York

Hand I, Angenendt J, Fischer M, Wilke C (1986) Exposure in vivo with panic management for agoraphobia: treatment rationale and longterm outcome. In: Hand I, Wittchen HU (eds) Panic and phobias. Empirical evidence of theoretical models and longterm effects of behavioral treatments. Springer, Berlin Heidelberg New York

Marks IM (1987) Fears, phobias and rituals. Panic, anxiety, and their disorders. Oxford University Press, New York

Iver Hand
Hans-Ulrich Wittchen

Foreword

Sources of Current Controversies in Treatment of Panic and Phobia

G. L. KLERMAN[1]

In reviewing advances in a scientific field, the conventional wisdom holds that progress occurs in a linear fashion through incremental new knowledge. This view of the history of science as a rational and progressive process has been challenged by many observers, notably Thomas Kuhn, the philosopher and historian of science at Princeton University, who views progress in a scientific field not so much as the rational accumulation of new knowledge arrived at by dispassionate scientists; rather, he believes that the history of a field is punctuated by periods of ferment and revolution during which competing theories and groups of scientists adhering to these theories (which Kuhn calls "paradigms") contend with each other until, subsequently, one paradigm emerges triumphant.

The field of anxiety is a current example of this process. For many decades, there was a consensus that anxiety in normal and clinical states was aligned on a continuum of severity. This view, which I have called the "continuum model," was accepted by otherwise competing theories - behavioral, psychodynamic, biological - and was embodied in most classifications of mental disorders and in textbooks of psychiatry and psychology.

[1] Professor of Psychiatry and Associate Chairman for Research, Department of Psychiatry, Cornell University Medical College, c/o Payne Whitney Clinic, 525 East 68th Street, New York, NY 10021, USA

During the 1960s and 1970s, the continuum model was challenged by a number of sources. This challenge resulted in revision of the USA classification as promulgated by the American Psychiatric Association in its third edition of the Diagnostic and Statistical Manual (DSM-III). Subsequently, controversies have erupted concerning the nature of anxiety disorders, their etiology and pathogenesis, and the most suitable and effective methods for their treatment. Currently, this controversy involves the conflicting views held by adherents of a biological paradigm and a behavioral paradigm.

In the midst of this controversy, the 1987 Ringberg Conference brought together many of the leading investigators in this field to share ideas and, hopefully, to reconcile differences and formulate a consensus as to the treatment of panic and phobias. While the goal of formulating a consensus was only partially realized, the papers in this volume capture the ferment in the field and offer the reader insight into efforts to resolve the controversies relating to treatment.

The Continuum Model and Its Discontents

It is of note that this continuum view was held by the advocates of three different theoretical paradigms - biological, psychoanalytic, and behavioral - which emerged between World War I and World

War II and which offered both competing explanations for the origin of anxiety and extensively different treatment recommendations. All three paradigms accepted the continuum model.

This continuum model was also the basis for the official diagnostic classification systems - the ICD 8 and 9 - developed by the World Health Organization (WHO), as well as the first and second editions of the Diagnostic and Statistical Manual of the American Psychiatric Association (DSM-I and DSM-II).

The continuum theory came under increasing criticism during the 1960s and 1970s. The discontent with the continuum model derived from two lines of investigation, psychopathological and therapeutic.

Psychopathological investigations, particularly in the United Kingdom, led to an increasingly differentiated view of anxiety states. Roth and his associates at Newcastle applied multivariate statistical techniques, particularly discriminant function and factor analysis, to interview data and rating scales involving large numbers of neurotic patients. These techniques generated evidence for the separation of anxiety states from depressive states and, within the depressive states, for the separation of endogenous depression from neurotic depression. Marks and Gelder proposed a three-way classification of phobias distinguishing among simple phobias, social phobias, and agoraphobia. The agoraphobic syndrome came under increasing clinical attention and the clinical utility of the syndrome was partially validated by factor analytic studies which identified a cluster of common situations precipitating agoraphobia, notably those involving public transportation, shops and markets, cinemas and theater, and other public gatherings.

Therapeutic investigations proceeded in two directions: first, the emergence of behavioral therapeutic techniques which challenged psychoanalysis and psychodynamic psychotherapy and, secondly, the demonstration of the efficacy of selected psychopharmacological agents for anxiety states.

Psychotherapeutic theory and practice, particularly in North America, had been strongly influenced by psychoanalytic and psychodynamic ideas and methods during and after World War II. After World War II, behaviorally derived techniques such as relaxation, desensitization, exposure in imagery, exposure in vivo, and flooding emerged. These treatments were supported by the growing advances in learning theory, particularly those following the ideas of B.F. Skinner. Many new techniques were developed and applied with increasing success to neurotic conditions such as anxiety states, phobias (including agoraphobia), obsessions and compulsions, and sexual dysfunctions. In many clinical centers, particularly in the United Kingdom and Australia and New Zealand, behavioral techniques became the standard forms of psychotherapy of neuroses.

In parallel, diverse psychopharmacological agents were applied to the treatment of anxiety states. The most widely prescribed group of anti-anxiety agents, the benzodiazepines, were mainly useful for situational generalized anxiety. The conventional wisdom among experienced psychopharmacologists was that the benzodiazepines have limited efficacy in agoraphobia and other phobic conditions, obsessions, compulsions, and dissociative states. In this context, a number of reports about atypical depression appeared in which anxiety and phobic symptoms were prominent, being responsive to monoamine oxidase (MAO) inhibitors.

The contributions of Donald Klein were of major importance. Klein documented the efficacy of imipramine against agoraphobia and elaborated upon his observations about the important role played by panic attacks in the psychopathogenesis of agoraphobia. Thus, by the latter part of the 1970s, the continuum view had no longer proven viable, and alternative views emphasized multiple clinical anxiety states and both psychotherapeutic and pharmacological treatments in the treatment of anxiety conditions.

The Impact of DSM-III

The promulgation in 1980 by the American Psychiatric Association of the DSM-III served as a watershed in the development of theory, research, and procedure about anxiety and anxiety disorders in general and panic and phobias in particular. The DSM-III broke with established tradition in a number of important ways; applied to anxiety disorders, two important features of the DSM-III are noteworthy.

First, the DSM-III discontinued the time-honored category of neurotic conditions. For eight decades, almost all diagnostic and classification systems of mental disorders distinguished between organic and functional states, and within the functional or nonorganic states, the major diagnostic separation was between psychoses and neuroses. The psychotic-neurotic distinction had implications for description, etiology, locus of treatment, and type of treatment. The psychoses were considered to be caused by constitutional or biological factors, manifested clinically by delusion, hallucinations, dementia, or other serious impairments of higher mental functions discontinuous with normal experience and justifying hospitalization, often involuntary hospitalization with civil commitment. Where treatments were available, they were almost always somatic treatments, such as electroconvulsive therapy, or, in earlier decades, insulin coma treatment, or such drastic interventions as lobotomy and other forms of psychosurgery.

In contrast, the neuroses were believed to be due to environmental causes, including psychological conflict at the conscious or unconscious level or to problems of learning and conditioning. Their treatment was expected to take place in outpatient settings, with hospitalization required only on infrequent occasions and for brief durations. When treatment was available, it would be psychotherapy, behavioral, psychodynamic, individual, or group.

Instead of a single overriding category of neurotic conditions, DSM-III proposed a series of new categories: "affective disorders," "anxiety disorders," "eating disorders," "psychosexual disorders," etc. The grouping together of different disorders into these categories did not represent any presumption as to a common etiology; rather, the categories were based on vigor presenting symptoms, in the case of anxiety disorders, presentations due to tension, anxiety, and fears.

Most controversial in the reclassification of anxiety disorders was the separation of panic disorder from generalized anxiety. The separation of anxiety neurosis into panic disorder and generalized anxiety had been incorporated in the Research Diagnostic Criteria (RDC) developed for use in the NIMH Collaborative Program on the Psychobiology of Depression and increasingly applied in clinical studies in the 1970s and also in the community epidemiological surveys. Furthermore, the pathogenic linkage between panic anxiety and agoraphobia was highlighted, and two forms of agoraphobia were included within the category of anxiety disorders - panic disorder with agoraphobia and agoraphobia without panic disorder. However, the DSM-III narrative clearly indicated that the expectation was that agoraphobia without panic attacks was to be considered as a nonexistent or, at best, rare condition.

For the most part, this controversy over the DSM-III approach has led to stimulating investigations in epidemiology, family and genetic disorders, and clinic psychopathology.

The most extensive and intense controversies have been in the area of treatment. The focus of controversy is now in the relative merits of behavioral and cognitive psychotherapeutic techniques versus psychopharmacological methods. Interpreting the content of these controversies is made difficult by the confounding of scientific and professional issues. The advocates of behavioral and cognitive techniques tend to be Ph.D. psychologists, while the advocates of psychopharmacological agents are the M.D. psychiatrists. Moreover, issues of the efficacy of specific treatments are related to general theories of causation, with the psychopharmacologists emphasizing a genetically determined abnormality of CNS chemistry as the predisposition and minimizing environmental and cognitive factors. In contrast, the behavior therapists emphasize the role of learning and situational and environmental cues and minimize the possible role of endogenous physiological abnormalities.

These therapeutic differences are often extended to issues of diagnosis, nosology, and classification. For the most part, the advocates of behavior therapy have been hesitant to accept the nosologic separation of panic anxiety from generalized anxiety and tend to emphasize the continuity of normal and clinical anxiety, regarding panic as the more intense form of anxiety. In contrast, the biological theorists emphasize the discontinuity between panic anxiety and normal states and the uniqueness of the subjective experience and biology of the panic attack.

Future Directions

As stated in their introduction, Wittchen and Hand, the organizers of the conference and the editors of this volume, had expected that the available evidence would allow a consensus to emerge. The opposing points of view are represented in this volume, and the alternative interpretations of available data are presented in articulate and reasoned fashion. The first part of their expectation was well realized: The individual papers capture the current diversity of the field. However, in the area of therapeutics, the main focus of this volume, it is evident that further research is necessary before the issues will be resolved. Carefully designed studies are needed in the following areas:

1. Evaluation of pharmacological treatments as compared with placebo controls
2. Carefully designed controlled studies of behavioral treatment as compared with creditable psychological controls
3. Comparative studies of drugs as related to psychological treatments
4. Studies of combined drug and psychological treatment
5. Long-term studies to assess relapse, recurrence, and psychosocial functioning
6. Studies to improve design and methodology

Seen in the context of both the historical background and the ongoing scientific disputes, this volume provides the reader with an excellent assortment of current investigations in Western Europe and North America. High-quality research is under way based on investigations from a variety of theoretical backgrounds and disciplines. One looks forward to future reports similar to this. The quality of investigations continues to improve, the issues become more sharply defined, and the results are more precisely interpreted. Until results of such studies are available, this volume provides the state of the art in anxiety research.

Contents

Part III: Specific Variables Affecting Mode of Treatment: Experimental Studies on Physiology and Cognition

Part IV: Specific Variables Affecting Treatment Outcome of Anxiety Disorders: Clinical, Psychosocial, and Interactional Factors

Epilogue:

List of Contributors

Prof. Dr. med MANFRED ACKENHEIL
Nervenklinik der Universität München
Nußbaumstraße 7
8000 München 2
Federal Republic of Germany

Dr. med. Dr. MARGOT ALBUS
Nervenklinik der Universität München
Nußbaumstraße 7
8000 München 2
Federal Republic of Germany

PAVLOS ANASTASIADES, B.Sc.
University of Oxford
Department of Psychiatry
Warneford Hospital
Oxford OX3 7JX
Great Britain

Prof. GAVIN ANDREWS, M.D.
Clinical Research Unit for
Anxiety Disorders
St. Vincent's Hospital
299 Forbes Street
Darlinghurst NSW 2010
Australia

JÖRG ANGENENDT, Dipl.-Psych.
Max-Planck-Institut für Psychiatrie
Kraepelinstraße 10
8000 München 40
Federal Republic of Germany

GORDON G. BALL, Ph. D.
Payne Whitney Clinic
(Cornell University)
525 E. 68th Street
New York, New York
U.S.A.

PROF. DAVID H. BARLOW, Ph.D.
Department of Psychology
State University of New York at Albany
1400 Washington Avenue
Albany, New York 12222
U.S.A.

PROF. DR. MED. OTTO BENKERT
Psychiatrische Klinik und Poliklinik
der Universität Mainz
Langenbeckstraße 1
6500 Mainz
Federal Republic of Germany

Dr. med. STEFAN BRAUNE
Nervenklinik der Universität München
Nußbaumstraße 7
8000 München 2
Federal Republic of Germany

Prof. Dr. med. Dr. rer. nat.
JOHANNES C. BRENGELMAN, Ph.D.
Max-Planck-Institut für Psychiatrie
Kraepelinstraße 10
8000 München 40
Federal Republic of Germany

HEIDRUN BÜTTNER-WESTPHAL, Dipl.-Psych.
Psychiatrische Universitätsklinik
Behavior Therapy Outpatient Unit
Martinistraße 52
2000 Hamburg 20
Federal Republic of Germany

Dr. med. RAIMUND BULLER
Psychiatrische Klinik und Poliklinik
der Universität Mainz
Langenbeckstraße 1
6500 Mainz
Federal Republic of Germany

JEROME A. CERNY, Ph.D.
Department of Psychology
State University of New York at Albany
1400 Washington Avenue
Albany, New York 12222
U.S.A.

Prof. DIANNE L. CHAMBLESS, Ph.D.
Department of Psychology
The American University
Asbury Building
Washington, D.C. 20016
U.S.A.

DAVID M. CLARK, Ph.D.
Department of Psychiatry
Oxford University
Warneford Hospital
Oxford OX3 7JX
Great Britain

Dr. phil. ANKE EHLERS, Dipl.-Psych.
Fachbereich Psychologie
Philipps-Universität Marburg
Gutenbergstraße 18
3550 Marburg/Lahn
Federal Republic of Germany

Prof. PAUL EMMELKAMP, Ph. D.
Akademisch Siekenhuis
Klinische Psychologie
Groningen Vakgroep
Oostersingel 59
9713 EZ Groningen
The Netherlands

Prof. Dr. rer. nat. ROLF ENGEL, Dipl.-Psych.
Nervenklinik der Universität München
Nußbaumstraße 7
8000 München 2
Federal Republic of Germany

PD Dr. WOLFGANG FIEGENBAUM, Dipl.-Psych.
Fachbereich Psychologie
Philipps-Universität Marburg
Gutenbergstraße 18
3550 Marburg/Lahn
Federal Republic of Germany

MARTINA FISCHER, Dipl.-Psych.
Psychiatrische Universitätsklinik
Behavior Therapy Outpatient Unit
Martinistraße 52
2000 Hamburg 20
Federal Republik of Germany

Prof. EDNA B. FOA, Ph.D.
The Medical College of Pennsylvania
Department of Psychiatry
3200 Henry Avenue
Philadelphia, Pennsylvania 19129
U.S.A.

ABBY FYER, M. D.
Office of Mental Health
New York State/Psychiatric Institute
722 West 168th Street
New York, New York 10032
U.S.A.

Prof. Dr. MICHAEL GELDER
University of Oxford
Department of Psychiatry
Warneford Hospital
Oxford OX3 7JX
Great Britain

BONNIE GITLIN, MSW
Payne Whitney Clinic
Cornell University
525 E. 68th Street
New York, New York
U.S.A.

EDWARD J. GRACELY, Ph.D.
The American University
Department of Psychology
Asbury Building
Washington, D.C. 20016
U.S.A.

ANN HACKMANN, M.Sc.
University of Oxford
Department of Psychiatry
Warneford Hospital
Oxford OX3 7JX
Great Britain

Dr. med. JOACHIM HALLMAYER
Psychiatrische Klinik und Poliklinik
Universität Mainz
Langenbeckstraße 1
6500 Mainz
Federal Republic of Germany

Prof. Dr. med. IVER HAND
Psychiatrische Universitätsklinik
Behavior Therapy Outpatient Unit
Martinistraße 52
2000 Hamburg 20
Federal Republic of Germany

Dr. med. L. HARTL
Max-Planck-Institut für Psychiatrie
Kraepelinstraße 10
8000 München 40
Federal Republic of Germany

Prof. M. A. VAN DEN HOUT, Ph.D.
Mental Health Sciences/
Experimental Psychopathology
University of Limburg
P.O. Box 616
6200 Maastricht
The Netherlands

ANNE JEAVONS, B.A.
University of Oxford
Department of Psychiatry
Warneford Hospital
Oxford OX3 7JX
Great Britain

STEPHEN C. JOSEPHSON, Ph.D.
Payne Whitney Clinic
Cornell University
525 E. 68th Street
New York, New York
U.S.A.

JANET S. KLOSKO, Ph.D.
Department of Psychology
State University of New York at Albany
1400 Washington Avenue
Albany, New York 12222
U.S.A.

CATHARINE KOEHLER, B.Sc.
University of Oxford
Department of Psychiatry
Warneford Hospital
Oxford OX3 7JX
Great Britain

Dr. med. WOLFGANG MAIER, Dipl.-Psych.
Psychiatrische Klinik und Poliklinik
Universität Mainz
Langenbeckstraße 1
6500 Mainz
Federal Republic of Germany

CHRISTA MANECKE, Dipl.-Psych.
Psychiatirsche Universitätsklinik
Behavior Therapy Outpatient Unit
Martinistraße 52
2000 Hamburg 20
Federal Republik of Germany

Dr. phil. JÜRGEN MARGRAF, Dipl.-Psych.
Fachbereich Psychologie
Philipps-Universität Marburg
Gutenbergstraße 18
3550 Marburg/Lahn
Federal Republic of Germany

Prof. Dr. ISAAC M. MARKS
Institute of Psychiatry
Maudsly Hospital
De Crespigny Park
London SE5 8AF
Great Britain

MERRYANNE MARTIN, Ph.D.
University of Oxford
Department of Experimental Psychology
South Parks RD
Oxford OX1 3PS
Great Britain

Prof. ANDREW MATHEWS, Ph.D.
Department of Psychology
St. George's Hospital Medical School
Cranmer Terrace
London SW17 ORE
Great Britain

Prof. MATIG R. MAVISSAKALIAN, M.D.
The Ohio State University
Department of Psychiatry
473 West 12th Avenue
Columbus, Ohio 43210-1228
U.S.A.

HUGH MIDDLETON, M.D.
University of Oxford
Department of Psychiatry
Warneford Hospital
Oxford OX3 7JX
Great Britain

CARMEN MORAN, M.D.
Clinical Research Unit for
Anxiety Disorders
St. Vincent's Hospital
299 Forbes Street
Darlinghurst NSW 2010
Australia

Dr. med. HELMUT PETER
Psychiatrische Universitätsklinik
Behavior Therapy Outpatient Unit
Martinistraße 52
2000 Hamburg 20
Federal Republik of Germany

Prof. WALTON T. ROTH, M.D.
Stanford University School of Medicine
Department of Psychiatry (116A3)
Palo Alto V.A. Medical Center
3801 Miranda Ave.
Palo Alto, California 94304
U.S.A.

PAUL M. SALKOVSKIS, Ph.D.
University of Oxford
Department of Psychiatry
Warneford Hospital
Oxford OX3 71X
Great Britain

CATHY SHEAR, M.D.
Payne Whitney Clinic
Cornell University
525 E. 68th Street
New York, New York
U.S.A.

MURRAY B. STEIN, M.D.
National Institute of Mental Health
NIMH, Intramural Program Building 10
9000 Rockville Pyke
Bethesda, Maryland
U.S.A.

Prof. GAIL STEKETEE, Ph.D.
Boston University
School of Social Work
264 Bay State Road
Boston, Massachusetts 02215
U.S.A.

PD Dr. med. FRIEDRICH STRIAN
Max-Planck-Institut für Psychiatrie
Kraepelinstraße 10
8000 München 40
Federal Republic of Germany

ROBIN B. TASSINARI, Ph.D.
Department of Psychology
State University of New York at Albany
1400 Washington Avenue
Albany, New York 1222
U.S.A.

THOMAS UHDE, M.D.
National Institute of Mental Health
NIMH, Intramural Program Building 10
9000 Rockville Pyke
Bethesda, Maryland
U.S.A.

Prof. Dr. phil. HANS-ULRICH WITTCHEN,
Dipl.-Psych., Universität Mannheim,
Klinische Psychologie and
Max-Planck-Institut für Psychiatrie
Unit of Evaluation Research
Kraepelinstraße 10
8000 München 40
Federal Republic of Germany

Dr. med. ANDREAS ZELLNER
Nervenklinik der Universität München
Nußbaumstraße 7
8000 München 2
Federal Republic of Germany

Acknowledgments

We are most grateful for the support of the Max Planck Gesellschaft and Professor Dr. Johannes C. Brengelmann, Director at the Max Planck Institute for Psychiatry (Department of Psychology), which allowed us to organize the conference on "Panic and Phobias II - Treatments and Variables Affecting Course and Outcome" at the Ringberg Castle, Oct. 28-31, 1987.

We would like to thank Rita Lindemann, Annemarie Pröbstl, and Elisabeth Schramm for their valuable assistance in the organization of the meeting at the Ringberg Castle and in the preparation of this volume. The excellent cooperation with Springer Verlag, allowing us to publish the outcome of this meeting within a very short period of time, is gratefully acknowledged.

Hamburg and Munich, April 1988

IVER HAND
HANS-ULRICH WITTCHEN

Part I

Psychological or Biological Treatments of Panic and Phobias: Current State of the Controversy

1. Natural Course and Spontaneous Remissions of Untreated Anxiety Disorders: Results of the Munich Follow-up Study (MFS)*

H.-U. WITTCHEN

Introduction: What is the Natural History of Untreated Anxiety Disorders?

Anxiety disorders obviously belong to the most frequent mental disorders both in the community (Robins et al. 1984; Myers et al. 1984; Lépine 1987; Marks 1987; Surtees et al. 1987; Wittchen et al. 1988; Wittchen and Burke, to be published) and in treatment settings (Goldberg 1982; Strian 1983; Marks 1987). They have also been studied extensively with regard to the effectiveness of psychological and pharmacological treatment methods. Little, however, is known about their natural course and the frequency of so-called spontaneous remissions in untreated anxiety disorders. This paper discusses some methodological reasons for this deficit and presents some new, still preliminary results on the natural course of untreated anxiety disorders from a general population survey.

Methodological Considerations

At first sight, the uncertainty about the natural course of different forms of anxiety disorders might be surprising, if one considers the large number of studies in this field, which range from anecdotal remarks to a few prospective long-term epidemiological studies (Table 1). But a closer look at these studies reveals quite a number of deficiencies that hamper considerably a clear answer to the question posed at the beginning of this paper:

Table 1. Sources of information for the evaluation of the natural course (history) of treated and untreated anxiety disorders

- Anecdotal remarks
- Case reports
- Studies on treatment effectiveness
- Follow-up studies (retrospective)
- Epidemiological studies
- Prospective long-term epidemiological studies

- Only very few studies have been conducted in an epidemiological setting with a representative data base, and to our knowledge only one has been done prospectively (Agras et al. 1969, 1972).
- There is a lack of studies with data on the natural course of anxiety disorders that have used a differentiated diagnostic subclassification as suggested by DSM-III and its revision DSM-III-R (APA 1987).
- Reliable diagnostic decisions are difficult to obtain in anxiety disorders without the use of standardized diagnostic procedures (Helzer et al. 1985; Barlow et al. 1986; Semler et al. 1987). The lack of studies using diagnostic instruments with a proven reliability might be regarded as a major problem for the generalization of findings across studies.
- Even large epidemiological studies like the NIMH Epidemiological Catchment Area Program (ECA), designed to cover several waves of

* This study is part of the Munich Follow-up Study (MFS). The MFS was supported by a grant from the Robert Bosch Foundation.

Table 2. Variables affecting course and outcome of disorders

Social, cultural, environmental	**Psychological**	**Biological**
Structure of the (mental) health system	Self-perception	Central and autonomous functions
Sociocultural norms	Individual life style	Degree and duration of biological dysfunctions
Environmental strains and stressors (work, etc.)	Former experience with anxiety and illness	"Spontaneous" remission of the biological dysfunction
Social and technical network/ integration	Goals and aspirations in life	Internal, biological conditioning ("kindling")
Living conditions and arrangements	Attitudes toward disorder	Effects of medication and other biological treatments
Life events and changes of life conditions	Attitudes toward therapy	Adverse therapy effects (biological)
	Emotional arousal and stability	Individual variation in the regeneration capacity of the disturbed functions
External Factors +	Internal factors +	Biological factors = **OUTCOME**

examinations over the years, have inherent problems, such as the issue of the validity of data that are collected by non-clinicians and the degree to which results can be generalized to "true" patient populations.

- There are also a number of specific methodological problems in the evaluation of the long-term course and outcome of a mental disorder, such as the specificity of instruments used for an adequate assessment of the long-term course of symptoms, avoidance behavior, social and psychological aspects, and the use of appropriate indicators of course and outcome.
- Finally, there is a lack of theoretical models that can offer an acceptable framework in which the long-term course can be studied appropriately. This applies particularly to key constructs like vulnerability, risk factors, full and partial remission, relapse, rebound phenomena, comorbidity, chronicity, and intervening biological, social, and psychosocial factors, all of which lack a precise and generally accepted definition. It is frequently forgotten in this context that there is a considerable number of variables – as summarized in Table 2 – potentially affecting remission and the development of chronicity.

Thus, our present knowledge about the natural course of anxiety disorders is heavily dependent on a few retrospective surveys (e.g. Marks and Herst 1970) and numerous treatment studies about the effectiveness of pharmacological and psychological interventions (see Mathews et al. 1981; Lydiard and Ballenger 1987; Sheehan 1987; Marks 1987). These types of studies usually include information about the length of illness history (prior to the index treatment) and follow-up results. These data cannot however be regarded as a sufficiently firm basis for our knowledge about the natural history of anxiety disorders because of the well-documented methodological problems of clinical follow-up studies (differences in the selection of patients, design, length of follow-up period, nosological concepts, diagnostic instruments used, and differences in the criteria for improvement) and because of theoretical considerations. The latter refer to the issue that notions or conclusions about the **natural course of an disorder in a stricter sense** should be based on representative samples – including untreated subjects with a disorder – to allow for a generalization of findings to nonclinical and varying clinical target populations. It is evident that such a requirement cannot be met in clinical treatment studies that primarily test the effectiveness of a given intervention strategy in a sample "of convenience."

Current Assumptions about the Natural Course of Treated Anxiety Disorders

In spite of these restrictions, clinical studies published so far also show a few rather consistent findings: Most **phobic disorders** (ICD-9: Phobia; DSM III: Social Phobia, Simple Phobia, Agoraphobia) seem to start early in the patient's life, often before age of 18 (Marks 1987; Wittchen and von Zerssen 1988), and they tend to persist over many years (Reich 1986). However, we find rather varying indications about the percentage of cases that develop marked avoidance behavior and social restrictions in everyday life. There is some consensus that agoraphobia can be regarded as a distinct syndrome, characterized by a higher average age of onset in the twenties, a less favorable long-term prognosis, and more severe social impairments as compared with social and other specific phobias (Marks 1987; Mathews et al. 1981). Most recent review papers (see Marks 1987; Chaps. 4, 24, this volume) provide rather clear evidence that most phobic disorders profit considerably from different pharmacological and psychological treatment methods. However, some studies also seem to indicate that, even when treatment significantly reduces the degree and severity of anxiety symptoms, avoidance behavior and symptom-related social consequences, mild - often subclinical symptoms of anxiety - tend to persist (Reich 1986; Krieg et al. 1987; Wittchen and von Zerssen 1988); complete remissions seem to be rare.

For pharmacological treatments (antidepressants, benzodiazepines, betablockers, etc.) - although they are quite effective in blocking acute symptoms of anxiety - there is increasing evidence that patients frequently relapse even after an adequate time period of treatment when the administration of the drug is discontinued (see Chaps. 4 and 5, this volume). Behavioral treatments, particularly different kinds of exposure treatments, seem to produce longer-lasting effects over several years (see McPherson et al. 1980; Mathews et al. 1981; Marks 1987).

Some studies even show further improvements for treatment responders during follow-up (Hand et al. 1986). Others, however, caution the generally more optimistic view of behavioral therapists by pointing to the problem of specific selection effects for clinical studies. In addition, it has been suspected that failures of behavior therapies do accumulate in agencies offering successful pharmacological treatments (see Chap. 2, this volume). Data reported by Fischer et al. (Chapter 19, this volume) do not however support this "impression".

Whereas the majority of clinical studies underline the persistence of symptoms and the development of chronicity in anxiety disorders, some authors also entertain a different point of view. Based on clinical experience, they suggest that many, if not most of the anxiety disorders in the community are short-lived, with a high rate of spontaneous remissions (Mathews et al. 1981; Eysenck 1960; Rachman 1973; Jablensky and Hugler 1982).

With regard to **anxiety states** (ICD-9: Anxiety Neurosis; DSM-III: Panic Disorder, Generalized Anxiety Disorder), it is more difficult to make any clear judgments. Reliable indications about their natural course are mainly restricted by the ongoing changes in classification and diagnostic criteria, as well as by the nature and the pattern of psychopathological features in "anxiety states" that often comprise phenomena of both, anxiety and depression (see DSM-III criteria for generalized anxiety disorder; Boyd et al. 1984; Barlow et al. 1986). Additionally, there is still considerable controversy (Jablensky 1985; Hand and Wittchen 1986), whether agoraphobias with panic attacks belong to panic disorder, as suggested by DSM-III-R, or to agoraphobia. Focussing on panic disorder with and without agoraphobia, rather similar results with regard to age of onset (in the late twenties) and the mode of onset (sudden or stuttering), as in agoraphobia, have been reported by some research groups (Mathews et al. 1981). The long-term course seems to be fluctuating, often being punctuated by partial remissions and frequent severe relapses of varying duration (Reich 1986). In the absence of treatment, partial rather than full remission is to be expected according to the results by Marks and Herst (1970). Further, there are indications that spontaneous panic attacks are correlated with general anxiety and depressed mood, with the attacks often diminishing over the years (Breier et al. 1986).

Aims of the Study

The rather inconclusive findings in the literature and the general lack of long-term community follow-up studies for anxiety disorders have stimulated our interest in using data from our prospective and retrospective 7-year Munich Follow-up Study (MFS) to investigate in more detail indicators for the natural course of untreated panic disorders, agoraphobia, simple and social phobia, and obsessive-compulsive disorders. Specifically, the following questions will be dealt with:

1. What is the age of onset of different kinds of anxiety disorders and their mean duration and severity?
2. What percentage of subjects with anxiety disorders receives some kind of intervention by general practitioners or other agencies?
3. Is there an increased risk for developing other mental disorders?
4. What are the typical patterns of the long-term course and outcome of anxiety disorders and their rate of spontaneous remissions.

Methods

Subjects and Design

To answer these questions, data from the epidemiological part of the MFS were used. For comparison, some epidemiological data from the ECA (Regier et al. 1984) were analyzed. The ECA data set used comprises the overall results from five sites (New Haven, Baltimore, Durham, St. Louis, and Los Angeles). For this analysis, only subjects with the same ages of 25–65 as the MFS and only whites were included (see Wittchen and Burke, to be published).

The MFS is a 7-year follow-up study of a general population sample originally consisting of 1366 subjects [wave 1: 1974; wave 2 ($n = 657$ subjects): 1981] and a cohort of former psychiatric inpatients of the Max Planck Institute of Psychiatry in Munich (not dealt with in this paper). Both groups (subjects and former inpatients) were studied within the same design and with the same instruments (Table 3). The MFS data on symptoms and diagnoses of anxiety are based on a two-stage procedure at wave 2 (1981). In this procedure, all subjects in the population were first examined with the full set of instruments by clinical psychologists or psychiatrists; then all high scorers and probable cases were independently reassessed once again by a psychiatrist in order to fully evaluate relevant psychopathological features and the illness history. The data reported here are based primarily on the results of the Diagnostic Interview Schedule (DIS) (Robins et al. 1981; Wittchen et al. 1985), clinical rating scales, and the clinical reexamination of all cases that scored high on the DIS- and/or met any DIS/DSM-III lifetime diagnosis (Wittchen et al. 1983).

Table 3. Some methodological aspects of the Munich Follow-up Study (MFS)

	MFS
General population sample	
Year of wave 1 (and sample size)	1974 ($n = 1501$)
Year of wave 2 (and sample size)	1981 ($n = 657$)
Patient sample	291 former inpatients with different diagnoses including 40 patients with anxiety disorders
Age groups	25–65 years
Case definition	Diagnostic Interview Schedule (DIS) Clinical diagnoses according to the ICD-9 Other clinical scales and comprehensive psychosocial evaluations by clinical interviewers (psychiatrists and psychologists
Data analysis for DSM-III diagnoses	DIS program and DIS variables 6-month, 12-month, and lifetime diagnoses

The clinicians also assigned diagnoses according to the International Classification of Diseases (ICD) and rated clinical course and outcome. Since the MFS has already been described in detail in several other reports (Wittchen and von Zerssen 1988; Wittchen et al. 1983, 1985; Wittchen 1986), further methodological details will not be described in this paper.

The analyses focus on five groups of Anxiety Disorders with the following DSM-III diagnoses: agoraphobia (with [1] and without panic attacks [2], simple or social phobia [3], panic disorder [4], and obsessive-compulsive disorder [5]. DSM-III diagnoses are based on the DIS (Version 2) and were calculated by not using the DSM-III exclusion criteria.

Indicators for the Natural Course

To assess indicators for long-term course and natural history, information was collected by a careful and structured assessment of the time period between the two waves (1974 and 1981), using all sources available to the clinical and nonclinical interviewer in order to cover psychopathological and psychosocial aspects. Specifically, the following indicators were chosen (Table 4):

Table 4. Some indicators for the natural course of anxiety disorders

- Age of onset
- Mean duration of illness
- Severity and psychosocial impairments
- Development of other mental disorders
- Remission rates (symptoms and social impairments)

1. **Age of onset** of the disorder, taken from the DIS, where the patient is asked at what age he first experienced the full clinical picture for one of the anxiety disorders.
2. **Length of illness,** calculated by subtracting the age at the first, from the age at the last manifestation of the disorder. The rating was based on a clinical consensus rating that took into account the age of onset and recency ratings from the DIS, as well as all additional sources of information available (treatment records of health insurance, results taken from the medical and hospital records, etc).
3. **Course of symptoms and characterization of the dominant pattern.** Because age of onset and length of illness are only imprecise "indicators" and not measures for the natural course, the clinical interviewers classified all cases according to the course of key syndromes, their

severity, and persistence. In this paper, cases were assigned to one of the following three types of course: chronic, episodic with no full remission, episodic with full remission. The latter type also includes the remitted cases.

Results

Prevalence of Anxiety Disorders and Comorbidity

Table 5 shows the weighted and adjusted DIS/DSM-III lifetime prevalence rates for anxiety disorders, as found in the ECA and the MFS. There are no significant differences between the two studies. In both studies, anxiety disorders belong to the most frequent mental disorders. There is a marked female preponderance, especially for DSM-III diagnoses of simple and social phobia (Wittchen et al. 1988; Wittchen and Burke, to be published; Myers et al. 1984; Robins et al. 1984). Altogether, 77 subjects in the general population survey fulfilled criteria for at least one of the DSM-III anxiety disorders.

For lifetime diagnoses, a considerable overlap within the anxiety disorders (Fig. 1) was found. Only 26 (33.8%) out of 77 cases had "pure" anxiety disorders. Only one case involving panic disorder and no case with obsessive-compulsive disorder had no other lifetime DIS/DSM-III diagnosis. The most frequent comorbidity patterns were agoraphobia and simple phobia, agoraphobia and depression, simple phobia and depression, and panic disorder with depression. As shown in Fig. 1, almost 40% of all cases with simple phobia and agoraphobia also fulfill the diagnostic criteria for panic disorder

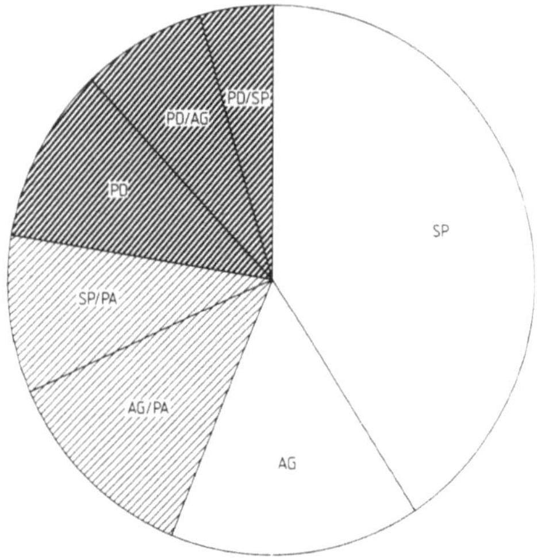

Fig. 1. Diagnostic overlap within the anxiety disorders. Simple Phobia (SP), Agoraphobia (AG); Agoraphobia with panic attacks (AG/PA); Simple Phobia with panic attacks (SP/PA); Panic Disorder (PD); Panic Disorder and Agoraphobia (PD/AG); Panic Disorder and Simple Phobia (PD/SP)

Table 5. Anxiety disorders: Lifetime and 6-month prevalence according to DIS/DSM-III in the MFS and rates for the ECA after adjusting for age and race

	Prevalence Lifetime				**Prevalence 6-Month**			
	MFS total		ECA total		MFS total		ECA total	
DIS/DSM-III diagnoses	(%)	(SE)	(%)	(SE)	(%)	(SE)	(%)	(SE)
Anxiety disorders	13.87	1.24	15.09	0.55	8.13	0.98	9.05	0.43
- Panic disorder	2.39	0.53	2.05	0.23	1.08	0.37	0.89	0.15
- Simple and social phobia	8.01	0.96	9.34	0.46	4.06	0.68	6.36	0.40
- Agoraphobia	5.74	0.85	4.83	0.35	3.59	0.68	3.40	0.29
- Obsessive-compulsive disorder	2.03	0.48	3.05	0.27	1.79	0.47	1.59	0.19
Overall prevalence (All DIS/DSM-III diagnoses)	32.06	1.73	31.88	0.79	14.59	1.29	17.60	0.55

(DSM-III) or at least criteria for one severe panic attack (DSM-III-R). Because of methodological problems (Barlow et al. 1986), rates for generalized anxiety disorder (GAD), and Obsessive-Compulsive Disorder were not included in Fig. 1. The overlap rate for obsessive-compulsive disorder with any other anxiety disorders was 40%, an additional estimation for comorbidity with GAD - thus not taking into account the DSM-III exclusion rules - based on a clinical judgment revealed 42% overlap with other anxiety disorders.

Comorbidity with other disorders was markedly lower for the cross-sectional (6-month) DIS/DSM-III diagnoses (lifetime, 66.2%, as compared with 42.0% for the 6-month criterion). Comorbidity with other mental disorders was found to be high as well, especially with affective disorders, medication- and alcohol abuse - less frequently with dependence. The analysis for the specific anxiety disorders reveals the highest comorbidity rates for cases with panic disorder: 71.4% met criteria for affective disorder, 28.6% for medication abuse, and 50% for alcohol abuse. The comorbidity rates for agoraphobia were slightly lower, with 65.4% for depression, medication abuse (23%), and drug abuse (23%). Simple phobia had a markedly smaller overlap with depression (43.8%) and with medication abuse (12.5%). Because of the high comorbidity rate with depression, the occurrence of major depression as well as the co-occurrence of agoraphobia with panic attacks are taken into account in some of the subsequent analyses.

Age of Onset of Anxiety Disorders and Mean Duration of Illness

The majority of anxiety disorders, especially simple and social phobias, begin early in the subject's life and persist over many years in adulthood. Panic disorders have a markedly later mean onsetz in the thirties.

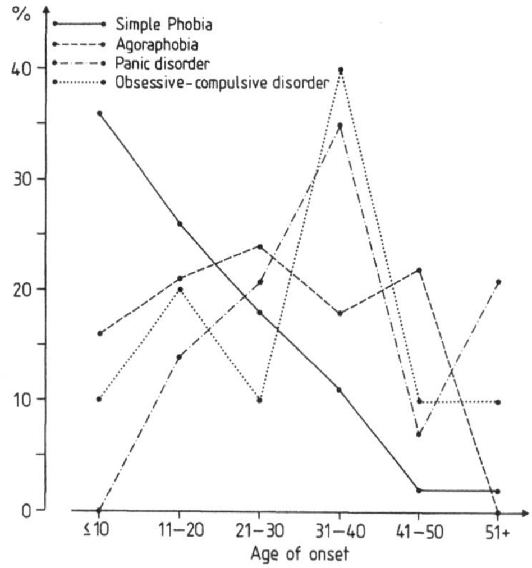

Fig. 2. Age of onset curves for anxiety disorders

Figure 2 indicates a continuous drop of cases of simple phobia in the higher age groups, whereas the rates for agoraphobia rise to a mean age of onset of 28 years. Agoraphobia thus lies between simple phobia and panic disorder. No clear indication for two peaks of onset was found for agoraphobia (Marks and Gelder 1965).

The calculation for the mean duration of illness (Table 6) reveals a rather long history of illness for almost all groups. The longest durations were found for simple phobia and agoraphobia; in accordance with the markedly later age of onset, duration of panic disorder was significantly shorter. The most frequent pattern of symptom course was **chronic and persistent.** Only few cases indicated an episodic course with almost symptom-free intervals, defined as being free of any anxiety symptoms (including avoidance behavior) over a period of more than 6 months. As expected from the literature, cases with panic disorders and agora-

Table 6. Anxiety disorders in the MFS: Mean duration (time in years elapsed between first and last occurrence) and symptom course

DSM-III Diagnosis	Mean duration		Course of symptoms					
			Chronic		Episodic		SFI	
	X (MD)	SD	(*n*)	*T*	(*n*)	*T*	(*n*)	*T*
Panic disorder ($n=14$)	(6.0)	*	(6)	++	(6)	++	(2)	–
Agoraphobia with panic attacks ($n=13$)	(10.0)	*	(8)	+++	(3)	+	(2)	–
Agoraphobia without panic attacks ($n=13$)	18.6	16.5	(8)	+++	(1)	–	(4)	+
Simple phobia ($n=32$)	24.3	13.8	(17)	++	(2)	–	(13)	++
Obsessive-compulsive disorder ($n=13$)	13.0	13.1	(3)	+	(6)	++	(4)	+

SFI = symptom-free intervals (6 months); T, overall tendency; ( )* = skewed distribution, median (MD)

phobia indicated more frequently exacerbations and were more often rated by the clinicians as serverely impaired than cases who had only simple and social phobia.

Psychosocial Severity and Treatment Status of Anxiety Disorders With and Without a Co-occurring Depression

Figure 3 summarizes for each type of anxiety disorder the degree of psychosocial impairments at the time of the follow-up examination, as measured with the Global Assessment Scale (GAS; Spitzer et al. 1978). The majority of simple and social phobias reveal at best minor impairments at this cross-sectional evaluation, whereas agoraphobia and panic disorders show rather often significant or marked dysfunctions in their social role behavior. The degree of psychosocial impairments is strongly related to the presence of depression (major depression/dysthymia). In accordance with the higher prevalence of co-occurring depression, cases with panic disorder and agoraphobia are more often markedly impaired in many social role areas (work, interaction with partner/spouse, restrictions in leisure time) than those with simple or social phobias. It is noteworthy that psychosocial impairments in the 4-week-period preceding the follow-up investigation were found in both, cases with a current (6-month) diagnosis of depression and in those with a past (lifetime) diagnosis of depression, (i.e., those who were at least partially remitted). This finding might indicate that the occurrence of depression in anxiety disorders has a strong and long-lasting impact the long-term course and outcome. No clear association was found between length of illness and degree of psychosocial impairments.

A similar association with depression was found for the variable treatment status in the follow-up interval. Whereas only a few of the cases with simple and social phobia without depression received some

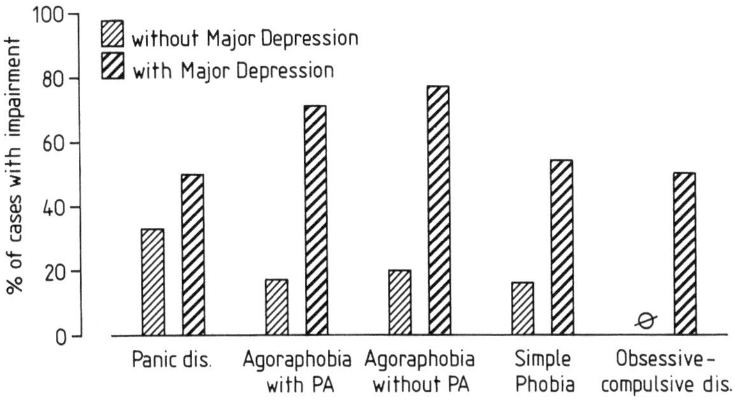

Fig. 3. Percentage of anxiety cases with and without a lifetime diagnosis of depression with psychosocial impairments

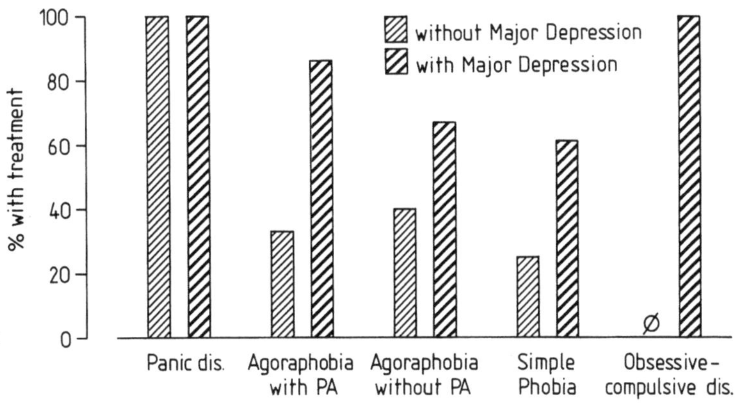

Fig. 4. Proportion of cases with and without lifetime depression having received at least once any therapeutic intervention

kind of professional intervention, all cases with panic disorder and two-thirds of all phobic cases with depression indicated having had some kind of professional intervention. Except for three cases with panic disorder and one with agoraphobia who had contacted a psychologist or psychiatrist, all the remaining indicated having received unspecific pharmacological prescriptions by their general practitioner only (almost exclusively tranquilizers and barbiturates, see Wittchen 1988). None of these treatments, however, proved to be adequate with regard to minimal dosage, the drug chosen, or standards of minimal duration of treatment.

Because the highest proportion of cases having received treatment was found for those with a lifetime diagnosis of depression, it can be suggested that the occurrence of depression in the course of anxiety disorders might be regarded as a **tracer condition** for treatment.

Long-Term Course and Remission Rates

The analysis of remission rates in Fig. 5., defined as the percentage of cases not fulfilling the diagnostic criteria for a DSM-III anxiety diagnosis in the 6-month and 12-month interval preceding the follow-up interview, reveals only very low remission rates for all groups.

To further illustrate the course of the disorder, the development of comorbidity,

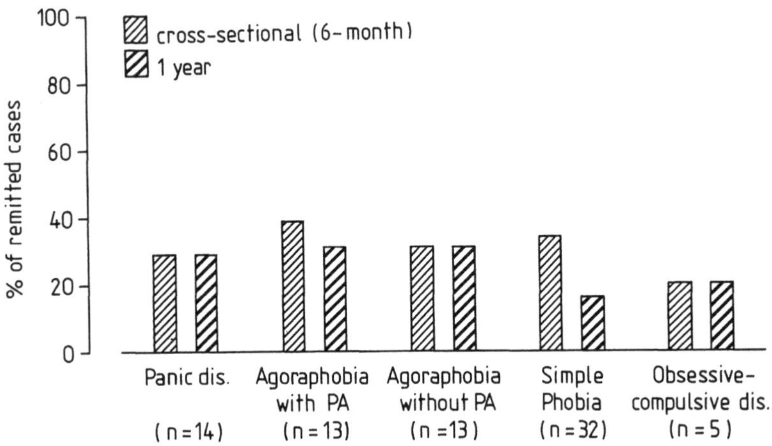

Fig. 5. Remission rates as measured by the presence at a 6-month and 1-year anxiety diagnosis

use of health services, and psychosocial outcome, Table 7 summarizes the cases by case results for a subsample of 38 of the 77 cases. These cases have been analyzed separately with respect to health service use in another publication (Wittchen 1988). Table 7 ranks cases fulfilling criteria for any of the anxiety disorders according to their outcome, based on the GAS score. Those with a poor outcome as measured by the GAS are ranked in the lower part of the table, those with a more favorable one in the upper part. The table also shows the diagnostic results and age of onset according to the DIS for wave I, the onset for additional diagnoses, and the cross-sectional DIS diagnoses at the time of follow-up investigation. In addition, health services use is indicated (HSU) in terms of number of visits to general medical services (GP, etc.), as well as whether the subject visited a psychiatrist or psychologist at least once [J] or received pharmacological treatment [(J)] by a GP (treatment status: TS).

From Table 7, a number of inferences can be made:

1. The majority of cases develop one or more other diagnosis **after** onset of the anxiety disorder. As discussed before this frequently involves major depression [MD] (or dysthymia [Dyst]), or stubstance abuse [AB].
2. Cases with a less favorable outcome frequently have more than one diagnosis and show marked to severe impairment in psychosocial functioning.
3. Panic disorder (PA) and depression (MD, Dyst) seem to be a combination rather frequently associated with poor outcome.
4. Substance abuse is a frequent complication of the long-term course of agoraphobia and panic disorders. Alcohol and medication abuse in 52% of cases with this diagnosis and the lower GAS scores for these subjects further underscore the unfavorable outcome pattern.
5. The majority of cases with agoraphobia and/or panic disorder display a significantly elevated average number of visits to general health services (The mean number of health service visits in a matched control group with no mental disorder is 62 visits in the 7-years interval).

Conclusion

Before drawing conclusions from our data, the main limitations of this study must be recalled. In our general population sample, we were able to identify 77 subjects with a lifetime diagnosis of an anxiety disorder. This is a rather small number to test hypotheses for subgroups;

Table 7. Long-term course and outcome at follow-up in a subsample of anxiety disorders (Wittchen 1988)

Case No.	Diagnoses and age at onset (years) (wave I/1974)	HSU (*n*)	TS	Additional diagnoses in the follow-up interval (age in years)	6-Month diagnoses at follow-up	GAS score
1		44	N	AG 42	AG	+
2	SP 19	62	N			+
3	SP 10	72	N			+
4	AG 10	14	N		AG	+
5	SP 10	44	N			+
6	MD 37, SP 37, AG 37	56	J			+
7	SP 10, AG 10	56	N		SP	+
8	SP 18	87	(J)	AB 31	AB	+
9	SP 30	21	N	AB 37	SP	+
10	SP 10, AG 10	75	N		SP, AG	+
11	SP 10, AG 10	159	J		SP, AG	+
12	SP 13	59	N	DYST	DYST	+
13	DYST 19, SP 10, OBS 16	72	J		SP, DYST	+
14	SP 10	29	N			+
15	SP 10, AG 10	36	N		SP, AG	+
16	SP 10	26	N		SP	+
17	MD 19, SP 19, AG 19, PA 19	64	J			+
18	AG 29	88	N		AG	+
19	SP 17	108	N		AG	+
20	AG 28	51	N			=
21	SP 41	46	N		SP	=
22	AG 25	240	J	OSB 61	AG, OSB	=
23	SP 19, AG 19	221	N		SP, AG	=
24		64	J	SP 39, MD ?	SP	=
25	MD 20, AB 22	26	N	SP 28, PA 28	MD	=
26	SP 10, AB 37	29	N	AB	AB	=
27	AG 41, PA 41	80	(J)		AG	=
28		80	(J)	AG 35, AB 35	AG, AB	–
29	SP 29	87	N	AB 56	SP	–
30	AG 30	56	N	MD 33	AG	–
31	SP 11	44	(J)	AB 52	SP, AB	–
32	AG 17	150	J	DYST	AG, DYST	–
33	SP 18	142	J	PA 50, MD 51	SP	–
34	SP 10	29	N	MD	SP	– –
35	AG 16	137	(J)	PA 56, AB 56	AG, PA	– –
36	MD 12, AG 10	79	N		AG	– –
37	MD 24, SP 18	240	(J)	AG 42, AB 43	MD, AG, AB	– –
38	PA 39, AG 39	164	(J)	MD 40	PD, AG	– –

HSU = health services use; TS = treatment status; SP = simple phobia; AG = agoraphobia; MD = major depression; DYST = dysthymia; OBS = obsessive-compulsive disorder; PA = panic disorder; AB = substance abuse; no or minor impairments (+); slight impairments (=); marked impairments (-); severe impairments (- -)

furthermore, this anxiety group is rather heterogenous, consisting of subjects with a variety of syndromes (panic, phobia, obsessions, depression, and substance abuse) all known to affect in themselves course and outcome. Therefore, it proved to be difficult to examine pure diagnostic groups in more detail.

Nevertheless, some major apparent findings can be summarized:

1. For **anxiety disorders in general**, our data indicate a chronic symptom pattern as the most frequent pattern of long-term course. This is underscored by the low rate of spontaneous and complete remissions in all groups. For subjects untreated by a specialist, there is a risk of 66.2% for the overall group with anxiety disorders to develop major depression, dysthymia, substance abuse or dependence, or other disorders after the first onset of anxiety. Furthermore, the findings indicate a significantly higher rate of visits to non-psychiatric health care services, especially to general practitioners and internal doctors.
2. The natural course of **simple phobias** is in the majority of cases chronic and can be characterized by the persistence of mild rather than severe symptoms of anxiety over decades. Only 16% remitted completely over the follow-up period of 7 years; thus, only very few spontaneous remissions could be observed. With regard to psychosocial impairments, rather variable results were found. Our findings suggest nevertheless that, in "pure" simple and social phobias, severe and stable psychosocial restrictions are rare or mostly transient. In more than one third of this group, however, the long-term course of the disorder was obviously "complicated" by the occurrence of depression and substance abuse. The onset of both, depression and substance abuse in these cases was clearly **after** the first manifestation of the phobia, in the majority of cases even more than 10 years later.
   These rates for depression and substance abuse are far in excess of those reported for men and women in the general population (Robins et al. 1984; Myers et al. 1984). At the current stage of the analysis, this finding is difficult to interpret further. One possibility that will be tested in cases with simple phobia is the role of life events (separations and divorce) triggering exacerbations.
3. The long-term course of **panic disorders** differs in most aspects from the pattern found in simple and social phobias. We found a later age of onset (consequently, a significantly shorter illness history), the highest comorbidity rates of all groups, the highest number of cases with treatment, the most severe psychosocial impairments, and the worst outcome. All cases of panic disorder, except for one, fulfilled DSM-III criteria for other disorders – mostly major depression (71.4%), alcohol abuse (50%), and drug abuse. The course of symptoms was either stable-chronic or chronic with episodic exacerbations. Although we report these findings with caution because of the low number of cases ($n = 14$), it should be pointed out that some other studies have found quite similar results. The chronic nature of the disorder is supported by several older treatment studies (Marks and Herst 1970; Errera and Coleman 1963; Roberts 1964), as well as the more recent investigation by Breier et al. (1986). The latter also found quite similar comorbidity rates.
4. For **agoraphobic cases**, rather variable results, were found that considerably hamper forming a clear conclusion. Generally, however, cases with agoraphobia with and without panic attacks were more severely impaired and had a markedly higher comorbidity rate for depression than other phobias.
   No differential findings were ascertained for agoraphobia with and without panic attacks. It should be pointed out that, like Weissman et al. (1986) and Angst and Dobler-Mikola (1985, 1986), we identified more cases of agoraphobia without panic attacks or without panic disorder than cases with these features. The dominant pattern

of long-term course for both groups was chronic, with slightly higher remission rates for agoraphobia with panic attacks than for cases with panic disorder.

5. The degree of psychosocial impairments in all groups was apparently related to the lifetime occurrence of a major depression. In contrast to the chronic and unremitting course of anxiety symptoms, the course of depressions was predominantly episodic, with full remissions. Nevertheless, it is remarkable that psychosocial dysfunctions were significantly more severe and frequent in all cases involving depression, even if the depression was fully remitted. This might be an indication for long-lasting psychosocial aftereffects of depression, which possibly remit much more slowly than the acute psychopathological features (Paykel et al. 1978; Wittchen et al. 1988). Help-seeking behavior also seems to be related to the occurrence of depression in anxiety disorders, especially in panic disorder and agoraphobia.

To conclude, our findings may be summarized by paraphrasing Klerman's phrase of a couple of years ago with regard to depressive disorders: **The anxiety patients in the community are poorly recognized and treated.** Without specific biological or psychological intervention or a combination of both, the majority of anxiety disorders in the community are persistent and chronic. There is a remarkably high long-term risk for developing psychopathological and psychosocial complications and a low probability for complete remission. It remains an open question not only whether we have succeeded thus far in developing efficient treatment strategies to change the obviously unfavorable pattern of **the natural course and outcome,** but also whether we are able to make our treatment methods available to those in need of help. Recent long-term follow-up studies of severely impaired inpatient samples (see review by Wittchen and von Zerssen 1988; Krieg et al 1987) or the rather low rate of cases having received any specific or adequate professional help in the health care system do not necessarily seem to justify a very optimistic outlook.

Acknowledgment. The author would like to thank Isaac Marks, Iver Hand, and Cecilia Essau for their helpful comments on an earlier draft of this paper.

References

American Psychiatric Association (1980) Diagnostic and Statistical Manual of Mental Disorders (DSM-III). APA, (revised 1987)

Agras WS, Sylvester D, Oliveau D (1969) The epidemiology of common fear and phobia. Compr Psychiatry 10:151–156

Agras WS, Chapin N, Oliveau DC (1972) The natural history of phobia: course and prognosis. Arch Gen Psychiat 26:315–317

Angst J, Dobler-Mikola A (1985) The Zurich study V: Anxiety and phobia in young adults. Eur Arch Psychiatr Neurol Sci 235:171–178

Angst J, Dobler-Mikola A (1986) Assoziation und Depression auf syndromaler und diagnostischer Ebene. In: Helmchen H, Linden M (eds) Die Differenzierung von Angst und Depression. Springer, Berlin Heidelberg New York London Paris Tokyo

Barlow DH, DiNardo PA, Vermilyea BB, Vermilyea J, Blanchard E (1986) Comorbidity and depression among the anxiety disorders. J Nerv Ment Dis 174:63–72

Boyd JH, Burke JD, Gruenberg E (1984) Exclusion criteria of DSM-III. Arch Gen Psychiatr 41:983–989

Breier A, Charney DS, Heninger GR (1986) Agoraphobia with panic attacks. Development, diagnostic stability, and course of illness. Arch Gen Psychiat 43:1029–1036

Errera P, Coleman JV (1963) A long-term follow-up study of neurotic phobic patients in a psychiatric clinic. J Nerv Ment Dis 136:267–271

Eysenck HJ (1960) The effects of psychotherapy: an evaluation. In: Eysenck HJ (ed) Handbook of abnormal psychology. Pitman, London

Goldberg RJ (1982) Anxiety: A guide to biobehavioral diagnosis and therapy for physicians and mental health clinicians. Medical Examination, New York

Hand I, Wittchen HU (eds) (1986) Panic and phobias: empirical evidence of theoretical models and long-term effects of behavioral treatments. Springer, Berlin Heidelberg New York Tokyo

Hand I, Angenendt J, Fischer M, Wilke C (1986) Exposure in vivo with panic management for agoraphobia: treatment rationale and long-term outcome. In: Hand I, Wittchen HU (eds) Panic and phobias: empirical evidence of theoretical models and long-term effects of behavioral treatments. Springer, Berlin Heidelberg New York Tokyo

Helzer JE, Robins LN; McEvoy LT, Spitznagel EL, Stoltzman RK, Farmer A, Brockington IF (1985) A comparison of clinical and Diagnostic Interview Schedule diagnoses. Arch Gen Psychiatry 42:657–666

Jablensky A (1985) Approaches to the definition and classification of anxiety and related disorders. In: Tuma AH, Maser JD (eds) Anxiety and the anxiety disorders. Lawrence Erlbaum, Hillsdale, NJ

Jablensky A, Hugler H (1982) Möglichkeiten und Grenzen psychiatrischer epidemiologischer Surveys für geographisch definierte Populationen in Europa. Fortschr Neurol Psychiatr 50:215-239

Krieg JC, Bronisch T, Wittchen HU, von Zerssen D (1987) Anxiety disorders: a long-term prospective and retrospective follow-up study of former inpatients suffering from an anxiety neurosis or phobia. Acta Psychiatr Scand 76:36–47

Lépine JP (1987) Epidémiologie des attaques de panique et de l' agoraphobie. In: Boulenger JP, (ed) L' attaque de panique: un nouveau concept? Goureau, Château de Loir

Lydiard RB, Ballenger JC (1987) Antidepressants in panic disorder and agoraphobia. J Affective Disord 13:135–168

Marks IM (1987) Fears, phobias, and rituals: panic, anxiety, and their disorders. Oxford University Press, New York

Marks IM, Gelder MG (1965) A controlled retrospective study of behavior therapy in phobic patients. Br J Psychiatry III:571–573

Marks IM, Herst ER (1970) A survey of 1200 agoraphobics in Britain. Soc Psychiatry 5:16–24

Mathews AM, Gelder MG, Johnston DW (1981) Agoraphobia: nature and treatment. Tavistock, London

McPherson FM, Brougham L, McLaren S (1980) Maintenance of improvement in agoraphobic patients treated by behavioral methods: a four-year follow-up. Behav Res Ther 18:620–627

Myers JK, Weissman MM, Tischler GL, Holzer CE, Leaf PJ, Orvaschel H, Anthony JC, Boyd JH, Kramer M, Stoltzman R (1984) Six-month prevalence of psychiatric disorders in three communities. Arch Gen Psychiatry 42:651–656

Paykel ES, Weissman MM, Prusoff BA (1978) Social maladjustment and severity of depression. Compr Psychiatry 19:121–128

Rachman S (1973) The effects of psychological treatment. In: Eysenck H (ed) Handbook of abnormal psychology. Basic Books, New York

Regier DA, Myers JK, Kramer M, Robins LN, Blazer DG, Hough RL, Eaton WW, Locke BZ (1984) The NIMH Epidemiological Catchment Area Program: historical context, major objectives and study population characteristics. Arch Gen Psychiatry 41:934–941

Reich J (1986) The epidemiology of anxiety. J Nerv D 174:129–136

Roberts AH (1964) Housebound housewives: a follow-up study of a phobic anxiety state. Br J Psychiatry 110:191–197

Robins LN, Helzer JE, Croughan J, Ratcliff KS (1981) National Institute of Mental Health Diagnostic Interview Schedule: its history, characteristics and validity. Arch Gen Psychiatry 38:381–389

Robins LN, Helzer JE, Weissman MM, Orvaschel H, Gruenberg E, Burke JD, Regier DA (1984) Lifetime prevalence of specific psychiatric disorders in three sites. Arch Gen Psychiatry 41:949–958

Semler G, Wittchen H-U, Joschke K, Zaudig M, von Geiso T, Kaisre S, von Cranach M, Pfister H (1987) Test-retest reliability of standardized psychiatric interview (DIS/CIDI). Eur Arch Psychiatr Neurol Sci 236:214–222

Sheehan DV (1987) Benzodiazepines in panic disorder and agoraphobia. J Affective Disord 13:169–181

Spitzer RL, Endicott J, Fleiss L (1978) The global assessment scale: a procedure for measuring overall severity of psychiatric disturbance. Arch Gen Psychiat 33:766–771

Strian F (1983) Angst: Grundlagen und Klinik. Springer, Berlin Heidelberg New York Tokyo

Surtees PG, Sashidharan SP, Dean C (1987) Affective disorders amongst women in the general population: a longitudinal study. Br J Psychiatry 148:176–186

Weissman MM, Leaf PS, Blazer DG, Boyd SH, Florio L (1986) The relationship between panic disorder and agoraphobia: An epidemiological perspective. Psychopharmacology Bulletin

Wittchen HU (1986) Epidemiology of panic attacks and panic disorders. In: Hand I, Wittchen HU (eds) Panic and phobias I. Springer, Berlin Heidelberg New York Tokyo

Wittchen HU (1988) Zum Spontanverlauf unbehandelter Fälle mit Angststörungen und Depressionen. In: Wittchen HU, von Zerssen D (eds) Verläufe behandelter und unbehandelter Depressionen und Angststörungen. Springer, Berlin Heidelberg New York Tokyo

Wittchen HU, Burke JD (to be published) DIS/DSM-III prevalence rates of mental disorders in the US and Germany

Wittchen HU, von Zerssen D, Ellmann R, Möller HJ (1983) Der Verlauf behandelter und unbehandelter psychischer Störungen: Methodik und erste Ergebnisse. In: Kommer D, Röhrle B (eds) Gemeindepsychologische Perspektiven (Cologne) 3:118–124

Wittchen HU, von Zerssen D (1988) Verläufe behandelter und unbehandelter Depressionen und Angststörungen. Springer Berlin Heidelberg New York Tokyo

Wittchen HU, Semler G, von Zerssen D (1985) A comparison of two diagnostic methods: clinical ICD diagnoses vs DSM-III and Research Diagnostic Criteria using the Diagnostic Interview Schedule (Version 2). Arch Gen Psychiatry 42:677–684

Wittchen HU, Hecht H, Zaudig M, Vogl G, Semler G, Pfister H (1988) Häufigkeit und Schwere psychischer Störungen in der Bevölkerung: eine epidemiologische Feldstudie.In: Wittchen HU, von Zerssen D (eds) Verläufe behandelter und unbehandelter Depressionen und Angststörungen. Springer, Berlin Heidelberg New York Tokyo

2. Biology and Pharmacological Treatment of Panic Disorder

T. W. UHDE and M. B. STEIN

Introduction

Considerable controversy exists regarding the etiologic nature of panic disorder. Predictably, proponents of psychological therapies posit psychological and experiential origins for panic disorder, while believers in psychopharmacological approaches put forward biological explanations. Who is correct?

During the past 25 years, a sizeable literature has emerged centering on biological approaches to the treatment of panic disorder with or without agoraphobia. The seminal contributions of Donald Klein (1964, 1967) focused attention on the phenomenology of the "panic attack" as being distinct from other forms of "neurotic" anxiety. Klein's observations that panic attacks responded specifically to treatment with the tricyclic antidepressant imipramine paved the way for an interest in the pharmacotherapy of panic disorder that continues unabated. While it is beyond the scope of this chapter to chronicle in detail the great number of controlled psychopharmacological studies in panic disorder that have been published to date, suffice it to say that medication treatments for panic disorder have been proven highly effective. (For complete recent reviews of this area, see Lydiard and Ballenger 1987; Sheehan 1987.) In this chapter, we will summarize our approach to the pharmacotherapy of patients with panic disorder and varying degrees of phobic avoidance, and we will highlight some of the controversial issues in this area.

In addition, we will bring together some of the current evidence supportive of a biological hypothesis for the nature of panic disorder. This evidence includes information based on the study of "biological markers" in patients with panic disorder, as well as on the evolving body of literature using challenge paradigms (including the use of lactate and caffeine to provoke panic attacks in the laboratory setting).

Overview of Issues in the Pharmacological Treatment of Panic Disorder

Pharmacological treatment is only one of several potentially efficacious treatments for panic disorder and agoraphobia. Behavioral interventions, particularly in vivo exposure, have a significant role to play in some patients with panic disorder and agoraphobia (Marks et al. 1983; Marks 1987; Mavissakalian and Barlow 1983). More recently, cognitive therapies have also been reported to be effective in the treatment of panic disorder (Clark 1986; Beck and Emery 1985), although more systematic study is required to firmly establish their efficacy.

Choice of Treatments: Medication or Not?

As might be expected, there is much ongoing debate about the relative roles each of these therapeutic modalities should play in the management of patients with panic disorder with or without agoraphobia. At the present time, remarkably little is known in answer to the crucial question, "Who does best with which kind of treatment?" Currently, the choice of an appropriate form of treatment rests more on the therapist's personal expertise and preference than on any well-considered selection process. Future studies that address the problem of optimal treatment selection for each individual patient are sorely needed. Progress in this area will require the collaboration of investigators with a variety of theoretical orientations and abilities.

Despite the absence of any general consensus in this field, we feel that the usefulness of pharmacotherapy in the treatment of panic disorder has been firmly established. Several recent studies suggest, moreover, that treatment modalities which combine medications with some degree of exposure therapy confer an added element of efficacy over medications alone (Mavissakalian et al. 1983; Telch et al. 1985). In practice this may be a moot point, as many practitioners seem to take the route of making suggestions regarding gradual in vivo exposure once patients begin to feel some beneficial effects from pharmacotherapy. We have found that many patients receiving antipanic medication require little more than basic education about their illness, including some explanation of the role that their own avoidance serves in the perpetuation of their fears, in order to overcome their avoidant behavior. Nonetheless, we not infrequently encounter patients who have apparently failed to benefit significantly from well-constructed, well-respected behavioral/cognitive therapy programs. These patients present to us as behavioral therapy "failures," and the majority seem to respond well to antipanic medications. Many of these individuals report to us that the behavioral and cognitive techniques they previously learned, while ineffective alone in helping them, acquire newfound relevance once medication begins to take effect in lessening their symptomatology. While highly uncontrolled and impressionistic, these clinical observations are in keeping with those studies that report additive effects of behavioral and pharmacological therapies (Solyom et al. 1981; Mavissakalian et al. 1983; Telch et al. 1985; Mavissakalian and Michelson 1986). No study, to our knowledge, has attempted to look specifically at the pharmacotherapy of patients who are "refractory" to nonpharmacological interventions, despite the fact that much natural selection probably occurs in reality. That is, many patients who come for medication therapy have already tried some sort of non-medication-based treatment. Conversely, it is not known whether or not there exists a subgroup of patients who might respond preferentially to behavioral therapies over medication therapies.

Do Patients Need to be Depressed?

Do panic disorder patients need to be dysphoric, demoralized, or depressed in order to respond to antipanic medications? Isaac Marks, a major contributor to the understanding and treatment of phobic disorders, maintains that tricyclic antidepressants are useful in the treatment of panic disorder (with or without agoraphobia) because they relieve dysphoria (Marks 1983, 1987). He contends that these drugs are not specifically "antiphobic," but are of some benefit because they influence the secondary depression that many agoraphobic patients experience. Despite Marks' contentions, many other studies indicate that the antipanic and antiphobic effects of tricyclic and monoamine oxidase compounds are not dependent on the antidepressant action of these medications (Zitrin et al. 1980; Sheehan et al. 1980; Ballenger et al. 1984). In our own clinical experience, we have successfully treated numerous nondepressed panic disorder patients with antidepressants (including tricyclics such as imipramine and monoamine oxidase inhibitors [MAOIs] such as phenelzine). Thus, the presence of a clinical depressive syndrome is not a prerequisite for the successful treatment of panic disorder with antidepressants. In fact, there is some evidence to suggest that patients with the dual diagnoses of panic disorder and major depression are actually more resistant to standard pharmacotherapeutic interventions than patients with panic disorder alone (Grunhaus et al. 1986). Panic disorder patients with obsessive-compulsive features, who also have a high prevalence of depression, also respond less well to standard antipanic agents (Mellman and Uhde 1987a).

Anticipatory Anxiety versus Panic Anxiety: Differential Pharmacotherapy?

Another unresolved issue in the pharmacotherapy of panic disorder is the topic of differential drug effects on "anticipatory anxiety" versus "panic anxiety." Klein's observations (1964, 1967) that some "anxious" patients experienced their anxiety in the form of panic attacks, and that these attacks could be prevented with imipramine (Klein 1964, 1981), served as the foundation for the pharmacological treatment of panic disorder. Klein postulated that panic anxiety responded preferentially to imipramine, while anticipatory anxiety responded better to benzodiazepines (such as diazepam or chlordiazepoxide). This led to the phenomenological distinction between panic disorder and generalized anxiety that can be seen today in most classification systems, including the Diagnostic and Statistical Manual of Mental Disorders in its current third revised editon (DSM-IIIR, American Psychiatric Association 1987). Although some current evidence favors this dichotomous distinction between panic and generalized (or anticipatory) anxiety (Klein et al. 1987), several recent findings have challenged this separation. Alprazolam, a triazolobenzodiazepine, has unequivocal effects in blocking panic attacks (Sheehan 1982; Chouinard et al. 1982). Initially, it was felt that alprazolam, a second-generation benzodiazepine, might have special properties that made it an exception to the rule that benzodiazepines were ineffective in treating panic anxiety. More recently, however, other traditional benzodiazepines such as lorazepam have been shown to be effective in treating panic (Charney et al. 1987), as has the anticonvulsant benzodiazepine compound, clonazepam (Chouinard et al. 1982; Spier et al. 1986). Presumably, it is by virtue of their higher relative potencies that these newer benzodiazepines are effective in treating panic, whereas diazepam is not. Moreover, evidence is accumulating suggesting that imipramine has beneficial effects in the treatment of generalized anxiety (Kahn et al. 1987).

Thus, the differential pharmacotherapy of panic versus generalized anxiety has been thrown into a state of flux, as have the sharp phenomenological lines along which these therapeutic interventions were originally based. Nevertheless, this model of panic anxiety as being distinct from anticipatory or generalized anxiety has been influential in the promotion of considerable interest and progress in the pharmacotherapy of anxiety disorders in general and panic disorder in particular. In fact, several family-pedigree (Crowe et al. 1983; Noyes et al. 1987) and twin studies (Torgerson 1983) provide strong support for the delineation of panic disorder from generalized anxiety on genetic, if not pharmacological, grounds.

An Approach to the Pharmacological Treatment of Panic Disorder

Predictors of Response to Pharmacotherapy

As we have indicated, the decision when to treat patients with medications for their panic disorder is often based on the clinician's individual preference and experience, as well as the patient's preference. Few, if any, clinical predictors of response to pharmacotherapy exist in the literature. Table 1 summarizes our clinical impressions about positive and negative predictors of successful response to pharmacotherapy in panic disorder. These are offered as suggestions that the clinician may wish to take into consideration in deciding on an appropriate treatment modality.

Table 1. Drug therapy of panic disorder

1. Predictors of *positive* response
   a) "Classic" panic attack
      - Unexpected
      - Recalls precise time, place and situation of first panic attack
   b) Typical course of illness
      Panic attacks → Anticipatory anxiety → Agoraphobia
   c) good premorbid (pre-attack) personality
2. Predictors of *poor* response
   a) "Atypical" panic attacks
      - Wish to die
      - Never unexpected
      - Predominance of psychosensory symptoms (especially severe derealization)
   b) Atypical course of illness
      - Gradual onset
      - Agoraphobia → Panic attacks
      - Thoughts → Panic
   c) Disturbed personality traits
      - Borderline personality traits: e.g., impulsivity, self-damaging acts
      - Obsessive-compulsive personality traits

Choice of Pharmacotherapeutic Agents

Once a decision has been made to employ pharmacotherapy, with or without some element of behavioral intervention, the choice of medication is again a matter of preference. The three classes of medications shown to be useful in the treatment of panic disorder include
a) the tricyclic antidepressants, with imipramine being the most frequently used,
b) the MAOIs, with phenelzine being the most frequently used, and
c) the benzodiazepines, with alprazolam being the most frequently used.

As in the pharmacotherapy of major depression, choice of the "best" agent for an individual patient is made by taking into consideration the relative side effects and clinical profiles of each drug. These are summarized in Table 2.

Imipramine

Generally, most clinicians choose to start treatment with either imipramine or alprazolam. Alprazolam may offer the relative advantages of more rapid symptom relief and fewer initial side effects (Sheehan 1987), but the problems with withdrawing this drug are considerable (Mellman and Uhde 1987b; Fyer et al. 1987). Imipramine has been used in psychiatry for over a quarter of a century, and its longevity and relative paucity of known long-term adverse effects lead us to uphold its status as the drug of first choice in the treatment of panic disorder. With few exceptions, we believe that patients should initially be given a therapeutic trial of imipramine. Clearly, some of these patients will not respond to imipramine, or will suffer from early side effects such as tachycardia, agitation, stimulation, or actual worsening of anxiety. These early side effects have been described in

Table 2. Selecting an antipanic medication: profile of clinical effects

	Imipramine	Phenelzine	Alprazolam	Clonazepam
Onset	Gradual (3–5 weeks)	Gradual (3–5 weeks)	Rapid (1-2 days)	Rapid (1–2 days)
Special diet	None	Required	None	None
Side effects (acute)	Many	Some	Few	Few
Side effects (chronic)	Few	Few	Few	Few
Antidepressant effects	Excellent	Excellent	Fair[a]	Unknown[b]
Overdose/toxicity	High	High	Low	Probably low
Inducing (disinhibition) (predisposed)	Low	Low	High	Unknown
Discontinuation symptoms	Low	Low	High	Now-moderate
Abuse potential	None	None	Low	Low

[a] While alprazolam exhibits good antidepressant effects in most studies, it has also been shown to precipitate depression in some patients with panic disorder (Lydiard et al. 1987)
[b] May worsen depression at higher doses (4–6 mg/day)

20%–30% of patients with panic disorder (Zitrin et al. 1978), and may lead to abrupt medication discontinuation if the patient and the physician are not prepared to anticipate and deal with these symptoms. It has been our experience, however, and that of others (Lydiard and Ballenger 1987), that these initial side effects can be alleviated or avoided altogether by the use of very low starting doses (e.g., 10 mg of imipramine b.i.d.), divided dosing, and very gradual dosage increases. Alternatively, clinicians may wish to make use of a combination of imipramine (10 mg q.i.d.) and alprazolam (0.25–0.50 mg q.i.d; Uhde 1986), thereby taking advantage of alprazolam's almost immediate anxiolytic properties, which may help counteract some of imipramine's initial side effects. If this combined approach is used, then the goal would be to gradually taper and then withdraw the alprazolam once therapeutic doses of imipramine (usually 100–300 mg/day) have been achieved.

Other Medications

If imipramine is not tolerated, there might be some merit to using alternative tricyclics such as nortriptyline or desipramine. These secondary amine tricyclics generally cause fewer problems with side effects such as sedation, dry mouth, and orthostatic hypotension but, surprisingly, their use in panic disorder has not been systematically studied to any great degree. A recent report from Lydiard (1987) does suggest that desipramine is effective in panic disorder, and this is consistent with our own experience. There may also arise situations where the clinician wishes to switch a patient from one antidepressant to another if a patient is having specific difficulties with a particular drug. For example, we have successfully switched a patient who developed hepatotoxicity on imipramine to the heterocyclic compound doxepin, with maintenance of the antipanic effects and normalization of liver transaminase enzymes. In another case, we switched a patient who had severe symptomatic postural hypotension on imipramine to the secondary amine tricyclic nortriptyline, with maintenance of the antipanic effects and normalization of blood pressure.

Alprazolam or clonazepam (Chouinard et al. 1982; Beaudry et al. 1986; Spier et al. 1986), both potent benzodiazepine antipanic agents, should probably be seen as second-line drugs in the treatment of panic disorder. The MAOIs are at least as effective, if not more effective, than the tricyclics (Sheehan et al. 1980), but carry with them the burden of dietary restrictions. For this reason MAOIs are generally relegated to third-line status. The MAOIs, however, may have a special role to play in the treatment of patients who experience panic attacks, rejection-sensitive dysphoria, and interpersonal hypersensitivity (Liebowitz et al. 1984b). General guidelines for treatment with each of these specific medications are given in Table 3.

Experimental Treatments

Our group has recently investigated the use of clonidine (Uhde et al. 1988b) and carbamazepine (Uhde et al. 1988a) in the treatment of panic disorder, with limited success. Clonidine exhibits potent acute anxiolytic effects in patients with panic disorder (Uhde et al. 1984), but these effects wane during chronic treatment, likely due to the occurrence of tolerance (Fig. 1). Carbamazepine, a tricyclic anticonvulsant recently found useful in the treatment of a variety of psychiatric and neuropsychiatric disorder (Uhde et al. 1985a), while helpful in a minority of patients, did not substantially improve the condition of most patients with panic

Table 3. Guidelines for pharmacotherapy of panic disorder

	Imipramine	Alprazolam	Clonazepam	Phenelzine
Starting dose	10–25 mg/day	0.25 mg t.i.d. or q.i.d.	0.125–0,25 mg b.i.d.	15 mg/day
Increase by	25 mg increments every 4–7 days as tolerated	0.50–1.0 mg increments every 2–4 days as tolerated	0.50 mg/week as tolerated	15 mg increments every 4–7 days as tolerated
Average therapeutic dose	100–200 mg/day	3.0–6.0 mg/day	2.0–4.0 mg/day	60–75 mg/day
Maximum dose	300 mg/day	10.0 mg/day q.i.d.	6.0 mg/day q.i.d. or b.i.d.	90 mg/day t.i.d. with last dose at supper time
Dosing schedule	Variable; may be given in divided doses with most at h.s. Individualize for each patient to minimize side effects. Note: Blood level determination may be helpful (imipramine + desipramine = 150–200 ng/ml therapeutic range)	–	–	Low monoamine diet required

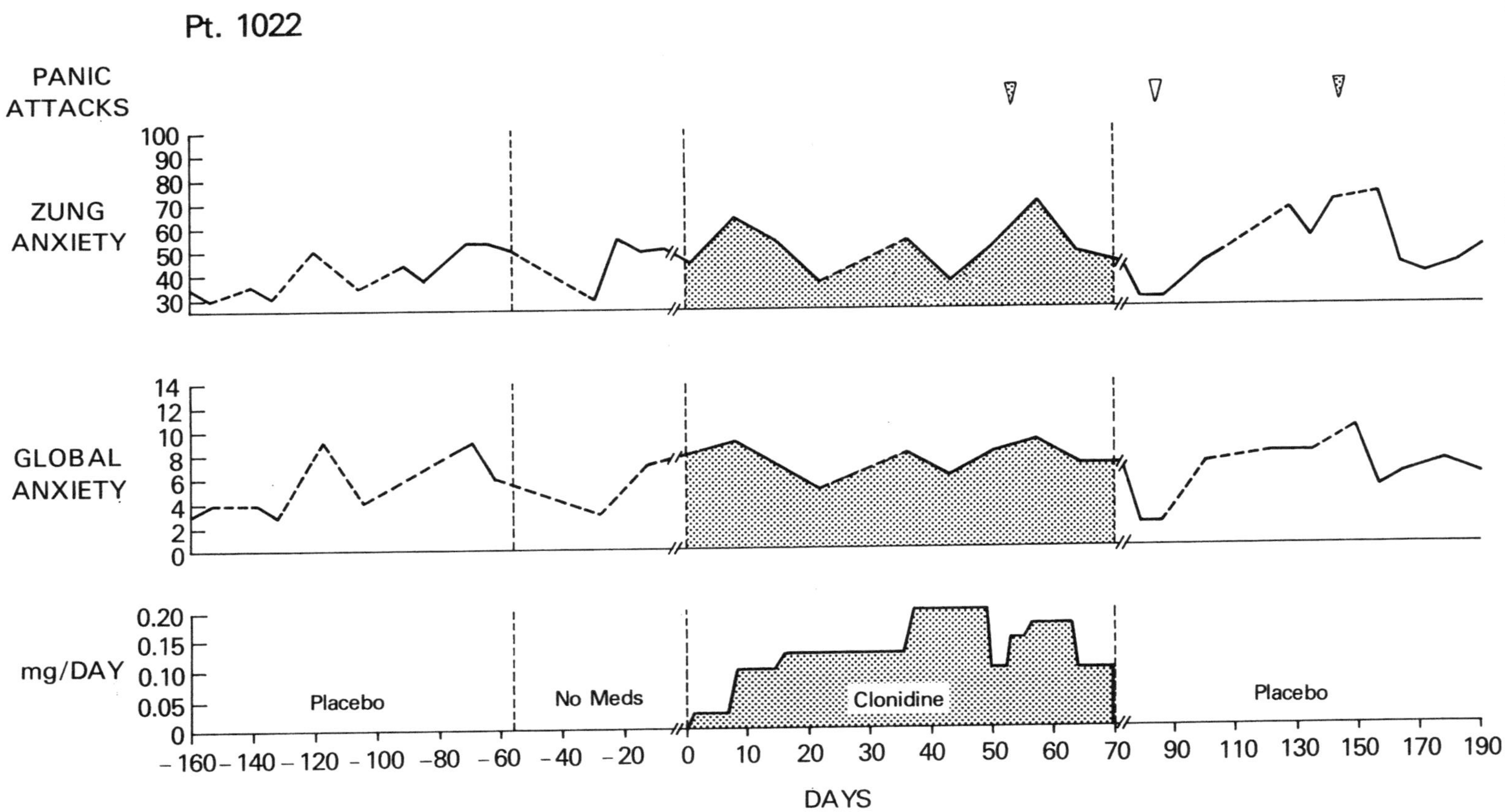

Fig. 1. Response of a 40-year-old patient with panic disorder to treatment with the alpha$_2$-agonist clonidine hydrochloride. During treatment with oral clonidine (in doses ranging up to 0.20 mg/day), this individual's anxiety varied little from her prior course on placebo. An apparent anxiolytic response occurred between days 8–22, but the patient's anxiety crept back up (days 23–36) despite the dosage being held constant. This may be an example of the tolerance that can occur to clonidine's anxiolytic effects

disorder (Uhde et al. 1988a). Carbamazepine may still have a role to play, however, in the treatment of patients with "atypical" panic attacks that include hostility, social withdrawal, and electroencephalographic abnormalities (Edlund et al. 1987). Our preliminary experience with verapamil, a calcium-channel blocker, has been promising (Klein and Uhde, in press). Verapamil may prove to be particularly useful in patients who also suffer from hypertension (Frohlich 1985), migraine (Solomon et al. 1983), or irritable bowel syndrome (Byrne 1987).

Long-Term Medication Treatment

Currently, considerable uncertainties exist regarding the long-term pharmacological treatment of panic disorder. Overall, the limited available data suggests that 20%–100% of patients relapse within 2 years of medication discontinuation. In the absence of any empirical guidance provided in the literature, our clinical approach is to treat patients for 6–12 months, and then to gradually withdraw the medication over 2–3 months. In patients who relapse, we reinstitute treatment for another 12–24 months, before reattempting discontinuation. Further investigatons are required to establish clinical and biological predictors of those patients who will or will not require longer-term pharmacotherapy. In addition, further studies are needed to determine whether or not concomitant behavioral therapies reduce the risk of relapse when medications are discontinued.

Evidence for Biological Disturbances in Panic Disorder

Biological Markers

The major psychiatric disorders such as schizophrenia and major depression have long been the subject of investigations into their biological underpinnings. Much interest has been generated in the study of "biological markers" for psychiatric illness, markers that are intended to demonstrate a physiological abnormality in these disorders. The best renowned of these markers is the dexamethasone suppression test (DST), which has gained fame in the study of major depressive illness (Carroll 1984). More recently, a similar line of research has led to an interest in the study of various biological indices in panic disorder. In this section, we will cite some of the studies that have examined biological indices in panic disorder, including the DST, the thyrotropin (TSH) response to thyroid releasing hormone (TRH), and several measures of noradrenergic function. Limitations in the knowledge gained from these studies will also be addressed.

The Dexamethasone Suppression Test and other Measures of Hypothalamo-Pituitary-Adrenal Axis Functioning

The dexamethasone suppression test (DST) was originally proposed as a diagnostic test for melancholic depression (Carroll 1984) based on observations about abnormalities in cortisol secretion patterns in depressed individuals (Sachar et al. 1973). While its preliminary brilliance as a diagnostic test has become tarnished with time (Arana et al. 1985), the DST remains of interest as a means to study the hypothalamo-pituitary-adrenal (HPA) axis in psychiatric disorders.

Several investigators have examined the DST in panic disorder (Curtis et al. 1982; Lieberman et al. 1983; Sheehan et al. 1983; Coryell et al. 1985; Avery et al. 1985; Peterson et al. 1985; Roy-Byrne et al. 1985; Bridges et al. 1986; Goldstein et al. 1987). While some of these studies are in disagreement, most suggest that patients with panic disorder have normal DSTs (i.e., demonstrate 4 p.m. plasma cortisol levels less than 5 μg/dl). Moreover, we found normal levels of urinary-free cortisol in 12 patients with panic disorder compared to 12 healthy controls (Uhde et al., in press). Nevertheless, two recent studies suggest that more subtle disturbances in HPA function, abnormalities that neither the DST nor urinary cortisol measures would necessarily detect, might be associated with panic disorder.

In collaboration with Phil Gold, our unit examined the adrenocorticotropic hormone (ACTH) response to corticotropin-releasing hormone (CRH) in panic disorder (Roy-Byrne et al. 1986a). In depression a blunted ACTH response to CRH has been found (Gold et al. 1986; Amsterdam et al. 1987), suggesting hypersecretion of CRH in depression with secondary down-regulation of pituitary CRH receptors. In 8 patients with panic disorder, we found a blunted ACTH response to CRH compared to 30 normal controls (Fig. 2). This response resembles that reported in depression (Gold et al. 1986; Amsterdam et al. 1987) with some noticeable differences. In depression, basal levels of cortisol are elevated, while basal levels of ACTH are normal (Gold et al. 1986; Amsterdam et al. 1987). However, in the patients with panic disorder, basal levels of both cortisol and ACTH are elevated, perhaps pointing to an acute disturbance in ACTH secretion in panic disorder.

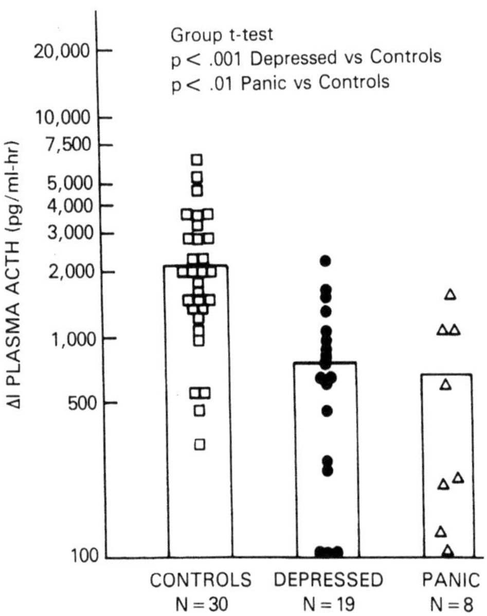

Fig. 2. Blunted ACTH response to CRH in 19 depressed patients and 8 panic disorder patients compared to 30 normal controls. The *bars* represent the mean responses for each group

In another recent report of HPA functioning in panic disorder, Goldstein and colleagues (1987) studied various aspects of the HPA axis in 24 outpatients with panic disorder in comparison with 38 outpatients with major depressive disorder and 61 normal controls. They found similarly low rates of DST nonsuppression in the panic disorder outpatients, depressed outpatients, and normal volunteers (all less than 15% nonsuppression rates). However, interestingly, they found nearly identically elevated rates of afternoon basal cortisol levels in the panic outpatients and depressed outpatients, compared to the normal controls. They conclude that an abnormality of the HPA system may be part of the panic disorder syndrome, as reflected by elevated basal cortisol levels (Goldstein et al. 1987).

Currently, the nature and meaning of these findings is unclear. Disturbances in the HPA system may indeed be a component of the panic disorder syndrome, although perhaps not intimately related to the pathogenesis of panic attacks themselves since elevations in serum cortisol are not found during in vivo exposure-induced panic attacks (Curtis et al. 1978) or lactate-induced panic attacks (Liebowitz et al. 1985). Alternatively, the perturbation in the HPA axis may be a nonspecific phenomenon related to the secondary effects of chronic or intermittent stress and arousal. This issue will be discussed in more detail later in this chapter.

The Thyroid-Releasing Hormone (TRH) Test and other Measures of Hypothalamo-Pituitary-Thyroid Axis Functioning

Another biological marker that has been studied in psychiatric patients over the past 15 years is the thyrotropin (TSH) response to thyrotropin-releasing hormone (TRH; Loosen and Prange 1982). Approximately 30% of depressed patients exhibit a diminished TSH reponse to the administration of TRH (Loosen and Prange 1982) compared to normal controls, an abnormality also observed in some patients with anorexia nervosa (Casper and Frohman 1982), bulimia nervosa (Gwirtsman et al. 1983), alcoholism (Loosen et al. 1979), and borderline personality disorder (Garbutt et al. 1983).

We have been extensively involved in the study of the hypothalamo-pituitary-thyroid (HPT) axis in patients with panic disorder. Our preliminary observations (Roy-Byrne et al. 1986b) on the TSH response to TRH are illustrated in Fig. 3. Four out of 12 panic disorder patients had an abnormally low (i.e., maximal change in TSH from baseline $\leqq 7$ μIU/ml) response, compared to none of 10 normal controls (Fisher's exact test, $P = 0.06$).

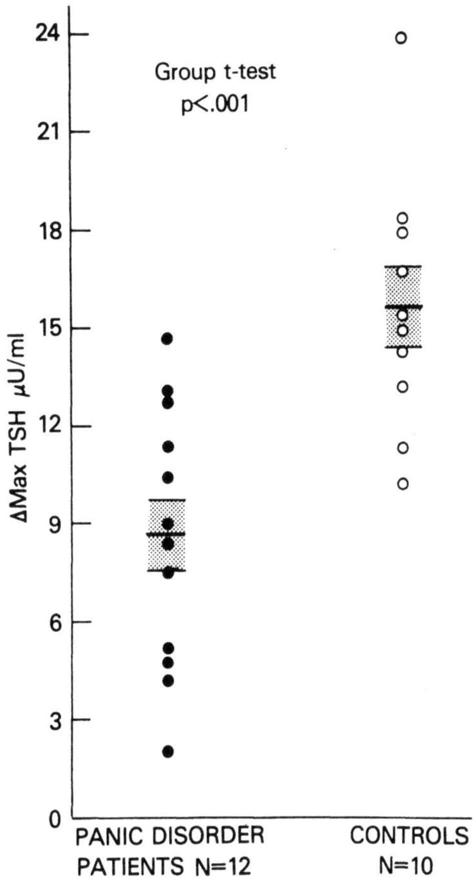

Fig. 3. Blunted TSH response to TRH in 12 patients with panic disorder compared to 10 normal controls. The *dark middle lines* represent the mean for each group; the *shaded areas* represent the SEM

At the present time, the mechanism involved in the blunted TSH response to TRH is poorly understood (Loosen 1985; Peabody et al. 1987). A "blunted" TSH reponse to TRH could be reflecting a disturbance in a variety of neuroendocrine parameters. A number of factors intrinsic and extrinsic to the HPT axis are involved in the regulation of this system. Factors extrinsic to the HPT axis itself include, but are not limited to, somatostatin, dopamine, norepinephrine, and cortisol (Visser 1985). Within the HPT system, elevated levels of serum T_3 and/or T_4 would, by way of normal autoregulatory feedback mechanisms, result in decreased pituitary secretion of TSH. This would be clearly reflected by a decreased TSH response to TRH stimulation. Conceivably, then, the decreased TSH secretion seen in response to TRH in panic disorder could represent a condition of "subclinical hyperthyroidism." However, our recent work suggests that this is an unlikely possibility. We have examined routine peripheral thyroid indices in 26 patients with panic disorder, compared to 26 normal controls (Stein and Uhde 1988). In this study, no evidence of thyroid hyperfunctioning (as measured by plasma levels of thyroxine, free thyroxine, triiodothyronine, and TSH) was found in the panic disorder patients as compared to the normal controls. This suggests that subclinical hyperthyroidism is an unlikely explanation for the blunted TSH response seen in some patients with panic disorder; the pathophysiological nature of this disturbance remains to be elucidated.

Other Biological Indices

Although too extensive to describe in detail here, a number of other biological indices have been found to be abnormal in panic disorder (for review see, Uhde et al. 1986a; Stein and Uhde, in press). As is the case for patients with major depression (Siever and Uhde 1984), patients with panic disorder have been shown to exhibit a blunted growth hormone response to intravenous clonidine (Charney et al. 1986; Uhde et al. 1986b), a finding possibly indicative of noradrenergic dysfunction. Similarly, other investigations have found abnormalities in noradrenergic receptors in patients with panic disorder (Cameron et al. 1984; Nesse et al. 1984; Uhde et al. 1985b). These data provide some support for a noradrenergic hypothesis of panic disorder (Redmond and Huang 1983; Ballenger et al. 1984; Uhde et al. 1984; Charney et al. 1986).

Finally, among the most intriguing of the biological findings in panic disorder have been the recent positron emission tomography (PET) studies (Reiman et al. 1986). This group of investigators, in studies that must still be classified as preliminary, have found that patients with panic disorder show some differences in cerebral blood flow compared to normal controls. These observations should stimulate interesting future research into brain anatomical and physiological correlates of panic.

Pharmacological Challenge Paradigms in Panic Disorder

A number of exogenously administered substances can provoke panic attacks in individuals with panic disorder. These substances include lactate, caffeine, isoproterenol, CO_2, and others (for reviews see, Uhde and Nemiah, in press; Uhde and Tancer, in press; Gorman et al., in press). The fact that these substances can induce panic attacks in susceptible individuals can be interpreted as evidence in favor of a biological diathesis for panic disorder.

Lactate Challenge in Panic Disorder

The sodium lactate model of panic disorder is probably the best known of the pharmacological challenge paradigms. Beginning with the now-classic observations of Pitts and McClure (1967), numerous investigations have been conducted looking at the behavioral and physiological response to infusions of sodium lactate in patients with panic disorder. This model has been thoroughly reviewed elsewhere (Gorman et al., in press; Margraf et al. 1986a) Briefly, it is known that approximately 50%–70% of patients with panic disorder will experience a panic attack that significantly resembles their naturally occurring attacks, during a lactate infusion. In comparison, 0%–30% of normal controls have panic attacks during this procedure.

While there may well be credibility to the notion that patients with panic disorder are displaying a metabolic or biological abnormality when they panic in response to lactate, this hypothesis has been criticized. Margraf and colleagues (1986a) suggest that patients with panic disorder exhibit elevated levels of baseline anxiety, and that lactate, or other substances administered in challenge paradigms, merely pushes patients over the "threshhold" for panic. They argue that normal controls start out with lower levels of baseline anxiety and, consequently, do not have panic attacks in response to the same net stimulus. Others argue that patients with panic disorder are acutely aware of their bodily sensations (such as heart rate), and that the challenge paradigms merely elicit the internal sensations to which patients have become sensitized, thereby causing patients to react with their characteristic response to these sensations, i.e., a panic attack.

The context-specific nature of panic induction under experimental conditions, including the mediating effects of patient's expectations (Clark 1986), and the influences of parameters outside of the immediate effects of the pharmacological agents themselves, will require further study.

Caffeine Challenge in Panic Disorder

Several investigators (Boulenger et al. 1984; Charney et al. 1985; Uhde and Boulenger, in press) have noted the increased sensitivity of caffeine of patients with panic disorder compared to normal controls. Patients with panic disorder subjectively report that caffeine can make them feel anxious, and they often have reduced their own caffeine intake in response to this awareness, prior to coming for treatment. In our experience, some patients with panic disorder benefit tremendously from a reduction in their caffeine intake, even before pharmacotherapy is initiated (Uhde, in press; Roy-Byrne and Uhde, in press).

Our group continues to investigate the usefulness of the caffeine challenge paradigm (Uhde and Boulenger, in press) as a model for panic disorder. In our clinical laboratory, 24 panic disorder patients and 14 normal controls were administered 480 mg of caffeine orally. Nine of the 24 patients and none of the normal controls experienced panic attacks in response to this pharmacological challenge. These findings, and those of Charney and associates (1985), suggest that patients with panic disorder may have an abnormality in the brain's adenosinergic system. Adenosine and its analogs function as major neuromodulators in the brain (for review, see Daly 1983). Caffeine and other related methylxanthine compounds (such as theophylline), are believed to function as antagonists at the adenosine receptor, and many of their clinical effects may be mediated through their actions at this site (Marangos and Boulenger 1985). Some recent evidence in humans (Boulenger et al. 1987) indirectly supports a role for adenosine receptor systems in caffeine-induced anxiety states. While preliminary, these observations suggest a potential role for disturbances in the adenosinergic system in patients with panic disorder. Further use of the caffeine challenge in patients with panic and other anxiety disorders promises to be an exciting avenue for future investigation.

Discussion

In this chapter, we have focused on some of the data that support a biological disturbance in panic disorder. A number of biological parameters are found to be abnormal in patients with panic disorder compared to healthy controls, including a variety of measures of HPA and HPT axis functioning. At the present time, however, it remains unclear as to whether or not these biological markers represent primary abnormalities that are intimately related to the pathogenesis of panic disorder, or whether or not they merely reflect the secondary effects of chronic anxiety or "stress". There is a paucity of studies that have followed these biological markers serially over time, and we therefore do not know if they remain abnormal or remit with treatment. In addition, no studies have yet been done to see if these same biological indices can become perturbed in normal volunteers by subjecting them to an equivalent degree of stress experienced by patients suffering from recurrent panic attacks. Therefore, at this time, these biological abnormalities remain intriguing pieces of an incompletely understood puzzle.

In the same vein, much attention has been paid to the use of panic induction (or "challenge") studies as models for a biological disturbance in panic disorder. Patients with panic disorder have been found to be hypersensitive to the effects of lactate (Liebowitz et al. 1984a, 1985), caffeine (Charney et al. 1985; Uhde and Boulenger, in press), and carbon dioxide (Woods et al. 1986), among other substances. While these studies have been criticized, particularly on methodological grounds (Margraf et al. 1986a, b), a biological vulnerability still remains a convincing and provocative hypothesis. There is no doubt that questions about the mechanisms involved in panic induction remain to be addressed. Confounding factors, such as the increased baseline anxiety seen in patients with panic disorder prior to panic induction, need to be further investigated. Similarly, greater attention needs to be paid to the potential mediating effects of cognitions in the precipitation of panic attacks (Hibbert 1984; Clark 1986). Nonetheless, two recent studies have highlighted the fact that panic attacks can occur at times when behavioral and cognitive cues are likely to be relatively inoperative.

Mellman and Uhde (1988) have shown that panic attacks not infrequently occur from sleep. In particular, attacks seem to arise out of stage 2 or 3 sleep, at a time when even dream mechanisms are not typically operative. Presumably, cognitions and attention to internal somatic cues are likely to be minimal, but not altogether absent, during these stages of sleep. Koenigsberg et al. (1987) have produced awakenings from sleep in patients with panic disorder using a sleep lactate infusion. These observations, while preliminary, suggest that a biological or physiological predisposition to panic may indeed be present in individuals who suffer from panic disorder.

Thus, it appears that neither biological nor cognitive/behavioral models can satisfactorily explain the overall phenomenon of panic. A complex set of somatic, experiential, psychophysiological, and cognitive variables may all be important parts in the equation that yields panic. None of these factors should be viewed as being mutually exclusive. In fact, we are of the belief that future studies that attempt to address the interplay of these variables will likely lead to the greatest advances in understanding panic and related anxiety disorders. For example, Breier et al. (1987) have shown in normal volunteers that the neuroendocrine and autonomic response to an acute acoustic stress may be mediated by cognitions, particularly those that relate to a sense of "control." When faced with the same net stress under controllable and uncontrollable conditions, subjects experienced the greatest anxiety, dysphoria, neuroendocrine hyperactivity, and autonomic hyperactivity when the stress was uncontrollable. To our knowledge, no comparable studies have yet been undertaken in patients with panic disorder, but the analogy is a tantalizing one. Perhaps patients with panic disorder do have an underlying biological abnormality that contributes to autonomic hyperactivity or increased arousal. This, when coupled with a cognitive schema that interprets certain physical sensations as "dangerous" or "uncontrollable" (Goldstein and Chambless 1978; Margraf et al. 1986b), may lead to the complete phenomenological picture of panic disorder.

In support of this hypothesis, we have observed patients experience the somatic equivalent of panic attacks (e.g., rapid onset of palpitations, derealization, tremulousness, dyspnea), but without any of the attendant fear or anxiety that is so prominent in panic attacks. Interestingly, such patients seem far less prone to develop avoidance behaviors and do not characteristically seek treatment for these symptoms (Stein and Uhde, unpublished observations). Presumably, such patients lack the necessary, psychological framework for perceiving their somatic sensations as threatening. Despite the presence of a hypothetical biological disturbance, as evidenced by these apparently unprovoked bouts of physical panic-like symptoms, these patients do not develop the full syndromal expression of panic disorder.

In summary, much remains to be learned about the etiology of panic disorder. Biological studies to date have only touched the surface, and may as yet have uncovered only epiphenomenal abnormalities. Future research strategies need to include provisions for the study of neuroendocrine, psychophysiological, and cognitive factors in individuals with panic attacks. Without doubt, pharmacological and nonpharmacological therapies all have something to offer patients with panic disorder. The goal for the research community will be to determine the common and different "active ingredients" in each of these treatments. Only through a multidimensional expedition into the complex jungle of biological, behavioral, and psychological explanations for panic disorder will we discover the true nature of the beast.

References

American Psychiatric Association (1987) Diagnostic and statistical manual of mental disorders, 3rd ed, revised. American Psychiatric Association, Washington

Amsterdam JD, Maislin G, Winokur A, Kling M, Gold P (1987) Pituitary and adrenocortical responses to the ovine corticotropin releasing hormone in depressed patients and healthy volunteers. Arch Gen Psychiatry 44:775–781

Arana GW, Baldessarini RJ, Ornsteen M (1985) The dexamethasone suppression test for diagnosis and prognosis in psychiatry. Arch Gen Psychiatry 42:1193–1204

Avery DH, Osgood TB, Ishiki DM, Wilson LG, Kenny M, Dunner DL (1985) The DST in psychiatric outpatients with generalized anxiety disorder, panic disorder or primary affective disorder. Am J Psychiatry 139:287–291

Ballenger JC, Peterson GA, Laraia M, Hucek A, Lake CR, Jimerson D, Cox D, Trockman C, Shipe JR Jr, Wilkinson C (1984) A study of plasma catecholamines in agoraphobia and the relationship of serum tricyclic levels to treatment response. In: Ballenger JC (ed) Biology of agoraphobia. American Psychiatric Press, Washington, pp 28–63

Beaudry P, Fontaine R, Chouinard G, Annable L (1986) Clonazepam in the treatment of patients with recurrent panic attacks. J Clin Psychiatry 47:83–85

Beck AT, Emery GD (1985) Anxiety disorders and phobias: a cognitive perspective. Basic, New York

Boulenger J-P, Uhde TW, Wolff EA, Post RM (1984) Increased sensitivity to caffeine in patients with panic disorders: preliminary evidence. Arch Gen Psychiatry 41:1067–1071

Boulenger J-P, Salem N Jr, Marangos PJ, Uhde TW (1987) Plasma adenosine levels: measurement in humans and relationship to the anxiogenic effects of caffeine. Psychiatry Res 21:247–255

Breier A, Albus M, Pickar D, Zahn TP, Wolkowitz OM, Paul SM (1987) Controllable and uncontrollable stress in humans: alterations in mood and neuroendocrine and psychophysiological function. Am J Psychiatry 144:1410–1425

Bridges M, Yeragani VK, Rainey JM, Pohl R (1986) Dexamethasone suppression test in patients with panic attacks. Biol Psychiatry 21:853–855

Byrne S (1987) Verapamil in the treatment of irritable bowel syndrome (letter). J. Clin Psychiatry 48:388

Cameron OG, Smith CB, Hollingsworth PJ, Nesse RM, Curtis GC (1984) Platelet alpha-2-adrenergic receptor binding and plasma catecholamines. Arch Gen Psychiatry 41:1144–1148

Casper RC, Frohman LA (1982) Delayed TSH release in anorexia nervosa following injection of thyrotropin-releasing hormone (TRH). Psychoneuroendocrinology 7:59–68

Carroll BJ (1984) Dexamethasone suppression test. In: Hall RCW, Beresford TPP (eds) Handbook of psychiatric diagnostic procedures. Spectrum, Jamaica, vol 1, pp 3–28

Charney DS, Heninger GR (1986) Abnormal regulation of noradrenergic function in panic disorders: effects of clonidine in healthy subjects and patients with agoraphobic and panic disorder. Arch Gen Psychiatry 43:1042-1054
Charney DS, Heninger GR, Jatlow PI (1985) Incdreased anxiogenic effects of caffeine in panic disorders. Arch Gen Psychiatry 42:233-243
Charney DS, Woods SW, Goodman WK, Krystal JH, Nagy LM, Heninger GR (1987) The efficacy of lorazepam in panic disorders. New Research Abstract 165. 140th Annual meeting of the American Psychiatric Association, Chicago, May 13, 1987
Chouinard G, Annable L, Fontaine R, Solyom L (1982) Alprazolam in the treatment of generalized anxiety and panic disorders: a double-blind placebo-controlled study. Psychopharmacology (Berlin) 7:229-233
Clark DM (1986) A cognitive approach to panic. Behav Res Ther 24:461-470
Coryell WM, Noyes R Jr, Clancy J, Crowe R, Chaudhry D (1985) Abnormal escape from dexamethasone suppression in agoraphobia with panic attacks. Psychiatry Res 15:301-311
Crowe RR, Noyes R, Pauls DL, Slymen D (1983) A family study of panic disorder. Arch Gen Psychiatry 40:1065-1069
Curtis GC, Nesse R, Buxton M, Lippman D (1978) Anxiety and plasma cortisol at the crest of the circadian cycle; reappraisal of a classical hypothesis. Psychosom Med 40:368-378
Curtis GC, Cameron OG, Nesse RM (1982) The dexamethasone suppression test in panic disorder and agoraphobia. Am J Psychiatry 139:1043-1046
Daly JW (1983) Role of ATP and adenosine receptors in physiologic process: summary and prospectus. In: Daly JW, Kuroda Y, Phillis JW, Shimizu H, Ui M (eds) Physiology and pharmacology of adenosine derivatives. Raven, New York, p 275
Edlund MJ, Swann AC, Clothier J (1987) Patients with panic attacks and abnormal EEG results. Am J Psychiatry 144:508-509
Frohlich ED (1985) Role of calcium entry-blocking drugs in hypertension: a symposium. Am J Cardiol 56:1H-111H
Fyer AJ, Liebowitz MR, Gorman JM (1987) Discontinuation of alprazolam treatment in panic patients. Am J Psychiatry 144:303-308
Garbutt JC, Loosen PT, Tipermas A, Prange AJ Jr (1983) The TRH test in patients with borderline personality disorder. Psychiatry Res 9:107-113
Gold PW, Loriaux LD, Roy A, Kling MA, Calabrese JR, Kellner CH, Nieman LK, Post RM, Pickar D, Gallucci W, Avgerinos P, Paul S, Oldfield EH, Cutler GB, Chrousos GP (1986) The corticotropin releasing factor stimulation test: implications for the diagnosis and pathophysiology of hypercortisolism in primary affective disorder and Cushing's disease. N Engl J Med 314-1329-1335
Goldstein AJ, Chambless DL (1978) A reanalysis of agoraphobia. Behav Ther 9:47-59
Goldstein S, Halbreich U, Asnis G, Endicott J, Alvir J (1987) The hypothalamic-pituitary-adrenal system in panic disorder. Am J Psychiatry 144:1320-1323
Gorman JM, Fyer MR, Liebowitz MR, Klein DF (in press) Pharmacologic provocation of panic attacks. Am J Psychiatry
Grunhaus L, Rabin D, Greden F (1986) Simultaneous panic and depressive disorder; response to antidepressant treatments. J Clin Psychiatry 47:4-7
Gwirtsman HE, Roy-Byrne PP, Yager J, Gerner RH (1983) Neuroendocrine abnormalities in bulimia. Am J Psychiatry 140:559-563
Hibbert GA (1984) Ideational components of anxiety. Br J Psychiatry 144:618-624
Kahn RJ, McNair DM, Frankenthaler LM (1987) Tricyclic treatment of generalized anxiety disorder. J Affective Disord 13:145-151
Klein DF (1964) Delineation of two drug-responsive anxiety syndromes. Psychopharmacologia 5:397-408
Klein DF (1967) Importance of psychiatric diagnoses in prediction of clinical drug effects. Arch Gen Psychiatry 16:118-126
Klein DF (1981) Anxiety reconceptualized. In: Klein DF, Rabkin JG (eds) Anxiety: new research and changing concepts. Raven, New York
Klein E, Uhde TW (in press) Verapamil in the treatment of panic disorder: a controlled study. Am J Psychiatry
Klein E, Uhde TW, Post RM (1986) Preliminary evidence for the utility of carbamazepine in alprazolam withdrawal. Am J Psychiatry 143:235-236
Klein DF, Ross DC, Cohen P (1987) Panic and avoidance in agoraphobia: application of path analysis to treatment studies. Arch Gen Psychiatry 44:377-385
Koenigsberg HW, Pollak C, Sullivan T (1987) The sleep lactate infusion: arousal and the panic mechanism. Biol Psychiatry 22:789-791
Lieberman JA, Brenner R, Lesser M, Coccaro E, Berenstein M, Kane JM (1983) Dexamethasone suppression tests in patients with panic disorder. Am J Psychiatry 140:917-919
Liebowitz MR, Fyer AJ, Gorman JM, Dillon D, Appleby IL, Levy G, Anderson S, Levitt M, Palij M, Davies SO, Klein DF (1984a) Lactate provocation of panic attacks: I. Clinical and

behavioral findings. Arch Gen Psychiatry 41:764-770

Liebowitz MR, Quitkin FM, Stewart JW, McGrath PJ, Harrison W, Rabkin J, Tricamo E, Markowitz JS, Klein DF (1984b) Penelzine versus imipramine in atypical depression: a preliminary report. Arch Gen Psychiatry 41:669-677

Liebowitz MR, Gorman JM, Fyer AJ, Levitt M, Dillon D, Levy G, Appleby IL, Anderson S, Palij M, Davies S, Klein DF (1985) Lactate provocation of panic attacks: II. Biochemical and physiological findings. Arch Gen Psychiatry 42:709-719

Loosen PT (1985) The TRH-induced TSH response in psychiatric patients: A possible neuroendocrine marker. Psychoneuroendocrinology 10:237-260

Loosen PT, Prange AJ Jr (1982) Serum thyrotropin response to thyrotropin-releasing hormone in psychiatric patients; a review. Am J Psychiatry 139:405-416

Loosen PT, Prange AJ, Wilson IC (1979) TRH (protirelin) in depressed alcoholic men: behavioral changes and endocrine responses. Arch Gen Psychiatry 36:540-547

Lydiard RB (1987) Desipramine in agoraphobia with panic attacks: an open, fixed-dose study. J Clin Psychopharmacol 7:258-260

Lydiard RB, Ballenger JC (1987) Antidepressants in panic disorder and agoraphobia. J Aff Disord 13:153-168

Lydiard RB, Laraia MT, Howell EF, Ballenger JC (1987) Emergence of depressive symptoms in patients receiving alprazolam for panic disorder. Am J Psychiatry 144:664-665

Marangos PJ, Boulenger J-P (1985) Basic and clinical aspects of adenosinergic neuromodulation. Neurosci Biobehav Rev 9:421-430

Margraf J, Ehlers A, Roth WT (1986a) Sodium lactate infusions and panic attacks: a review and critique. Psychosom Med 48:23-51

Margraf J, Ehlers A, Roth WT (1986b) Panic attacks: theoretical models and empirical evidence. In: Hand I, Wittchen H-U (eds) Panic and phobias. Springer, Berlin Heidelberg New York

Marks IM (1983) Are there anticompulsive or antiphobic drugs? Review of the evidence. Br J Psychiatry 143:338-347

Marks IM (1987) Behavioral aspects of panic disorder. Am J Psychiatry 144:1160-1165

Marks IM, Gray S, Cohen D, Hill R, Mawson D, Ramm L, Stern RS (1983) Imipramine and brief therapist-aided exposure in agoraphobics having self-exposure homework. Arch Gen Psychiatry 40:153-162

Mavissakalian M, Barlow DH (eds) (1983) Phobia: psychological and pharmacological treatment. Guilford, New York

Mavissakalian M, Michelson L (1986) Agoraphobia: relative and combined effectiveness of therapist-assisted in vivo exposure and imipramine. J Clin Psychiatry 47:117-122

Mavissakalian M, Michelson L, Dealy RS (1983) Pharmacological treatment of agoraphobia. Imipramine versus imipramine with programmed practice. Br J Psychiatry 143:348-355

Mellman TA, Uhde TW (1987a) Obsessive-compulsive symptoms in panic disorder. Am J Psychiatry 144:1573-1576

Mellman TA, Uhde TW (1987b) Withdrawal syndrome with gradual tapering of alprazolam. Am J Psychiatry 143:1464-1466

Mellman TA, Uhde TW (1988) Electroencephalographic sleep in panic disorder: a focus on sleep-related panic attacks. Submitted for publication

Nesse RM, Cameron OG, Curtis GC, McCann DS, Huber-Smith MJ (1984) Adrenergic function in patients with panic anxiety. Arch Gen Psychiatry 41:771-776

Noyes R Jr, Clarkson C, Crowe RR, Yates WR, Mohesney CM (1987) A family study of generalized anxiety disorder. Am J Psychiatry 144:1019-1024

Peabody CA, Whiteford HA, Warner MD, Faull KF, Barchas JD, Berger PA (1987) TRH stimulation test in depression. Psych Res 22:21-28

Peterson GA, Ballenger JC, Cox DP, Hucek A, Lydiard RB, Laraia MT, Trockman C (1985) The dexamethasone suppression test in agoraphobia. J Clin Psychopharmacol 5:110-102

Pitts FN Jr, McClure JN (1967) Lactate metabolism in anxiety neurosis. N Engl J Med 277:1329-1336

Redmond D Jr, Huang Y (1983) Current concepts II. New evidence for a locus coeruleus-norepinephrine connection with anxiety. Life Sci 25:2149-2162

Reiman EM, Raichle ME, Robins E, Butler FK, Herscovitch P, Fox P, Perlmutter J (1986) The application of positron emission tomography to the study of panic disorder. Am J Psychiatry 143:469-477

Roy-Byrne PP, Uhde TW (in press) Exogenous factors in panic disorder: Clinical and research implications. J Clin Psychiatry

Roy-Byrne PP, Bierer LM, Uhde TW (1985) The dexamethasone suppression test in panic disorder: comparison with normal controls. Biol Psychiatry 20:1237-1240

Roy-Byrne PP, Uhde TW, Post RM, Gallucci WM, Chrousos GR (1986a) The corticotropin-releasing hormone stimulation test in patients

with panic disorder. Am J Psychiatry 143:896–899
Roy-Byrne PP, Uhde TW, Rubinow DR, Post RM (1986b) Reduced TSH and prolactin responses to TRH in patients with panic disorder. Am J Psychiatry 143:503-507
Sachar EJ, Hellman L, Roffwarg HP, Halpern F, Fukashima D, Gallagher T (1973) Disrupted 24-hour patterns of cortisol secretion in psychotic depression. Arch Gen Psychiatry 28:19–24
Sheehan DV (1982) Panic attacks and phobias. N Engl J Med 307:156–158
Sheehan DV (1987) Benzodiazepines in panic disorder and agoraphobia. J Affective Disord 13:169–181
Sheehan DV, Ballenger JC, Jacobson G (1980) Treatment of endogenous anxiety with phobic, hysterical and hypochondriacal symptoms. Arch Gen Psychiatry 37:51–59
Sheehan DV, Claycomb JB, Surman OS, Baer L, Coleman J, Gelles L (1983) Panic attacks and the dexamethasone suppression test. Am J Psychiatry 140:1063–1064
Siever LJ, Uhde TW (1984) New studies and perspectives on the noradrenergic receptor system in depression: effects of the alpha-2-adrenergic agonist clonidine. Biol Psychiatry 19:131–156
Solomon GD, Steel JG, Spaccavento LJ (1983) Verapamil prophylaxis of migraine: a double-blind, placebo-controlled study. JAMA 250:2500–2502
Solyom C, Solyom L, Lapierre Y, Pecknold J, Morton L (1981) Phenelzine and exposure in the treatment of phobias. Biol Psychiatry 16:239–247
Spier SA, Tesar GE, Rosenbaum JF, Woods SW (1986) Treatment of panic disorder and agoraphobia with clonazepam. J Clin Psychiatry 47:238–242
Stein MB, Uhde TW (1988) Thyroid indices in panic disorder. Submitted for publication
Stein MB, Uhde TW (in press) Panic disorder and major depression: Lifetime relationship and biological markers. In: Ballenger JC (ed) Neurobiological aspects of panic disorder. Liss, New York
Telch MJ, Agras WS, Taylor B, Roth WT, Gallen CC (1985) Combined pharmacological and behavioral treatment for agoraphobia. Behav Res Ther 23:325–335
Torgerson S (1983) Genetic factors in anxiety disorders. Arch Gen Psychiatry 40:1085–1092
Uhde TW (1986) Treating panic and anxiety. Psychiatr Ann 16:536–541
Uhde TW (in press) Caffeine: Practical facts for the psychiatrist. In: Roy-Byrne PP (ed) Anxiety: new research findings for the clinician. APA Press, Washington, DC
Uhde TW, Boulenger J-P (in press) Caffeine model of panic. In: Lerer B, Gershon S (eds) New directions in affective disorders
Uhde TW, Nemiah JC (in press) Panic and generalized anxiety disorders. In: Kaplan HI, Sadock BJ (eds) Comprehensive textbook of psychiatry, 5th ed. Williams and Wilkins, Baltimore
Uhde TW, Tancer ME (in press) Pharmacological challenge paradigms in panic disorder. In: Tyrer P (ed) Proceedings of the British Association for Psychopharmacology symposium on anxiety. Oxford University Press, London
Uhde TW, Boulenger J-P, Post RM, Siever LJ, Vittone BJ, Jimerson DC, Roy-Byrne PP (1984) Fear and anxiety: relationship to noradrenergic function. Psychopathology 17 (Suppl 3):8–23
Uhde TW, Ballenger JC, Post RM (1985a) Carbamazepine: Treatment of affective illness and anxiety syndromes. In: Pichot P, Berner P, Wolf R, Than K (eds) Psychiatry: the state of the art, vol 3. Plenum, New York, pp 474–484
Uhde TW, Boulenger J-P, Roy-Byrne PP, Geraci MF, Vittone BJ, Post RM (1985b) longitudinal course of panic disorder: clinical and biological considerations. Prog Neuropsychopharmacol Biol Psychiatry 9:39–51
Uhde TW, Roy-Byrne P, Post RM (1986a) Panic disorder and major depressive disorder: biological relationship. In: Shagass C, Josiassen RC, Bridger WH, Weiss KJ, Stoff D, Simpson GM (eds) Biological psychiatry 1985. Elsevier, New York, pp 463–465
Uhde TW, Vittone BJ, Siever LJ, Kaye WH, Post RM (1986b) Blunted growth hormone response to clonidine in panic disorder patients. Biol Psychiatry 21:1081–1085
Uhde TW, Stein MB, Post RM (1988a) Lack of efficacy of carbamazepine in the treatment of panic disorder. Submitted for publication
Uhde TW, Stein BM, Vittone BJ, Siever LJ, Boulenger J-P, Klein EM, Mellman TA, Post RM (1988b) Behavioral and physiological effects of acute and chronic response to clonidine in panic disorder. Submitted for publication
Uhde TW, Joffe RT, Jimerson DC, Post RM (in press) Normal urinary-free cortisol and plasma MHPG in panic disorder: clinical and theoretical implications. Biol Psychiatry
Visser TJ (1985) Regulation of the release of TSH. Front Horm Res 14:100–136
Woods SW, Charney DS, Loke J, Goodman WK, Redmond DE, Heninger GR (1986) Carbon dioxide sensitivity in panic anxiety: ventilatory and anxiogenic responses to carbon dioxide in healthy subjects and patients with panic anxiety before and after alprazolam treatment. Arch Gen Psychiatry 43:900–909

Zitrin CM, Klein DF, Woerner MG (1978) Behavior therapy, supportive psychotherapy, imipramine and phobias. Arch Gen Psychiatry 35:307-316

Zitrin CM, Klein DF, Woerner MG (1980) Treatment of agoraphobia with group exposure in vivo and imipramine. Arch Gen Psychiatry 37:63-72

3. The Mutually Potentiating Effects of Imipramine and Exposure in Agoraphobia

M. MAVISSAKALIAN

Introduction

This paper will focus on six controlled studies which have investigated the relative and combined effects of behavioral and pharmacological treatments of agoraphobia (Zitrin et al. 1980, 1983; Marks et al. 1983; Mavissakalian et al. 1983; Telch et al. 1985; Mavissakalian and Michelson 1986a). The pharmacological agent in all of these studies is the tricyclic drug imipramine and, therefore, conclusions drawn from this review are more likely to generalize to some (e.g., phenelzine, chlorimipramine, zimeledine, desimipramine, and trazodone) but not all (e.g., benzodiazepines, in particular, aprazolam) pharmacological agents which have been reported to be effective in the treatment of panic disorder/agoraphobia. The behavioral treatment in the six studies includes instructions and encouragement for self-directed exposure to phobic situations with or without therapist-assisted in vivo exposure sessions. Five of the studies have compared imipramine plus exposure vs placebo plus exposure and, therefore, assess whether imipramine enhances the effects of exposure. Two of the studies have compared imipramine with and without exposure and thus assess the opposite question: Does exposure enhance the effects of imipramine? Finally, the choice of agoraphobia is fortunate in these studies because this complex disorder encompasses both panic and phobic symptomatologies and thus provides a natural clinical context in which to study the differential effects of exposure (which targets phobic avoidance/anxiety) and of imipramine (which presumably changes the central "endogenous" processes mediating panic attacks). Given that both pharmacological and behavioral approaches have their advocates (see the papers by Uhde in this volume and by Hand et al. in the previous volume *Panic and Phobias* 1986), it would be of the utmost importance to determine the relative efficacy ot these treatments in panic disorder/agoraphobia. Unfortunately, only the study by Telch et al. (1985) can be said to have addressed the most basic question of differential efficacy between exposure and imipramine by directly comparing these two treatments. In this study, to which we will return later, ten patients received imipramine with antiexposure instructions ("giving the drug time to work before attempting to confront feared situations") for 8 weeks at which point the antiexposure instructions were lifted and patients were informed that "the medication had had sufficient time to build up in their system and that they should try to venture out into previously feared situations." However, no other systematic intervention was provided to this group which represents a pure imipramine condition group to be contrasted with nine patients who where assigned to double-blind placebo and who received three therapist-assisted prolonged in vivo exposure sessions in groups between the absence of statistically significant dose effects on panic measures was not due to a lack of commensurate levels of response on these measures in patients receiving high imipramine doses, but rather to the substantial improvement/response rates for panic obtained in placebo and low-dose patients. We concluded that non-pharmocological factors, primarily exposure, had accounted for most of the improvement in panic in our study.

In addition to the dose-response relationship obtained in this study, other observations were made that would provide compelling evidence in favor of a specific pharmacological effect of imipramine in agoraphobia. First, we obtained a positive relationship between plasma imipramine levels and improvement in agoraphobia in a subsample of 15 of these patients whose steady-state imipramine dose approximated a weight-adjusted fixed protocol of 2.5 mg/kg/day, suggesting that in this study response in agoraphobia was dependent on dose as well as the bio-availability of imipramine (Mavissakalian et al. 1984). Second, the frequency and duration of self-practice did not differ significantly among the various experimental treatment groups or between patients receiving placebo, low dose or high dose of imipramine (Mavissakalian and Michelson 1986b; Mavissakalian, in press, a). Indeed, it appeared that imipramine had a significant effect in the reduction of phobic anxiety experienced during an equivalent amount of in vivo exposure, which in turn suggests that the drug may have enhanced the therapeutic process of habituation underlying exposure treatment (Mavissakalian and Michelson 1986a). Finally, along with others (Zitrin et al. 1980, 1983; Sheehan et al. 1980) we found no evidence to support the contention of Marks et al. (1983) that the benefit of imipramine in agoraphobia is primarily due to its antidepressant action.

We also analyzed the long-term differential effects of imipramine and exposure in our sample in a prospective 2-year study (Mavissakalian and Michelson 1986b). At the last treatment session (12th week), drugs were tapered and discontinued over 10 to 14 days, but the double-blind condition was maintained until patients came to the clinic for their 1-month posttreatment follow-up assessment. The 1-month data were therefore used to assess short-term outcome and the net effects of protocol treatments. Subsequently, patients were seen at 6 months, 1 year, and 2 years after treatment. Cross-sectional analyses based on available data revealed significant improvement from pretreatment levels at each follow-up assessment on virtually all measures. Results from the 1-month posttreatment assessment revealed that both imipramine and flooding had significant effects on phobic measures and that both treatments, particularly imipramine, had enhanced the net therapeutic benefits derived from programmed practice as judged by the distribution of high end-state functioning patients across the experimental treatment groups, e.g., imipramine plus flooding (n = 14), 64%; imipramine plus programmed practice (n = 17), 65%; flooding (n = 17), 47%; and programmed practice (n = 14), 29% ($X^2 = 4.46$; $P = 0.03$). However, there were no significant differential treatment findings at subsequent follow-up assessments.

Further analyses were performed on 25 patients who had completed all follow-up assessments to examine longitudinal patterns of maintenance or change over the entire follow-up period. Results revealed no significant flooding, imipramine, or repeated measures (time) effects on any measure. There were significant imipramine × time interaction effects, however, on clinician-rated global severity and self-rated severity, indicating a tendency for reversals in patients previously treated with imipramine in contrast to further improvement in patients treated with exposure alone at between 1 and 6 months of the follow-up period. Although neither the worsening in patients treated with imipramine, nor the improvement noted in patients receiving behavioral treatments alone were statistically significant, the differential pattern of maintenance was probably responsible for the disappearance of long-term treatment differences. Indeed, the reversals obtained following the withdrawal of imipramine support the notion of a direct effect which weakens upon discontinuation of the drug. However, it should be emphasized that the group mean change scores during follow-up were quite small and did not signify a return to pretreatment levels. Indeed, the most impressive finding from the data was the stability of gains achieved during treatment which were attributed to the emphasis placed on self-directed exposure during treatment. Interestingly, the exposure principle was still viewed by most patients as a useful coping strategy at the 2-year follow-up, which raises the possibility that it may have protected further or greater deterioration in patients treated with imipramine.

Does Exposure Enhance the Therapeutic Effects of Imipramine?

In a study specifically designed to investigate this question (Mavissakalian et al. 1983), 18 agoraphobics were randomly assigned either to imipramine (I) or imipramine plus programmed practice (I + BT). Three patients dropped out leaving seven patients in I and eight in I + BT. The administration of drug was open starting with imipramine 25 mg p.o. at bedtime with dose increments of 25 mg every second day until a tolerable maintenance dosage or a maximum of 200 mg/day was reached. The average steady-state dose of imipramine was 125 mg (range, 50 to 200 mg) in both groups. In the I group patients were not given behavioral instructions. Their treatment approximated the busy clinical practice of prescribing a medication known for its beneficial effects on mood and panic and its known clinical usefulness in agoraphobia. Patients in the I + BT group were given behavioral rationale and instructions emphasizing the role of habitual avoidance behavior in maintaining their condition and the crucial role of systematic self-directed exposure in treatment and met individually with a clinical psychologist for programmed practice. The results at the end of 3 months of treatment revealed statistically and clinically greater improvement, primarily on phobic measures in the I + BT group. Group differences, however, were relatively minimal on panic and anxiety measures, including an operationalized definition of spontaneous panic attacks, which improved highly and equally in both groups. The results also suggested that the clinical practice of prescribing imipramine to agoraphobics can lead to improvement, although in the absence of a placebo control it was hard to judge the specificity and significance of the changes due to imipramine proper. Furthermore, the possibility that a certain degree of exposure to phobic situations may have taken place in these patients whose primary aim, after all, was to be able to enter hitherto avoided situations remained an open question.

As already mentioned, Telch et al. (1985) have attempted to control for such inadvertent self-exposure by instructing patients in one of their imipramine groups to refrain from entering novel phobic situations (e.g., imipramine with antiexposure instructions). At the end of 8 weeks of treatment this group had improved significantly on anticipated as well as actual anciety experienced during the behavioral test and on dysphoric mood. However, no significant improvement had occurred in major clinical measures of phobia and panic. Comparisons between this group and the group receiving imipramine with exposure instructions revealed that the latter was significantly more improved on several measures of phobia as well as the anticipated and actual anxiety experienced during the behavioral test. However, the results at the 26-week assessment in their study are more clinically relevant. Thus, when antiexposure instructions were lifted and patients were "allowed" to face their feared situations if they wished, while being maintained on imipramine, significant improvement on measures of phobia occurred, but patients who had received systematic exposure in addition to imipramine evidenced superior improvement in panic and phobias. The evidence from these two studies, therefore, strongly suggests that the prescription of imipramine without specific instructions for or against self-directed exposure can have therapeutic effects, but that these are enhanced to a statistically and clinically significant degree by the addition of systematic exposure treatment. Consideration of these findings together with the negative results with counter-exposure instructions seems to suggest that some exposure may be necessary for imipramine's antiphobic and even antipanic effects in agoraphobia.

Summary and Conclusions

The most basic question of the relative efficacy of exposure and imipramine treatments of agoraphobia cannot be addressed at present. However, the available controlled studies demonstrate that the effects of exposure and imipramine are mutually potentiating and thus provide strong empirical support for combining behavioral and pharmacological approaches in the treatment of this disorder. Indeed, the combination of programmed practice and imipramine $\geqq$ 150 mg/day could be recommended as an effective and cost-efficient treatment that would yield marked response in three out of four patients suffering from agoraphobia with panic. It is also of substantial clinical interest that gains achieved during the combined treatment remain impressively stable following discontinuation of medication and that concurrent treatment with imipramine does not seem to affect negatively the long-term outcome of exposure treatments.

The review also cautions against the polarization between behavioral and pharmacological therapies because the evidence from the controlled studies does not support the premise of differential antipanic and antiphobic effects with imipramine and exposure, respectively. Indeed, both treatments induced significant improvement in phobias and the antiphobic effects were mutually potentiating, the combined treatment being consistently superior to the individual counterparts. In this regard, our findings that response in agoraphobia was dependent on dose, as well as the bio-availability of imipramine, coupled with evidence suggesting that imipramine's antiphobic effects were not mediated through its antidepressant action nor through increased frequency or procedurally improved self-directed exposure are of particular interest and suggest that imipramine may have a specific and direct facilitative effect on fear reduction in agoraphobia.

It is more difficult to provide a consensus summary on the differential antipanic effects of imipramine and exposure based on these studies. In our studies, (Mavissakalian et al. 1983; Mavissakalian and Michelson 1986a), the mutually potentiating effects of exposure and imipramine on phobic measures were not replicated on panic measures primarily because of a ceiling effect, e.g., substantial improvement in panic with imipramine or exposure. On the other hand, in the study by Telch et al. (1985) neither treatment alone exerted a significant improvement on panic, but their combination did. Finally, exposure treatment induced improvement in panic in the studies by both Marks et al. (1983) and Zitrin et al. (1980, 1983), but imipramine failed to enhance this response in the former, while it had a significant effect in the latter two studies. Undoubtedly, the different measures of panic utilized in the various studies may account for some of these inconsistencies. Be it as it may, the fact that panic improves with exposure treatment taken together with the finding that antiexposure instructions can block the antipanic effect of the drug calls into question the assumption that the specific effect of imipramine in agoraphobia is the blocking of "spontaneous" panic attacks (Klein 1981). Since some degree of exposure seems to be necessary for imipramine's antipanic and antiphobic effects to become manifest, and the more systematic the exposure the better, and in light of our findings that imipramine had a significant effect on the reduction of phobic anxiety experienced during an equivalent amount of in vivo exposure (Mavissakalian and Micheson 1986a), it is plausible to suggest that the mechanism of action of imipramine consists of facilitating the therapeutic process of habituation underlying fear reduction. The suggestion is consistent not only with the recent improvement in the American classification of panic disorder (DSM-IIIR 1987), which recognizes the fear of panic as an important phenomenological and diagnostic factor, but also the increasing number of studies demonstrating that behavioral treatments based on exposure to internal, cognitive, physiological stimuli accompanying anxiety can be very effective in treating panic attacks (Barlow 1986; Clark 1986).

References

American Psychiatric Association, Committee on Nomenclature and Statistics (1987) Diagnostic and statistical manual of mental disorders. Revision of 3rd edn. American Psychiatric Association, Washington DC

Barlow DH (1986) Behavioral conception and treatment of panic. Psychopharmacol Bull 22:802-806

Clark DM (1986) A cognitive approach to panic. Behav Res Ther 24:461-470

Cohen SD, Monteiro W, Marks IM (1984) Two-year follow-up of agoraphobics after exposure and imipramine. Br J Psychiatry 144:276-281

Garakani H, Zitrin CM, Klein DF (1984) Treatment of panic disorder with imipramine alone. Am J Psychiatry 143:348-355

Klein DF (1981) Anxiety reconceptualized. In: Klein DF, Rabkin JG (eds) Anxiety: new research and changing concepts. Raven, New York

Marks IM (1981) Cure and care of neuroses. Wiley Interscience, New York

Marks IM, Gray S, Cohen D et al (1983) Imipramine and brief therapist-aided exposure in agoraphobics having self-exposure homework. Arch Gen Psychiatry 40:153-162

Mavissakalian M (1982) Pharmacological treatment of anxiety disorders. J Clin Psychiatry 43:487-491

Mavissakalian M (in press a) Initial depression and response to imipramine in agoraphobia. J Nerv Ment Dis

Mavissakalian M (in press b) Differential Efficacy Between Tricyclic Antidepressants and Behavior Therapy of Panic Disorder. In: Ballenger G (ed) Clinical aspects of panic disorder. Liss, New York

Mavissakalian M, Michelson L (1986a) Relative and combined effectiveness of therapist-assisted in vivo exposure and imipramine. J Clin Psychiatry 47:117-122

Mavissakalian M, Michelson L (1986b) Two year follow-up of exposure and imipramine treatment of agoraphobia. Am J Psychiatry 143:1106-1112

Mavissakalian M, Perel J (1985) Imipramine in the treatment of agoraphobia: dose response relationships. Am J Psychiatry 142:1032-1036

Mavissakalian M, Michelson L, Dealy RS (1983) Pharmacological treatment of agoraphobia: imipramine vs imipramine with programmed practice. Br J Psychiatry 143:348-355

Mavissakalian M, Perel JM, Michelson L (1984) The relationship of plasma imipramine and N-desmethylimipramine to improvement in agoraphobia. J Clin Psychopharmacol 4:36-40

Sheehan DV, Ballenger J, Jacobsen G (1980) Treatment of endogenous anxiety with phobic, hysterical and hypochondrical symptoms. Arch Gen Psychiatry 37:51–59

Telch MJ, Agras WS, Taylor CB et al (1985) Combined pharmacological and behavioral treatment for agoraphobia. Behav Res Ther 23:325–335

Zitrin CM, Klein DF, Woerner MC (1980) Treatment of agoraphobia with group exposure in vivo and imipramine. Arch Gen Psychiatry 37:63–72

Zitrin CM, Klein DF, Woerner MG (1983) Treatment of phobias - I. Comparison of imipramine hydrochloride and placebo. Arch Gen Psychiatry 40:125–138

Part II

Pharmacological, Cognitive, and Behavorial Treatments of Panic and Phobias: Current State of Research

4. Effects of Discontinuation of Antipanic Medication

A. J. FYER

Introduction

A number of pharmacologic treatments have been established as effective in blocking the recurrent panic attacks experienced by patients with panic disorder or who have agoraphobia with panic attacks. However, the immediate and long-term posttreatment course in this patient group has only begun to be systematically investigated. Among patients commonly seen in treatment settings, panic attacks have a pattern of lifetime episodic recurrence (Breier et al. 1985; Uhde et al. 1985). Therefore, questions concerning issues such as the occurrence of withdrawal symptoms during drug discontinuation, the rates of and risk factors for post-discontinuation relapse, and the consequences of continuous long-term treatment are of both clinical and theoretical importance.

This paper reviews the currently available discontinuation and follow-up data on three types of medications commonly used for treatment of recurrent panic: tricyclic antidepressants (TCA), monoamine oxidase inhibitors (MAOI) and high-potency benzodiazepines (BZD). The term *discontinuation* will be used to refer to studies which examine symptoms *during* medication tapering. *Follow-up* will refer to studies which assess the clinical course *after* medication has already been tapered to zero.

When a drug is discontinued two types of symptoms may occur: those which represent a re-emergence of the illness which had been suppressed by the treatment *(relapse)* and those which are a direct consequence of the tapering process *(withdrawal symptoms)*. Among anxiety disorder patients there may be some difficulty in distinguishing these two phenomena since there is some overlap between the common symptoms of anxiety and of withdrawal. For this reason most controlled medication trials define withdrawal conservatively as the occurrence during medication discontinuation of *new* symptoms which were not previously reported by the patient either before or during treatment. Additional characteristics which distinguish withdrawal from relapse are its diminution with time and the stereotyped nature of the syndromes associated with tapering of different classes of drugs. In contrast, relapse closely resembles the patient's previous illness and is either constant or increases as the time off drug lengthens. The term rebound is used to describe relapse in which the patient's symptoms are significantly worse during or after the tapering than they were before treatment (Fontaine et al. 1984).

These guidelines are useful in making the necessary clinical decisions. However, given the current lack of knowledge concerning the etiology of anxiety disorders and of the mechanisms by which drugs alleviate these symptoms, there are often situations in which it is difficult to distinguish between relapse and withdrawal. This, in turn, limits significantly the interpretation of discontinuation study results.

Discontinuation of Antidepressant

Tricyclic Antidepressants

There are no reported controlled studies of tricyclic antidepressant (TCA) discontinuation in panic disorder patients. Clinical reports suggest that withdrawal symptoms are not usually seen during gradual TCA tapering (Fyer et al. 1984; Zitrin et al. 1983). Studies of other patient groups suggest that abrupt discontinuation of high doses of TCA may in a small percentage of patients be accompanied by a transitory influenza-like syndrome (Kramer et al. 1961; Dilsaver and Greden 1984). Typical symptoms are nausea, headache, giddiness, coryza, chills, and weakness.

Four studies have examined the posttreatment course in patients with panic disorder and/or agoraphobia with panic attacks who had received a therapeutic trial of the TCA imipramine. However, results are contradictory. Interpretation of the data is complicated by variations in the definition of relapse as well as by the fact that all subjects also participated in some form of psychotherapy while on medication.

Two studies found relatively low relapse rates. Zitrin and Klein (1983) followed-up patients who had participated in a controlled 26-week trial of imipramine combined with either supportive or behavioral psychotherapy for 2 years after discontinuation of medication. Relapse was defined as the return of avoidance behavior. In agoraphobic patients relapse rates were 19% for patients who received imipramine plus behavioral psychotherapy, 31% for those who received imipramine plus supportive psychotherapy, and 14% for those on placebo and behavioral psychotherapy. Relapse rates in mixed phobic (panic disorder) patients in each of these treatment groups were 23%, 38%, and 11% respectively. There were no significant differences between treatments or diagnostic groups for relapse rate at 2 year follow-up.

Mavissakalian and Michelson (1986) have reported results consistent with these in a 2-year follow-up study of 62 agoraphobic patients who participated in a 12-week, 2 × 2 comparative trial of imipramine and therapist-assisted flooding. Two types of analyses were done. The first was a cross-sectional examination of treatment outcome, the second a longitudinal study of the course of treatment effects in the subgroup of patients for whom a full (2-year) data set was available. This subgroup could not be considered as representative of the total sample since only 25 of the 62 patients were included. In addition, comparison at each time point of the patients in the whole sample to those in the longitudinal subgroup indicated that the latter had significantly fewer symptoms.

In the cross-sectional data there was a significant positive effect of imipramine on the severity of phobic anxiety and depression at 1 month. There were no significant between-group effects at 6-month and 1-year follow-up. At 2 years, follow-up patients in both flooding groups (imipramine and placebo) were significantly better with respect to agoraphobic symptoms. There were no other significant between-treatment effects at this time.

High end-state functioning was defined as a score of less than 2 (equivalent to well or very mildy symptomatic) on three out of four measures of phobic and panic anxiety. Of the patients who were judged to have achieved high end-state functioning, approximately half in each treatment group were well (i.e., maintained these gains) over the 2 years. Approximately two-thirds were considered to be either well or fairly well. Of the 14 imipramine-treated patients who achieved high end-state functioning at 12 weeks and for whom there were complete longitudinal data, 10 (71%) maintained this level of improvement throughout the 2-year study period.

In contrast, Sheehan (1986), in a 26-week comparative trial of imipramine phenelzine, alprazolam, and placebo, reported that over 70% of patients in all treatment groups relapsed within 1 year of discontinuation. However, in this study relapse was defined as the occurrence of at least two separate episodes in which the return of either unexpected anxiety or avoidance caused the patient to telephone the clinic and request restarting of medication. It is not clear whether patients were instructed to attempt stoically to weather a perhaps transient flare-up of recurrent symptoms or to view restarting medicine as the requisite course.

The fourth study, by Cohen et al. (1984), was a 2-year follow-up of 40 of the 45 agoraphobic patients who had participated in a comparative trial of imipramine vs. placebo and therapist-aided exposure vs. relaxation (Marks et al. 1983). All treatment groups maintained significant improvement over baseline as measured by mean scores on global, panic, and avoidance scales. There were no significant between-treatment differences in outcome. Neither a comprehensive criterion for relapse nor the number of patients who maintained recovery is reported. In addition, a number of patients had additional treatment during the follow-up period. The effect of this on follow-up outcome is not reported. Therefore, direct comparison with the results of the three previously discussed studies is difficult.

Additional data on the posttreatment effects of TCAs are available from a sodium lactate infusion study of remitted panic patients conducted at our center (Fyer et al. 1984; Sandberg unpublished data). A number of investigators have reported that intravenous infusion of 0.5 *M* racemic sodium lactate at a dose of 10 mg/kg body weight over 20 min will provoke a panic attack in individuals who have experienced previous recurrent panic. In contrast, normal and psychiatric controls who do not have a history of panic attacks do not panic when given the sodium lactate challenge (Leibowitz et al. 1984; Cowley et al. 1987; Pitts and McClure 1967;). Clinical blockade of panic by TCAs is accompanied by development of invulnerability to lactate-induced panic when use of the medication is ongoing (Liebowitz et al. 1984).

In the current experiment, patients with the DSM III diagnosis of panic disorder or agoraphobia with panic attacks who panicked during pretreatment sodium lactate infusion were treated openly with a TCA (imipramine or desmethylimipramine) and maintained on the drug until they had been panic-free for at least 4 weeks. At this point sodium lactate was reinfused. None panicked. Patients were then maintained on imipramine until they had been panic-free for at least 6 months. At that point they were tapered off the TCA and sodium lactate was reinfused 1–6 months later while still in clinical remission (panic free). Of the 14 patients studied to date, 6 (43%) panicked during the posttreatment infusion. Due to the small sample size this rate of panic does not differ significantly from that of either the normal control subjects or panic patients before treatment.

To investigate whether there was a relationship in panic patients between time off medication and vulnerability to lactate-induced panic, the median time off medication (in days) was calculated and patients were divided into two groups depending on whether their time off medication at posttreatment reinfusion was greater or less than the median. The rate of panic at posttreatment infusion was calculated and compared for these two groups. A significantly greater rate of panic at reinfusion was found for patients in whom lactate was reinfused at a time point greater than the median (5/7 or 71%) than among those in whom reinfusion was at less than the median time off medication (1/7 or 14%; $p < 0.03$, Wilcoxon test). The significant relationship between length of time after discontinuation of TCA and vulnerability to lactate-induced panic at posttreatment reinfusion suggests that successful treatment with TCAs is accompanied by a beneficial pathophysiological change which tends to decay slowly after the medication itself is discontinued.

Monoamine Oxidase Inhibitors

Only two follow-up studies have been reported of MAOI treatment in patients with panic disorder or agoraphobia with panic. Systematic data on possible withdrawal symptoms are not available.

As discussed above, Sheehan (1985) reported a 70% relapse rate in the first year following phenelzine discontinuation in patients who had received a successful 26-week course of treatment. Kelly et al. (1970) conducted a retrospective study of a large series of phenelzine-treated phobic anxiety patients. Of these, 30% relapsed shortly after tapering, 30% remained well, and 30% were not tapered due to concern for the clinical consequences.

Discontinuation of Benzodiazepines

Until recently BDZs were considered to be effective for generalized but not panic anxiety. However, during the past several years the high-potency BDZ alprazolam has been demonstrated to be an effective antipanic agent (Ballenger 1986; Liebowitz et al. 1986; Chouinard et al. 1982). Newly completed studies suggest that other BZDs may also have some panic-blocking capabilities (Speier et al. 1986; Dunner et al. 1987). BZD discontinuation is commonly associated with withdrawal symptoms in both mixed anxiety and other patient groups (Schopf 1983).

Anecdotal reports indicate that seizures, delirium, and severe agitation, similar to those that occur after short-acting barbiturates, can accompany abrupt discontinuation of moderate to high dose (4–10 mg/day) of alprazolam (Levy 1984; Noyes et al. 1985; Breier et al. 1984b). Three gradual discontinuation studies suggest that both withdrawal and relapse are a common problem during alprazolam tapering in panic disorder patients.

Mellmann and Uhde (1986) conducted a double-blind study of gradual discontinuation of alprazolam treatment in 10 hospitalized patients (eight panic disorder, two bipolar affective disorder). Patients were clinically assessed before treatment, during tapering, and after withdrawal. In addition, plasma cortisol levels, heart rate, blood pressure, and body temperature were measured at each stage. The postwithdrawal period was defined as one in which the patients had returned to their pretreatment clinical condition. Tapering rate varied between patients, with a mean rate of 0.19 mg/day (± 0.09). The average pretaper daily dose of alprazolam was 4.95 mg (± 3.22) and the mean length of time on the drug was 11.7 months (± 5.8).

All subjects were found to have significantly greater anxiety during the withdrawal period than after the withdrawal period. Plasma cortisol levels were also significantly increased during withdrawal and there was a trend toward a more rapid heart rate. There were no significant differences between the withdrawal and postwithdrawal periods in sleep time, diastolic blood pressure, or body temperature.

Pecknold and Swinson (1986) reported a systematic study of discontinuation in patients with panic disorder or agoraphobia with panic attacks who had participated in an 8-week blind treatment trial comparing alprazolam to placebo. The frequency of panic attacks was assessed from patients' diaries, which were completed on a weekly basis. Withdrawal symptoms were measured with a symptom and side effect scale and a more specialized BDZ withdrawal scale, which were completed at each visit. Results are somewhat difficult to interpret due to the high drop-out rate and the absence of explanation of the criteria used to categorize a subject as a drop-out. Only 54 (33 alprazolam, 21 placebo) of the 107 (58 alprazolam, 49 placebo) patients who completed the treatment trial also completed the 4-week taper and 2-week follow-up. A return of panic symptoms was noted during tapering in most patients in both the alprazolam and placebo responder groups. Nine (28%) of the alprazolam but only one (5%) of the placebo patients had rebound panic (i.e., a return of panic symptoms to the level of a 50% increase over pretreatment baseline). Specific comparisons are not given for milder degrees of relapse.

Withdrawal symptoms were defined as those which were newly occurring during the taper or posttaper periods. A significant increase in withdrawal symptoms for the alprazolam as compared to the placebo group was found during the last taper and first posttaper weeks. However, by the end of the second posttaper week the scores for the alprazolam group had dropped so that this difference was no longer significant. The number of patients experiencing withdrawal in each group is not given.

In a third study, Fyer et al. (1987) systematically discontinued medication in 18 of 30 panic disorder patients who had participated in an open trial of alprazolam. The mean time on alprazolam prior to tapering was 29.4 weeks for treatment responders ($n = 16$) and 14.8 weeks for nonresponders ($n = 2$). Alprazolam was tapered at a rate of 10% of the daily dose every 3 days, with the goal of discontinuing treatment in a maximum of 30 days. The mean pretaper daily doses of alprazolam were 5.25 mg for responders and 6 mg for nonresponders.

Of the 17 evaluable patients, only four completed alprazolam discontinuation (to zero dose) following the protocol. An additional four subjects were able to reach a zero dose in 7–13 weeks by slowing the rate of taper. The remaining nine subjects either refused to complete the tapering (n =2) or required adjunctive medication before they would consent to discontinuation of the alprazolam ($n = 7$).

Patients kept daily diaries of panic attacks and anxiety symptoms throughout the treatment and discontinuation periods. Using this measure, 15 of the 17 patients had a return of or increase in panic attacks during the tapering. In eight, relapse was considered mild and in seven, severe.

Withdrawal symptoms were defined as complaints newly occurring during the taper period and rated on either a symptom and side effect checklist or the BDZ withdrawal scale. Of the 17 subjects, 14 reported at least two new withdrawal symptoms during the tapering. Nine patients were considered to have a clinically significant withdrawal syndrome with either 1–2 weeks of serious discomfort or persistent moderate discomfort over 3–4 weeks. Neurological examinations and EEG studies conducted at baseline and weekly during tapering indicated no significant abnormalities. The most common withdrawal symptoms were similar to those reported in previous studies of BZD tapering in other patient groups: malaise, weakness, insomnia, tachycardia, dizziness, lightheadedness, faintness, confusion, sweating, and depression.

Discussion

Answers to the major clinical and theoretical questions concerning short- and long-term consequences of discontinuation of medication in panic patients are largely unknown. Current data on drug discontinuation and outcome in patients with panic disorder or agorphobia with panic attacks are incomplete and to some extent inconsistent. Variations in the operational definitions of relapse and withdrawal as well as the absence of any uniform assessment methodology limit cross-study comparisons.

Three of the four available follow-up studies indicate that many imipramine-(IMI) treated patients remain panic-free and/or functionally well for at least 2 years after discontinuation of medication. However, in all these studies during the acute treatment period the patients received some form of structured psychotherapy concomitantly with IMI. Therefore, additive or interactive effects of the psychological intervention on follow-up outcome cannot be ruled out.

Prospective or retrospective data from follow-up studies of MAOI treatments of panic patients are too week to allow any conclusions. Since these medications are extremely effective antipanic agents, further work in this area is of great importance.

The several open systematic studies of alprazolam discontinuation indicate that relapse and a withdrawal syndrome similar to that seen with other BZDs are common problems in the treatment of panic patients with this medication. Individuals taking alprazolam must be cautioned against abrupt discontinuation. New withdrawal symptoms appear to resolve in 2–3 weeks after tapering. However, neither controlled short-term nor long-term follow-up studies have been reported. It is therefore not known whether the recurrence of panic symptoms during tapering represents a persistant relapse or transient flare-up.

Only one systematic follow-up study directly contrasting panic patients treated with different types of antipanic medications has been reported. Sheehan (1986) found no difference in the rate at which patients treated with IMI, phenelzine, or alprazolam experienced recurrence of anxiety or avoidance. Unfortunately, neither the methodology of the follow-up, the timing or characteristics of withdrawal symptoms during tapering, nor the specific patterns of symptom recurrence associated with each drug were included in this report. Further blind controlled studies directly contrasting different antipanic medications in large groups of patients are needed to determine whether there are differences in the short-term discontinuation response and/or the long-term outcome. It is also important to find out, if relapse occurs, how simple it is to treat and the most effective methods by which to do so.

Follow-up data for a drug vs. psychotherapy comparison are only available for IMI. None of the three reported studies found significant differences in long-term outcome (2 years) for patients treated with IMI and psychotherapy as compared to placebo and psychotherapy. However, the small sample sizes, high attrition rates, and the nonsystematic additional treatment during follow-up limit the interpretation of these data. Further studies are needed both to answer the basic question of the comparative, overall, long-term effects of medication and psychotherapy as well as to determine: (a) whether either treatment has specific advantages for particular types of patients, and (b) whether combined treatment provides more benefits than each type alone.

References

Ballenger JC (1986) Pharmacotherapy of the panic disorders. J Clin Psychiatry 47 [6 Suppl]:27–31

Breier AW, Charney DS, Heninger GR (1985) The diagnostic validity of anxiety disorders and their relationships to depressive illness. Am J Psychiatry 142:787–790

Breier A, Charney DS, Nelson JC (1984) Seizures induced by abrupt discontinuation of alprazolam. Am J Psychiatry 141(12):1606–1607
Chouinard G, Annable L, Fontaine R, et al. (1982) Alprazolam in the treatment of generalized anxiety and panic disorders: a double-blind, placebo controlled study. Psychopharmacology 77:229–223
Cohen SD, Monteiro W, Marks IM (1984) Two-year follow-up of agoraphobics after exposure and imipramine. Br J Psychiatry 144:276–281
Charney DS, Woods SW, Goodman WK et al. (1986) Drug treatment of panic disorder: the comparative efficacy of imipramine, alprazolam, and trazodone. J Clin Psychiatry 47:12
Dunner DL, Ishiki D, Avery DH et al. (1986) Effect of alprazolam and diazepam on anxiety and panic attacks in panic disorder: controlled study. J Clin Psychiatry 47(9):458–460
Dilsaver SC, Greden JF (1984) Antidepressant withdrawal phenomena. Biol Psychiatry 19(2):237–255
Fontaine R, Chouinard G, Annable L (1984) Rebound anxiety in anxious patients after abrupt withdrawal of benzodiazepine treatment. Am J Psychiatry 141:848–852
Fyer AJ, Liebowitz MR, Gorman JM et al. (1987) Discontinuation of alprazolam treatment in panic patiens. Am J Psychiatry 144(3):303–308
Fyer AJ, Liebowitz MR, Gorman JM, Davies SO, Klein DF (1985) Lactate vulnerability of remitted panic patients. Psychiatry Res 14:143–148
Kelly D, Guirguis W, Frommer E et al. (1970) Treatment of phobic states with antidepressants. Br J Psychiatry 116:387–398
Kramer JC, Klein DF, Fink M (1961) Withdrawal symptoms following discontinuation of imipramine therapy. Am J Psychiatry 118:549–550
Levy AB (1984) Delirium and seizures due to abrupt alprazolam withdrawal: case report. J Clin Psychiatry 45:38–39
Liebowitz MR, Fyer AJ, Gorman JM et al. (1984) Lactate provocation of panic attacks. I. Clinical and behavioral findings. Arch Gen Psychiatry 41:764–770
Liebowitz MR, Fyer AJ, Gorman JM et al. (1986) Alprazolam in the treatment of panic disorders. J Clin Psychopharmacol 6(1):13–20
Mavissakalian M, Michelson L (1986) Agoraphobia: relative and combined effectiveness of therapist-assisted in vivo exposure and imipramine. J Clin Psychiatry 47(3):117–122
Mellman TA, Uhde TW (1986) Withdrawal syndrome with gradual tapering of alprazolam. Am J Psychiatry 143(11):1464–1466
Noyes R Jr, Clancy J, Coryell WH et al. (1985) A withdrawal syndrome after abrupt discontinuation of alprazolam. Am J Psychiatry 142:114–116
Pecknold JC, Swinson RP (1986) Taper withdrawal studies with panic disorder and agoraphobia. Psychopharmacol Bull 22(1):173–176
Pitts FM, McClure JN (1967) Lactate metabolism in anxiety neurosis. N Engl J Med 22:1329–1336
Schopf J (1983) Withdrawal phenomena after long-term administration of benzodiazepines a review of recent investigations. Pharmacopsychiatr 16:1–8
Sheehan D (1986) One-year follow-up of patients with panic disorder and withdrawal from long-term anti-panic medications. Read before the UpJohn Panic Disorder Biological Research Workshop, Washington, D.C., April 16, 1986
Spier SA, Tesar GE, Rosenbaum JF et al. (1986) Treatment of panic disorder and agoraphobia with clonazepam. J Clin Psychiatry 47(5): 238–242
Uhde TW, Boulenger JP, Roye-Byrne PP et al (1985) Longitudinal course of panic disorder. Prog Neuropsychopharmacol Biol Psychiatry 9:39–51
Zitrin CM, Klein DF, Woerner MG et al. (1983) Treatment of phobias: I. Comparison of imipramine hydrochloride and placebo. Arch Gen Psychiatry 40(2):125–138

5. Comparison of Alprazolam and Cognitive Behavior Therapy in the Treatment of Panic Disorder: A Preliminary Report*

J. S. Klosko, D. H. Barlow, R. B. Tassinari, and J. A. Cerny

Introduction

Pharmacological treatments are well established for panic disorder. Clinical evidence exists for the effectiveness of tricyclic antidepressants, monoamine oxidase inhibitors, and benzodiazepines (Barlow, in press). However, many of these reports are uncontrolled, open clinical trials conducted with heterogeneous groups of patients. More rigorous controlled trials seem to demonstrate that tricyclic antidepresants, in particular imipramine, can confer a significant advantage on psychologically based exposure therapies. Studies by Zitrin et al. (1980, 1983) have examined the separate and combined effects of imipramine and group in vivo exposure (Zitrin et al. 1980) or imaginal exposure (Zitrin et al. 1983). Generally, behavioral treatments produced improvement, but imipramine conferred an advantage on these behavioral treatments. Similar results have been reported by Telch et al. (1985) and Mavissakalian and Michelson (1986). Only Marks et al. (1983) have reported thát no particular advantage was conferred by adding imipramine to exposure-based treatments.

Despite these generally positive results, the specific effect of imipramine is not yet clear. While Zitrin et al. (1980, 1983) found some weak evidence for a specific antipanic effect, other studies have not supported these findings. Instead, studies reporting a therapeutic effect of imipramine (e.g., Mavissakalian and Michelson 1986; Telch et al. 1985) observed a generally anxiolytic effect. That is, panic improved equally in all groups, but anxiety reduction was greater in the group receiving imipramine. In fact, Telch et al. (1985) found no effects whatsoever from imipramine when exposure was specifically prevented, suggesting a necessary interaction between pharmacological and psychological methods for treatment.

Benzodiazepines were generally considered to be less effective than antidepressants, although Noyes et al. (1984) found diazepam at very high doses (5 to 40 mg/day) to be effective for panic disorder and agoraphobia with panic. More recently it has been suggested that triazolobenzodiazepines such as alprazolam may be useful for panic and panic disorder. Now there is evidence supporting the effectiveness of alprazolam in treatment of panic disorder.

A number of uncontrolled clinical trials of alprazolam have reported success (Alexander and Alexander 1986; Liebowitz et al. 1986). Chouinard et al. (1982) conducted a double-blind study of subjects with generalized anxiety disorder or panic disorder. Fifty subjects – 30 who fulfilled Research Diagnostic Criteria (RDC) for generalized anxiety disorder, and 20 who met RDC criteria for panic disorder –

* This study was submitted in partial fulfillment of the requirements for a Ph. D. at SUNY-Albany by Janet S. Klosko and was supported in part by the Upjohn Company and the National Institute of Mental Health

were assigned to 8 weeks of treatment with alprazolam or placebo. Dosage of alprazolam ranged from 0.25 to 3 mg/day. In addition, from week 5 onwards, 18 subjects (12 receiving alprazolam and 6 receiving placebo) attended behavior therapy sessions four times weekly for 4 weeks.

The authors report a subset of results separately for subjects with generalized anxiety disorder and with panic disorder. For both groups alprazolam was significantly superior to placebo at weeks 1 and 2 for Hamilton anxiety rating scale scores. There were no significant differences at weeks 4 and 8. The authors attribute the lack of significance at these times to improvement in placebo subjects. Now a large-scale cross-national study has demonstrated the effectiveness of alprazolam with panic disorder. Over 250 patients were randomly assigned to either an alprazolam or a placebo condition. Approximately 60% of patients in the alprazolam condition were panic free at 8 weeks, compared to 30% in the placebo condition (Ballenger et al., in press). Significant therapeutic benefits from alprazolam were often seen during the 1 week of administration.

Cognitive-Behavioral Treatment

Behavioral treatments for phobic disorders, particularly agoraphobia, have demonstrated effectiveness (Barlow and Beck 1984). Such treatments generally involve graduated exposure to feared situations. Unlike treatments for phobias, behavioral treatments for anxiety states such as panic disorder are largely untested. Exposure treatments, which target avoidance behavior, would seem of little benefit to patients with panic disorder, whose symptoms are mostly physiological and cognitive, although up to 40% of patients with agoraphobia with panic seem to be panic-free immediately following exposure treatment (Barlow, in press). Behavioral treatments for panic disorder have evolved only recently (Barlow, in press). Typically these treatments target both somatic and cognitive aspects of anxiety and panic.

A number of clinical replication series suggest the effectiveness of cognitive-behavioral treatment for panic attacks. Klosko and Barlow (1987) reported a series of 32 patients, 16 with panic disorder and 16 with agoraphobia with panic attacks. Only subjects with panic disorder had received cognitive-behavioral treatment directly targeting panic attacks. 80% of subjects with panic disorder, and 40% of subjects with agoraphobia, reported zero panic attacks in the 2-week period posttreatment. Gitlin et al. (1985) administered cognitive-behavioral treatment to 11 subjects with panic disorder; 10 of the 11 subjects reported they were panic-free throughout a 5-month period posttreatment. Clark et al. (1985) and Salkovskis et al. (1986) administered respiratory control training of subjects with panic disorder with and without agoraphobia. Results showed nearly complete elimination of panic attacks posttreatment, continuing through a follow-up period of 2 years. Beck (in press) reports results of cognitive-behavioral treatment of panic attacks in 28 subjects; panic attacks were completely eliminated posttreatment, and at 3-month follow-up. Finally, Ost (personal communication) eliminated panic in 8 patients with panic disorder using an applied relaxation procedure.

Despite the impressive results, the above-mentioned reports were uncontrolled clinical trials. In the first controlled study evaluating behavioral treatments for panic disorder (Barlow et al. 1984), 11 subjects with panic disorder and 9 with generalized anxiety disorder were assigned to treatment or waiting-list control groups. Treatment was cognitive-behavioral, and consisted of EMG biofeedback, progressive relaxation training (Bernstein and Borkovec 1973), and cognitive therapy (Beck and Emery 1979). Compared with controls, treated subjects improved significantly on clinical, psychophysiological, and self-report anxiety measures, including daily self-monitoring measures of background anxiety and episodes of high anxiety and panic. Subjects with panic disorder and generalized anxiety disorder responded equally well to treatment. At follow-up, subjects in the treatment group continued to improve.

Although there is evidence supporting the effectiveness of both pharmacological and cognitive-behavioral treatments of panic disorders, the evidence for pharmacological approaches is far stronger. The present study examined the effectiveness of two treatments, pharmacological treatment with alprazolam, and cognitive-behavior therapy. The study used a between-groups design, with four groups:

a) alprazolam;
b) medication placebo;
c) cognitive behavior therapy; and
d) waiting list.

To assess for possible differential expectancy effects, treatment credibility was measured. Anxiety and panic were assessed with psychophysiological, clinical and self-report measures, including daily self-monitoring of anxiety and panic. In addition, assessment were made across a wide range of other variables, such as depression and phobic symptoms. Assessment, measurement, and pharmacological treatment were administered according to the Upjohn cross-national panic study protocol. This ensured the compatibility of patients in these two studies.

Method

Subjects

Subjects were drawn from the pool of patients presenting to the Phobia and Anxiety Disorders Clinic at the State University of New York at Albany. All patients received a consensus DSM-III primary diagnosis of panic disorder, with a clinician's severity rating of at least 4 on a 0 to 8 scale, by two independent administrators of the anxiety disorders interview schedule (ADIS; DiNardo et al. 1983), revised (ADIS-R; DiNardo et al. 1985). We have demonstrated previously that panic disorder can be diagnosed reliably using the ADIS (DiNardo et al. 1983). ADIS administrators were senior clinic staff, including upper-level clincial psychology graduate students and licensed clinical psychologists. At least 15 male and female patients between 18 and 65 years of age were assigned to each of the four conditions.

Exclusion Criteria

Subjects who had begun either psychotherapy, or therapeutic doses of pharmacotherapy, for anxiety symptoms in the past 6 months were excluded. In addition, subjects who met any of the following criteria also were excluded:

1. Subjects who presented acute suicidal ideation
2. Females who were of childbearing potential who were not taking adequate contraceptive precautions, or who were pregnant or lactating
3. Subjects with history of epilepsy or seizures
4. Subjects with distinctly abnormal laboratory values or uncontrolled renal, hepatic, cardiac, pulmonary, endocrinological, or collagen disease, determined by history, medical report, and clinical laboratory determinations
5. Subjects with psychotic disorder, or drug-induced psychosis, within the past 6 months, defined by DSM-III criteria for psychotic disorders and substance abuse
6. Subjects with history of dementia
7. Subjects with current or lifetime history of bipolar disorder
8. Subjects with primary diagnoses of bipolar disorder or cyclothymic disorder. Subjects with current or lifetime history of major depression were excluded if they met the following criteria:

a) depression predominated over panic attacks in the current episode or over the individual's lifetime history (as determined by clinical judgment);
b) in the current episode, major depression preceded panic disorder chronologically

9. Subjects with melancholia
10. Subjects with history of alcoholism within the past 6 months, defined by DSM-III ciriteria for alcohol abuse
11. Subjects who were not available for weekly treatment sessions or follow-up
12. Subjects who were currently taking medication containing alpha or beta blockers
13. Subjects who had been on 4 mg or more of alprazolam for any 3-week period, and who had been determined to be nonresponders
14. Subjects with evidence of hypersensitivity to benzodiazepines
15. Subjects with history of obsessive compulsive disorder, defined by DSM-III criteria
16. Subjects with history of treatment for anxiety symptoms with cognitive therapy or relaxation training

Finally, subjects who had been receiving treatment for anxiety symptoms for more than 6 months with beta blockers, tricyclic antidepressants, or benzodiazepines were excluded unless they agreed to stop taking the drug for the duration of the study. Subjects who had been receiving treatment for anxiety symptoms for more than 6 months with psychotherapy were excluded unless they agreed to stop treatment for the duration of the study.

Measures

Psychophysiological, self-report, clinical assessment, and medical assessment measures were administered to all subjects pre- and posttreatment or waiting list. A subset of self-report measures was administered to all subjects throughout treatment or waiting list. Results from major clinical assessment and self-monitoring measures will be presented in this report.

Subjects engaged in daily self-monitoring for 2 weeks pre- and posttreatment or waiting list, and throughout treatment or waiting list, using a form called the „Weekly Record" constructed in our clinic. The Weekly Record provided information about levels of anxiety and related variables, such as depression and pleasant feelings. A set of procedures has also been developed to maximize compliance with recording, including instruction, review, and feedback. Subjects are instructed to record on the diary current levels of anxiety, depression, and pleasant feelings on 0 to 8 scales, four times each day. Such data served as measures of "background" levels of these variables. In addition, subjects are instructed to record on the diary the following information about each discrete episode of anxiety they experience that day which they rate 4 or higher on the 0 to 8 scale:

1. Date and time of onset and offset of the anxiety episode
2. Maximum level of anxiety during the episode
3. Level of anxiety at time of offset of the episode
4. Whether or not the subject considers this episode of anxiety a panic attack. [Subjects are instructed to define a panic attack as the sudden onset of intense apprehension, fear, or terror, accompanied by characteristic physiological panic symptoms (DSM-III, American Psychiatric Association 1980). The attack had to peak within 10 min]
5. Whether the subject considers the context of the episode stressful or nonstressful
6. The symptoms the subject experiences during the panic attack

Data from this record provided information on anxiety episodes and panic attacks, both "spontaneous" and situational. "Spontaneous" attacks were defined as episodes of intense anxiety that began suddenly, reached a peak within 10 min, were accompanied by physiological symptoms of panic, and occurred unexpectedly or in situations which subjects rated as nonstressful. Situational attacks were defined in similar fashion, except they occurred in situations which subjects rated as stressful.

In addition, there is space on the diary for patients to describe the situation in which the episode occurred, relevant behavior, and cognitions, and any comments they may have had. Data from this portion of the diary provide information about the phenomenology of anxiety and panic. Records of relevant cognitions provide a measure of frequency of anticipatory anxiety episodes, particularly anticipation of panic. Finally, such data point to environmental, physiological, and/or cognitive cues that reliably precede spontaneous panic attacks.

Clinical Assessment Measures

Clinical assessments of severity were obtained from the ADIS by assessors who were blind to the group assignment of patients at posttest.

Design

The study used a between-groups design to compare two treatments. The design included the following phases:

1. Pretreatment or waiting list assessment and recruitment
2. Medical assessment and procedures
3. Treatment or waiting list
4. Posttreatment or waiting-list assessment

All subjects underwent pretreatment or waiting list assessment and recruitment. Only subjects in the three active treatment groups (alprazolam, placebo, and cognitive-behavior therapy) underwent medical assessment and procedures. Subjects were assigned randomly to one of four treatment groups. Participation in each group lasted 15 weeks. All subjects who completed treatment underwent posttreatment or waiting-list assessment.

Treatment

In order to start treatment, subjects had to report at least one panic attack in the week prior to beginning treatment. The panic attack may have been spontaneous or situational, and its occurrence was determined by use of the Weekly Record.

The four treatment groups were as follows:

1. Alprazolam Treatment Group. Subjects in the alprazolam treatment group received 15 sessions of treatment in weekly meetings with a psychiatrist with experience in treating panic disorder with alprazolam.
Treatment followed a protocol adapted from one outlined by the Upjohn Company for phase 1 of Cross National Panic Study 4412 (Ballenger et al., in press). Subjects monitored themselves with the Weekly Record throughout the 15-week period.
The psychiatrist presented subjects with a rationale for treatment, and monitored physical condition and dosage levels. He made dose and regimen adjustments following a schedule provided by the Upjohn Company, or until the subject no longer experienced panic attacks. If panic attacks recurred upward dosing was resumed. In case of side-effects, dosage was stabilized or reduced until the subject better tolerated the medication. A resumption of upward dosing was then employed until 6 mg (6 × mg capsules) per day were reached or the subject again experienced side-effects. At least three attempts were made to titrate the medication upward to at least 6 mg per day. Dosage was advanced to a maximum of 10 capsules per day if panic attacks were still present and side-effects did not preclude such an advance, and if the psychiatrist believed therapeutic benefit might ensue.
The psychiatrist limited interactions with subjects to discussion of clinical history, explanation of panic disorder, description of what might be expected from medication treatment, discussion of medication effects and side-effects, and general sup-

port. General support included attempts to put subjects at ease and convey acceptance, to encourage subjects to be hopeful about treatment outcome, and to answer questions about anxiety and medication. Occasionally advice was offered, such as to socialize more, or to engage in activities that might distract one from anxious feelings. In addition, subjects were permitted to vent their self-doubts, and feelings such as anger and frustration. General support did not include discussion of specific psychological themes, clarification of subjects' feelings towards others or toward the psychiatrist, interpretation of interpersonal events or styles of interaction, attempts to uncover suppressed feelings, attempts to correct distorted cognitive sets, behavioral instructions (including instructions to expose oneself to fearful situations), nor psychological explanations of anxiety. All sessions with subjects were either tape-recorded and spot-checked for treatment integrity, or observed by a study investigator.

At the beginning of each visit the study psychiatrist recorded all reported side-effects on the Systematic Assessment For Treatment Emergent Events (SAFTEE-UP) form provided by the Upjohn Company. Alprazolam for the following week was administered by a clinic staff member, in the presence of the psychiatrist, at each weekly visit. The staff member collected the previous week's bottle, and recorded the amount of medication returned and dispensed on the drug distribution record. The staff member completed the vital signs medication record provided by the Upjohn Company.

If treatment was terminated due to severity of side-effects or potential harm to the subject, the subject was considered a dropout from the study, and was tapered off medication. Subjects who left the study were considered dropouts as well. Attempts were made to administer post-treatment assessments to all dropouts at time of termination, and reason for dropout was recorded.

At the beginning of the 13th week of treatment, attempts were made to taper medication at a rate no faster than 1 capsule every 3 days.

2. Placebo Treatment Group. Subjects in the placebo treatment group underwent procedures identical to subjects in the alprazolam treatment group. The only difference was that they received placebo rather than drug. Clinic staff members were blind to treatment conditions of subjects in medication groups.

3. Cognitive-Behavior Therapy Treatment Group. Subjects in the cognitive-behavior therapy treatment group received 15 sessions of treatment in weekly meetings with a senior clinic staff member. Treatment followed the protocol outlined in Barlow and Cerny (in press). The first session of this protocol included presentation of a rationale for treatment and education about panic disorder. The next 14 sessions were composed of the following components: Cognitive therapy, based upon the model for therapy described by Beck and Emery (1979, 1985); training in progressive muscle relaxation, based upon the model described by Bernstein and Borkovec (1973); exposure to external anxiety cues; and exposure to internal anxiety cues and panic symptoms.

The cognitive therapy component of treatment included presentation of didactic material, self-monitoring of automatic thoughts and self-statements, hypothesis testing, and behavioral experiments in the form of graduated homework assignments, from low to high anxiety.

The relaxation component of treatment began with a tension-relaxation phase, in which subjects were taught to tense and relax muscle groups. Exercises were gradually reduced from 16 to 4 muscle groups. Following this phase, subjects were taught relaxation by recall, in which they recalled sensations of muscle release in muscle groups. Finally, subjects were taught cue-controlled relaxation, in which they learned to associate the subvocalized word "relax" with muscle relaxation. Subjects were instructed to practice relaxation at home twice per day, and to maintain records of such practice. Subjects were encouraged to use cognitive and relaxation skills learned in treatment in their daily lives; the protocol contains procedures to enhance generalization.

The treatment component of exposure to external anxiety cues consisted of graduated in vivo exposure to phobic or otherwise stressful situations. Subjects and therapists together constructed hierarchies of feared situations, from low to high anxiety items. Subjects exposed themselves systematically to the situations through structured homework assignments.

The treatment component of exposure to internal anxiety cues and panic symptoms was developed by clinic staff through experience in treatment of panic disorders. It consisted of exposure to internal cognitive and physiological cues of anxiety and panic. These symptoms were induced through: imagery of anxiety-provoking situations and sensations; voluntary hyperventilation; physical exertion (i.e., running in place, spinning one's head); or other idiosyncratic methods for eliciting frightening physical symptoms, accompanied by deliberate catastrophic interpretations. Exposure proceeded up a hierarchy of feared cognitions and somatic sensations, both in sessions with the therapist, and in homework assignments which subjects carried out between sessions. A detailed description of the treatment protocol can be found in Barlow and Cerny (in press).

All therapy sessions were tape-recorded and spot-checked for treatment integrity.

4. Waiting-List Control Group. Subjects in the waiting-list control group were placed on a 15-week waiting list for treatment. They were told that they might contact the clinic by telephone during this time if they felt the need, and that we would contact them occasionally by telephone. Subjects came to the clinic pre- and post-waiting list for assessment. Following posttreatment assessment, subjects entered treatment, although they did not remain part of this study.

Posttreatment or Waiting-List Assessment. Subjects who completed treatment or waiting list attended two assessment sessions. The first session consisted of a structured interview, including part of the ADIS, by a senior clinic staff member who was blind to the subject's experimental condition, and the battery of self-report questionnaires. In addition, subjects were given blank Weekly Record forms, and instructed to record for 2 weeks, starting the next day. The second session consisted of the physiological assessment and collection of completed Weekly Records.

Results

Fifty-seven subjects completed this study. Subjects were considered dropouts if they had been randomly assigned to a treatment group and had attended at least the first treatment session or completed at least the first week of waiting list. Of 18 subjects who began the placebo condition, 7 dropped out. This was a significantly greater number than observed in the other three conditions which were not significantly different from each other (χ^2 [3, $n = 69$] = 8.74, $P < 0.05$).

Table 1 displays pretreatment demographic characteristics of completers of the four treatment groups. This table reveals that groups were relatively well matched.

Table 1. Demographic characteristics of treatment groups

	Group							
Variable	1 Alprazolam ($n = 16$) n	(%)	2 Placebo ($n = 11$) n	(%)	3 Therapy ($n = 15$) n	(%)	4 Waiting List ($n = 15$) n	(%)
Sex								
Male	4	(25.0)	4	(36.4)	4	(26.7)	3	(20.0)
Female	12	(75.0)	7	(63.6)	11	(73.3)	12	(80.0)
Marital status								
Married	11	(68.8)	5	(45.5)	6	(40.0)	9	(60.0)
Single	1	(6.3)	5	(45.5)	8	(53.3)	5	(33.3)
Separated	0	(0.0)	0	(0.0)	0	(0.0)	1	(6.7)
Divorced	4	(25.0)	1	(9.1)	1	(6.7)	0	(0.0
Widowed	0	(0.0)	0	(0.0)	0	(0.0)	0	(0.0)
Age (years)								
M	38.25		39.00		31.33		38.53	
SD	6.93		15.47		8.01		12.63	

Table 2 presents pretreatment diagnostic characteristics of treatment groups. The overwhelming majority of the subjects were diagnosed as having panic disorder with no more than limited avoidance, although a total of five subjects presented with more extensive agoraphobic avoidance. Global clinical severity ratings of panic disorder diagnoses were not significantly different among groups. Due to the extensive exclusionary criteria described above, patients presented with few comorbid diagnoses with the exception of additional anxiety disorders or additional affective disorders that were considered secondary to the primary panic disorder diagnosis.

The major results of the study are presented in Table 3. Due to severity of withdrawal effects, only one subject in the alprazolam group was assessed medication free. The remaining 15 subjects were permitted to resume stable dosage levels which approximated their therapeutic levels prior to posttest assessment. Of study completers, 30 subjects recorded 0 panic attacks in the 2-week period posttreatment. The distribution of subjects reporting 0 panic attacks across groups is presented in Table 3; a chi-square analysis of these relative frequencies was significant as indicated. Separate chi-squares upon all pairs of groups showed that the therapy group was significantly different from the placebo group and from the waiting-list group. Therapy and alprazolam were not significantly different from each other. Table 4 presents global clinical severity ratings of panic disorder at posttest for both study completers as well as the total sample including dropouts. These ratings were made by independent assessors blind to the group assignment of individual patients. A similar pattern of results is evident among these data. For study completers, an initial ANOVA with treatment group as the grouping factor and posttreatment clinical rating as the dependent measure was significant (F [3, 53] = 4.12, $P < 0.01$). One-way ANOVA with Duncan's multiple range test showed that the alprazolam and therapy treatment groups were significantly more improved then the waiting-list group.

Table 2. Pretreatment diagnostic characteristics of treatment groups

Variable	Group 1 Alprazolam ($n = 16$) n (%)	Group 2 Placebo ($n = 11$) n (%)	Group 3 Therapy ($n = 15$) n (%)	Group 4 Waiting list ($n = 15$) n (%)
Diagnosis (n and %)				
Panic disorder, uncomplicated	5 (31.3)	3 (27.3)	2 (13.3)	2 (13.3)
Panic disorder, limited avoidance	9 (56.3)	7 (63.6)	13 (86.7)	11 (73.3)
Panic disorder, extensive avoidance	2 (12.5)	1 (9.1)	0 (00.0)	2 (13.3)
Additional diagnoses				
Anxiety	11 (68.8)	5 (45.5)	8 (53.3)	9 (60.0)
Depression	2 (12.5)	2 (18.2)	1 (6.7)	4 (20.7)
Bipolar	0 (00.0)	0 (00.0)	0 (00.0)	0 (00.0)
Adjustment	0 (00.0)	0 (00.0)	0 (00.0)	0 (00.0)
Somatoform	0 (00.0)	0 (00.0)	0 (00.0)	0 (00.0)
Alcohol abuse	0 (00.0)	1 (9.1)	0 (00.0)	0 (00.0)
Personality	0 (00.0)	0 (00.0)	0 (00.0)	0 (00.0)
Global clinical severity ratings of panic disorder diagnoses				
M	5.38	5.36	5.00	5.47
SD	0.885	0.674	0.845	0.990

Table 3. Posttreatment panic attack measures of treatment groups

Measure	Group 1 Alprazolam ($n = 16$) n (%)	Group 2 Placebo ($n = 11$) n (%)	Group 3 Therapy ($n = 15$) n (%)	Group 4 Waiting list ($n = 15$) n (%)
Frequency of panic attacks				
With zero panic attacks	8 (50.0)[a, b]	4 (36.4)[b]	13 (86.7)[a]	5 (33.3)[b]
With panic attacks	8 (50.0)	7 (63.6)	2 (13.3)	10 (66.7)

[a, b] Groups sharing the same superscripts are not significantly different. Therapy vs placebo: $X^2 = 5.05$, $P < 0.05$; therapy vs. waiting list: $X^2 = 6.80$, $P < 0.01$

Table 4. Posttreatment clinical assessment measures of treatment groups: global clinical ratings

Measure	Group			
	1 Alprazolam	2 Placebo	3 Therapy	4 Waiting list
Study completers *(n)*	16	11	15	15
Global clinical rating				
M	3.56[a]	3.55[a, b]	2.73[a]	4.80[b] ($P<0.05$)
SD	1.90	1.51	1.53	1.47
End-state functioning	*n* (%)	*n* (%)	*n* (%)	*n* (%)
Nonclinical severity	8 (50.0)[a, b]	5 (45.5)[a, b]	11 (73.3)[a]	3 (20.0)[b] ($P<0.05$
Clinical severity	8 (50.0)	6 (54.5)	4 (26.7)	12 (80.0)
Total sample *(n)*	17	18	18	16
End-state functioning	*n* (%)	*n* (%)	*n* (%)	*n* (%)
Nonclinical severity	8 (47.1)[a, b]	5 (27.8)[a, b]	11 (61.1)[a]	3 (18.8)[b]
Clinical severity	9 (52.9)	13 (72.2)	7 (38.9)	13 (81.3)

[a, b] Groups sharing the same superscripts are not significantly different

Another method of analyzing the data was to ascertain the number of patients who obtained posttreatment global clinical ratings below clinical severity. Patients were classified in the range of nonclinical severity (high end-state functioners) if they obtained ratings less than 4. Low end-state functioners on the other hand reflected a score of 4 or more. Approximately one-half of the study completers obtained high end-state functioning. A chi-square analysis of patients with high and low end-state functioning across treatment groups revealed a significant difference (chi-square [3, 57] = 8.62, $P <$ 0.05). Separate chi-squares upon all pairs of groups demonstrated that the therapy group was significantly different from the waiting-list group (chi-square [1, 30] = 6.56, P 0.01). This was the only significant difference among the chi-squares.

Since the placebo group had a disproportionate number of dropouts, it may be that anlyses of end-state functioning that include only study completers represent a distortion of results. Classifying dropouts as low end-state functioners alters the overall percentage of patients who attain high end-state functioning, but does not change the pattern of results. Once again, therapy is superior to waiting list and this is the only significant difference among groups.

Discussion

The results of this report would confirm uncontrolled clinical trials, suggesting that an effective nondrug treatment for panic disorder exists. Fully 85% of the patients in this study receiving cognitive-behavioral therapy were panic free at the end of treatment.

While this was not significantly different from those who were panic free with alprazolam, statistical power considerations might have prevented significant findings between treatment conditions in this particular study. Similar considerations might account for the lack of statistical differentiation between alprazolam and placebo in this study. In the Upjohn cross-national study (Ballenger et al., in press) approximately 60% of the patients were panic free compared to 30% on placebo. These results are not substantially different from alprazolam-placebo comparisons in this study. Thus, it would seem that the results in the much larger multicenter study on the effects of alprazolam and placebo were essentially replicated in this study.

The very high dropout rate in the placebo condition observed in this study also replicates a finding in the larger multicenter study (Ballenger et al., in press). Alprazolam was well tolerated in this study as it was in the larger study. Only one subject dropped from treatment in the alprazolam group and this was not because of side-effects of medication.

Although many patients in this study were panic free and a significant number achieved high end-state functioning, residual anxiety, particularly over the possibility of future panic attacks remained. An essential step, not possible in this study, will be to follow-up initial treatment effects over a number of years. Preliminary data from a large ongoing study on cognitive behavioral treatment of panic in our Center suggests very positive results at 1- and 2-year follow-up. Specifically, continuing improvement on global clinical ratings and broad-based measures of anxiety is observed over time (Craske and Barlow 1987). Measures reflecting the number of patients panic free remain relatively stable at very high levels over time. Confirmation of these positive findings awaits full follow-up data.

The purpose of this study was not to explore the separate and combined effects of drug and cognitive behavioral treatments. An important future goal will be to examine the interactive effects of these treatments to determine the possible benefits of this strategy. For example, alprazolam seems to act very quickly, often producing significant relief within the first week (Ballenger et al., in press), while cognitive behavior therapy may take between 3 and 6 weeks before significant benefit is obtained. On the other hand, results from follow-up mentioned above suggest that cognitive behavioral treatment may be long-lasting (Craske and Barlow 1987). Meanwhile, preliminary examination of the effects of alprazolam withdrawal in patients treated for panic disorder are somewhat discouraging due to withdrawal effects and/or a return of symptoms (Fyer et al. 1987). It is possible that these disappointing results may be avoided by an extremely slow withdrawal regimen (Fontaine et al. 1984). More information on strategies for maintenance with drug treatment is necessary. In any case, these considerations might suggest beginning a patient on alprazolam and cognitive behavior therapy simultaneously and then withdrawing the patient from alprazolam slowly as cognitive behavioral therapy begins to take effect. On the other hand, evidence exists from a variety of sources suggesting that benzodiazepines (unlike tricyclic antidepressants) may interfere with the effects of cognitive behavioral therapy for panic and anxiety (Barlow, in press). A full explication of this process awaits further study.

References

Alexander P, Alexander D (1986) Alprazolam treatment for panic disorders. J Clin Psychiatry 48:301–304

Ballenger JC, Burrows G, DuPont R, Lesser I, Noyes R, Pecknold J, Riskin A, Swinson R (in press) Alprazolam in panic disorder and agoraphobia; results from a multi center trial. I.

Efficacy in short-term treatment. Arch Gen Psychiatry
Barlow DH (in press) Anxiety and its disorders. Guilford, New York
Barlow DH, Beck JG (1984) The psychosocial treatment of anxiety disorders. current status, future directions. In: Williams JBW, Spitzer RL (eds) Psychotherapy research: where are we and where should we go? Guilford, New York
Barlow DH, Cerny JA (in press) Psychological treatment of panic. Guilford, New York
Barlow DH, Cohen AS, Waddell MT, Vermilyea BB, Klosko JS, Blanchard EB, DiNardo PA (1984) Panic and generalized anxiety disorders: nature and treatment. Behav Res Ther 15:431-449
Beck AT (in press) Cognitive approaches to panic disorder: theory and therapy. In: Rachman S, Maser JD (eds) Panic: psychological perspectives. Erlbaum, Hillsdale
Beck AT, Emery G (1979) Cognitive therapy of anxiety and phobic disorders. Center for Cognitive Therapy, Philadelphia
Beck AT, Emery G (1985) Anxiety and the anxiety disorders. Erlbaum, Hillsdale
Bernstein DA, Borkovec TD (1973) Progressive relaxation training. Ill: Research Press, Champaign
Chouinard G, Annable L, Fontaine R, Solyom L (1982) Alprazolam in the treatment of generalized anxiety and panic disorders: a double-blind placebo-controlled study. Psychopharmacology 77:229-233
Clark DM, Salkovskis PM, Chalkley AJ (1985) Respiratory control as a treatment for panic attacks. J Beh Ther Exp Psychiatry 16:23-30
Craske MG, Barlow DH (1987) Behavioral treatment of panic: a controlled study. 21st Annual convention of the Association for the Advancement of Behavior Therapy. Boston, November 1987
DiNardo PA, O'Brien GT, Barlow DH, Waddell MT, Blanchard EB (1983) Reliability of DSM-III anxiety disorder categories using a new structured interview. Arch Gen Psychiatry 40:1070-1078
DiNardo PA, Barlow DH, Cerny J, Vermilyea JA, Vermilyea BB, Himadi W, Waddell M (1985) The anxiety disorders interview schedule - revised. Center for Stress and Anxiety Disorders, New York
Fontaine R, Chouinard G, Annable L (1984) Rebound anxiety in anxious patients after abrupt withdrawal of benzodiazepine treatment. Am J Psychol 141:848-852
Fyer A, Liebowitz M, Gorman J, Compeas R, Levin A, Davies S, Goetz D, Klein D (1987) Discontinuation of alprazolam treatment in panic patients. Am J Psychiatry 144:303-308
Gitlin B, Martin M, Shear K, Frances A, Ball G, Josephson S (1985) Behavior therapy for panic disorder. J Nerv Men Dis 173:742-743
Klosko JS, Barlow DH (1987) The treatment of panic in panic disorder and agoraphobia: a clinical replication series. Behav Res Ther Unpublished manuscript
Liebowitz MR, Fyer A, Gorman J, Campas R, Levin A, Davies S, Goeth D, Klein D (1986) Alprazolam in the treatment of panic disorders. J Clin Psychopharamcol 6:13-20
Marks IM, Grey S, Cohen SD, Hill R, Mawson D, Ramm L, Stern RS (1983) Imipramine and brief therapist-aided exposure in agoraphobics having self-exposure homework: a controlled trial. Arch Gen Psychiatry 40:153-162
Mavissakalian M, Michelson L (1986) Agoraphobia: relative and combined effectiveness of therapist-assisted in vivo exposure and imipramine. J Clin Psychiatry 47:117-122
Noyes R, Anderson DJ, Clancy J, Crowe RR, Slymen DJ, Ghoneim MM, Hinrichs JV (1984) Diazepam and propranolol in panic disorder and agoraphobia. Arch Gen Psychiatry 41: 287-292
Salkovskis PM, Jones DRO, Clark DM (1986) Respiratory control in the treatment of panic attacks: replication and extension with concurrent measurement of behavior and pCO_2. Br J Psychiatry 148:526-532
Telch MJ, Agras WS, Taylor CB, Roth WT, Gallen C (1985) Combined pharmacological and behavioural treatment for agoraphobia. Behav Res Ther 23:325-335
Zitrin CM, Klein DF, Woerner MG (1980) Treatment of agoraphobia with group exposure in vivo and imipramine. Arch Gen Psychiatry 37:63-72
Zitrin CM, Klein DF, Woerner MG, Ross DC (1983) Treatment of phobias: I. Comparison of imipramine hydrochloride and placebo. Arch Gen Psychiatry 40:125-138

6. Cognitive-Behavioral Treatment of Panic

M. K. SHEAR, G. G. BALL, ST. C. JOSEPHSON, and B. GITLIN

Introduction

The delineation of panic as distinct from other forms of anxiety is central to constructing the syndrome currently defined as panic disorder. This syndrome includes panic attacks, anticipatory anxiety and phobic fear, and avoidance. A panic episode is characterized by the sudden onset and rapid escalation of a sense of fear, usually focused on fear of physical or mental collapse. The hallmark of panic is a sense of actual or impending loss of control. Some panic episodes are described as unexpected, without any apparent trigger. Panic may also occur in reaction to confrontation with a feared situation, thought, image, or internal bodily sensation.

Patients who have recurrent panic attacks usually develop anticipatory fear of having another episode. This fear may be unfocused, general and persistent, or it may be episodic and directed toward specific situations in which panic is particularly feared. These situations are usually ones where panic has actually happened, or where panic consequences would seem particularly severe (e.g., the patient may feel alone and helpless or trapped and unable to escape in the event panic occurs). Patients who focus anticipatory anxiety on specific situations develop phobic avoidance of the situation(s). According to the most recent American Psychiatric Association diagnostic criteria (DSM-IIIR, 1987), phobic avoidance in response to panic episodes is designated agoraphobia. All panic disorder patients are classified on an agoraphobic dimension as none, mild, moderate, or severe. It is not known why patients develop varying degrees of agoraphobia. Proposed explanations include illness duration, illness severity, and personality characteristics.

DSM-IIIR criteria for panic disorder include the occurrence of one or more unexpected panic attacks followed by either three attacks in a 3-week period or persistent fear of panic lasting at least 1 month. Some degree of agoraphobia is almost always present. This diagnosis represents a revision of previous (DSM-III) criteria in that patients who were diagnosed as having agoraphobia with panic attacks are now subsumed under the panic disorder category. This important change is meant to focus attention on the central role of panic attacks in the agoraphobic syndrome and to highlight the importance of treating panic specifically in these patients.

The panic disorder diagnostic category was proposed initially by psychopharmacologists who noted the central role of seemingly spontaneous panic episodes in the pathogenesis of agoraphobia (Klein 1964). Klein and his colleagues observed that treatment with imipramine resulted in blocking of the panic episodes and facilitated recovery from phobic morbidity. These findings have been replicated and extended in a number of studies

(Zitrin et al. 1983; Sheehan et al. 1980; Mavissakalian and Michelson 1983). We now know that several classes of medication are effective in blocking panic attacks. These include trcyclic antidrepressants, monoamine oxidase inhibitors, and some benzodiazepines.

Most of the studies reporting medication efficacy have been conducted using patients who met criteria for agoraphobia with panic attacks. Importantly, these studies used panic as an outcome measure, and commented on significant antipanic effects. Recent open trials of medication in panic disorder patients without avoidance support this finding (Garalamo et al. 1984; Gloger et al. 1981). Clearly, medication is an acceptable form of treatment for panic, but there are several problems with its use. Side-effects occur and may be troublesome, debilitating, or even dangerous. Some patients refuse to take medication, or tolerate it poorly. Withdrawal symptoms and/or relapse may occur on discontinuation. Some patients are demoralized by taking medication. Others have a strong preference for avoiding medication use. The panic disorder population tends to be young and predominantly female. Commitment of this population to long-term medication use seems undesirable. Moreover, medication is particularly problematic during childbearing years.

Patients with panic attacks are frequently seen in general practice by psychotherapists. Traditional psychotherapy has been used clinically and does not appear to be successful, although no formal treatment trials have been conducted. Behavioral treatment of agoraphobia has been used and tested with promising results (Barlow and Wolfe 1981; Chambless and Goldstein 1981; Marks et al. 1983). However, initial studies of behavioral therapy efficacy did not focus on panic as an outcome measure. Some reviews of behavioral treatment efficacy in agoraphobic patients with panic attacks reveal incomplete antipanic effects (Klosko and Barlow, unpublished manuscript; Michelson et al. 1985). More recent studies (see Hand et al. 1986, Fiegenbaum this volume) suggest that treatment using flooding associated with high levels of anxiety may provide effective treatment for panic with good long-term stability. In addition, specific cognitive-behavioral techniques have now been developed to treat panic (see Clark and Barlow, this volume). We also developed such a treatment and began to use it in a clinical setting in the early 1980s. We have now completed two pilot studies which support the efficacy of this treatment. These will be summarized below.

Study I

Retrospective Chart Review and Follow-Up

Subjects

The study included eleven patients who met DSM III criteria for panic disorder (see Gritlin et al. 1986). There were five men and six women. Four had no phobic avoidance. Seven had mixed phobias (e.g., subways, buses, trains, site of first panic, physical exertion). These phobias were relatively mild in that they were inconsistent and easily reversible on therapist instructions. Mean frequency of panic episodes in the 3 weeks prior to treatment was 4.8 per week with a range of 0.06–21. Mean duration of illness was 3.4 $\pm$ 5.8 years. None of the patients was diagnosed as agoraphobic, and none met criteria for major depression. Six patients were taking medication intermittently for panic attacks. Medications used included benzodiazepines, betablockers, or nitroglycerin (one patient) although none had documented cardiologic illness.

Treatment Procedures

Treatment was conducted in group (five patients) or individual (six patients) formats. The group treatment was time limited (12 weeks) and the individual treatment was variable (mean length, 16 weeks). Techniques consisted of three components:

a) education and reassurance about the physiologic and psychologic aspects of panic;
b) training in panic management techniques; and
c) exposure to anxiety-provoking situations.

Patients were presented with an ethological model in which panic is conceptualized as a normal biobehavioral response meant to occur on acutal confrontation with immediate danger. In pathological conditions panic occurs in the absence of actual danger, for reasons which have not yet been fully elucidated. Patients were told that we do know that physiologic changes occur during panic (Shear et al. 1984; Shear et al., 1987), but that these changes appear to be mild and transient and to represent little or no real danger. Techniques of panic management included breathing retraining using slow abdominal breathing techniques, progressive muscular relaxation, and cognitive reframing of the panic experience. Patients were encouraged to view panic attacks as a series of unpleasant sensations rather than a global indication of catastrophic danger. Panic management techniques were practised and reviewed using exposure to anxiety-provoking situations or sensations (e.g., those provoked by exercise, hyperventilation, etc.).

Results

Ten of the eleven patients were free of panic attacks for more than 2 weeks at the time of termination. All patients who had taken medication prior to treatment had stopped taking it. One patient with a 20-year history of symptoms continued to have some phobic avoidance and situational panic attacks at the time of termination from the time-limited group treatment. The number of panic episodes decreased from a pretreatment mean of three per week to one per week. The other ten patients remained panic free during the follow-up period which ranged from 3 to 12 months. The majority of patients (64%) reported that education about the nature of the panic episodes had been most helpful to them and that abdominal breathing was the next most helpful aspect of the treatment.

Study II

Prospective Treatment Trial Using Structured Clinical Rating Scales and Sodium Lactate Vulnerability as Outcome Measures

The results presented here include only the clinical outcome measures.

Subjects

Twenty-four patients enrolled in the study and twenty-one completed to termination criteria. Two patients dropped out before week 3. One refused to do the exposure practice because he felt it would not help him, and one started a new business and said he would not have time to practice. The third patient dropped out at week 5 because of a need to have knee surgery. Fifteen female and six male subjects completed the study. All met DSM-III criteria for panic disorder (n = 17) or agoraphobia with panic attacks (n = 4). Fourteen of the panic disorder patients had limited phobic avoidance. Three had uncomplicated panic disorder. Mean age of the sample was 33 years ± 9.2. Mean illness duration was 7 years ± 7.3. No patient met criteria for major depression at the time of the study. One patient had a past history of major depression, and one patient had a history of bipolar disorder. All patients were free of psychotropic medication at the time of the sodium lactate infusion. One patient had been taking lorazepam 0.5 mg twice a day before entering the study. This patient resumed this dose of medication following the sodium lactate test and tapered the medication during the first 4 weeks of treatment. All other patients were drug free during the treatment trial.

Assessment Procedures

Diagnoses were confirmed using the structured interview for DSM-III (SCID) (Spitzer and Williams 1983). Patient and clinician symptom rating scales and global severity and disability scales were completed pretreatment and posttreatment. In addition, global rating scales were completed by patients and therapists on a weekly basis. Panic attack frequency, duration, and intensity were rated by clinicians using the Sheehan panic and anxiety scale. This scale includes full-blown spontaneous panic episodes (three or more symptoms) and limited symptom episodes (one or two symptoms). Situational panics are rated as situational surges which do not distinguish number of symptoms. Patients also completed self-report questionnaires describing panic frequency, duration, and intensity. Phobic symptoms were measures using the Marks and Mathews brief fear questionnaire (Marks and Mathews 1979), the fear survey schedule (Geer 1965) and the SCL 90 (Derogatis et al. 1973), phobic avoidance scale. Measures of generalized anxiety include clinician-rated Hamilton anxiety scale (Hamilton 1959) and patient-rated Spielberger Trait Anxiety (Spielberger et al. 1970) and the SCL 90 somatization and anxiety subscales. Patients rated depression using the Beck (Beck et al. 1961) Depression Inventory and SCL 90 depression subscales.

Treatment Procedures

Treatment was done in weekly individual sessions lasting until the patient was either free of panic symptoms and significant phobic avoidance for 1 month or had completed 24 weeks of treatment. A treatment manual was used and all treatments were reviewed weekly in a group supervision session. Treatment was conducted in three phases. During the first phase (three sessions) the therapist presented the model of panic outlined above (study 1) and a rationale for the treatment approach. The patient was educated in the use of a weekly diary and the concept of a hierachy of phobic situations was introduced. Breathing exercises and relaxation training were introduced. During the second phase of the treatment (variable length) the therapist and patient developed and planned graded exposure exercises. These were carried out using imaginal and in vivo techniques. Most of the exposure practice was self-directed. Panic management techniques were practiced and then applied during exposure experiences. The diary was reviewed at each session. Success in coping with panic was reinforced and problems identified and addressed. Therapist-assisted in vivo exposure was used when there was a problem which we could not solve without observing the patient.

Exposure exercises were directed at providing contact with stimuli which were reported to be panicogenic. These included both internal sensations and external situations in keeping with our view that panic patients are vulnerable to both types of triggers. Examples of exposure to internal sensations include exercise, hyperventilation, tensing or putting external pressure on throat or abdominal areas, daydreaming, sauna, exciting movies or sports events, drinking coffee, and going on amusement park rides. Examples of exposure to external situations include standard agoraphobic stimuli sich as subways, tunnels bridges, buses, trains, theaters, restaurants, stores, crowds, and walking or travelling far from home. Some patients also had prominent secondary social fears and were exposed to social situations.

Patients were instructed to record exposure exercises as well as unexpected panic attacks in the weekly diaries. The therapists reviewed with the patient thoughts, physical sensations, and behaviors associated with panic episodes and helped the patient find ways to alter panic-enhancing reactions. Patients were encouraged to accept the fact that they may not be able to control the onset of a panic episode, but they can modify the responses that magnify the initial sensation.

Results

Statistical Analyses

The general approach to analysis of pre-post differences among treatment completers was conduction of paired sample *t*-tests, with scores on pre- and posttreatment measures as dependent variables. Test were two-tailed. The level of significance was set at 0.005, to adjust for the number of tests conducted.

Global Ratings

On the clinical global index of severity scale, subjects obtained pretreatment mean severity ratings of almost 4 (moderately ill) on a 0 to 7 scale; posttreatment they obtained mean ratings somewhat higher than 2 (borderline mentally ill). T-test was significant (t [18] = 5.08, $P <$ 0.005). Posttreatment, clinicians rated subjects a mean of 1.89 on the 0 to 7 global improvement scale, or between much improved and very much improved.

Self-report ratings of clinical severity included the three global indices of distress of the SCL 90. On the global severity index, which indicates depth or level of disorder, subjects obtained pretreatment mean *t*-scores slightly above the 40th percentile, near the norm for outpatients; posttreatment, they obtained *t*-scores at approximately the 16th percentile; that is, 84% of outpatients were likely to score as more severe. T-test was significant ([14] = 4.59, $P < 0.005$). On the symptom distress index, an intensity measure corrected for number of symptoms endorsed, subjects obtained pretreatment mean *t*-scores at approximately the 30th percentile for outpatiens; posttreatment they obtained scores at approximately the 10th percentile. T-test was significant (t [14] = 4.63, $P < 0.005$). Finally, on number of positive symptoms subjects endorsed, pretreatment they obtained mean *t*-scores at approximately the 50th percentile, the norm for outpatients; while posttreatment they obtained scores at about the 20th percentile. T-test was significant (t [14] = 3.68, $P < 0.005$).

Measures of Panic

In accord with clinical ratings of spontaneous panic attack frequency, derived from the panic and anxiety attack scales, subjects were grouped as treatment responders (zero spontaneous panic attacks in the month before treatment ended), partial responders (between 50% and 100% decrease in number of attacks from the month before treatment started to the month before treatment ended), and nonresponders (less than 50% decrease in number of attacks). Seventeen subjects, or 81%, reported zero spontaneous panic attacks posttreatment, and were treatment responders; one subject was a partial responder, and three subjects were nonresponders. Two nonresponders reported a greater number of spontaneous panic attacks in the month before treatment ended than they reported in the month before treatment began; the third reported a decrease in number of attacks of 29.4% (from 17 to 12 attacks per month).

Panic frequency, severity, intensity, and duration were also measured. Pretreatment, subjects reported a mean of 12.52 spontaneous full-blown attacks per month; according to DSM-IIIR, this placed the study sample within the range of severe panic attacks. Posttreatment, subjects reported a mean of one panic attack per month. T-test was significant (t [20] = 3.72, $P < 0.005$). Subjects reported mean pretreatment intensity of attacks of 5.43 on the 0 to 10 scale; posttreatment they reported mean intensity of 1.38. T-test was significant (t [20] = 4.53, $P < 0.005$). Finally, subjects reported mean pretreatment duration of attacks of 12.86 min; posttreatment they reported mean duration of 1.47 min. T-test was nonsignificant, probably due to large variation in duration of attacks reported across subjects pretreatment.

Subjects also exhibited decreases in frequency, intensity, and duration of partial spontaneous attacks. T-tests were significant for frequency of partial attacks (t [19] = 3.73, $P < 0.005$).

Measures of Phobic Avoidance

Ratings on the Marks and Mathews brief fear questionnaire were relatively low since the patient population had a high level of panic but not phobic morbidity. Scores on the agoraphobia, blood and injury, and social fears subscales approached, but did not reach, significant pre-post treatment change; however, total scale scores were significant (t [20] = 3.16, $P < 0.005$). Results of other self-report measures of phobic avoidance were significant: These included the fear survey questionnaire (t [13] = 4.35, P 0.005); and the phobic avoidance subscale of the SCL 90 (t [14] = 3.71, $P < 0.005$).

Measures of Generalized Anxiety

Clinical assessment measures of generalized anxiety showed significant decrement in the Hamilton anxiety scale. T-tests were significant for total scores (t [17] = 4.91, $P < 0.005$), and for scores on the somatic subscale (t [16] = 3.53, $P < 0.005$), and the cognitive subscale (t [16] = 4.65, $P < 0.005$). Results were significant for all self-report measures of generalized anxiety as well. These measures included the trait scale of the state-trait anxiety inventory (t [11] = 4.05; $P < 0.005$); and SCL 90 somatization (t [14] = 4.18; $P < 0.005$) and anxiety (t [14] = 6.18; $P < 0.005$) subscales.

Measures of Depression

Pretreatment, subjects scored relatively low on depression scales; means fell within borderline to mildly depressed ranges. Although subjects exhibited improvement on depression scores from pre- to posttreatment, t-tests were not significant at the 0.005 level.

Discussion

Results of this clinical replication series as well as other reported studies (Jannoun et al. 1982; Beck, in press; Clark et al. 1985; Klosko and Barlow 1987), are promising in demonstrating good efficacy of cognitive behavioral treatment. In addition, three controlled studies from Barlow's group support the antipanic effectiveness of cognitive behavioral treatment (Barlow et al. 1984; Klosko 1987; Waddell et al. 1984).

These studies compared active treatment to a waiting-list control. One (see Barlow, this volume) also used a drug and placebo comparison.

Nevertheless, a number of questions related to clinical efficacy remain unanswered. For example, what is the relative effectiveness of the active treatment compared to nonspecific therapeutic contact? How important are each of the different components of the treatment package to overall outcome? Specifically, patients in our first study reported that education about panic symptoms was the most helpful aspect of the treatment. Were they right? How important is exposure compared to cognitive therapy? If exposure is essential, is exposure to internal sensations sufficient to treat panic or is exposure to external situations also necessary? What would be the outcome of a head to head randomized prospective study comparing cognitive behavioral treatment with an effective medication trial? Is there any benefit in combining medication and cognitive behavioral treatment of panic? What is the maintenance of treatment gains over short-term and long-term follow-up periods? What is the effect of cognitive behavioral treatment on biological measures of panic including effects on pharmacologic challenge tests and on baseline physiologic measures such as heart rate and blood gas? Studies in our center as well as others are underway to begin to answer these questions.

The development of theoretical models of panic grows out of clinical experience with patients. These models help to guide future research in understanding and treating panic disorder patients. There are currently three main models of panic disorder psychopathology being proposed by cognitive behavioral scientists. These include:

a) the cognitive model, articulated by Clark (1986), suggesting that panic occurs because of cognitive misinterpretation of bodily sensations;
b) the emotion theory model, articulated by Barlow (in press) which presents panic as equivalent to fear (pathological panic occurs because of abnormal accessibility of the relevant emotional schema which can be entered through activation of specific cognitive, behavioral, or physiologic channels); and
c) the ethological model articulated by Marks (1987) in which panic is seen as equivalent to phobic anxiety which is provoked in different patient groups by different phobic stimuli. This model focuses on the fact that there are typical stimuli for agoraphobic panic just as there are for animal phobic panic, height phobia panic, etc. Panic is seen as a secondary symptom which is not of central importance to the agoraphobic syndrome.
d) Another model of agoraphobia is presented by Bowlby (1973), who suggests that the anxiety experienced by this patient group is related to a fear of lack of resources for fighting danger. The agoraphobic patient differs from other phobic patients in that the latter fear harm from specific external situations while the agoraphobic is more generally fearful of failure and loss of control on confrontation with danger. The situations which trigger agoraphobic anxiety are not ones where there is fantasied harm. The patient does not fear that the restaurant or theater or bus will attack him. Rather, the agoraphobic experiences a heigthened sense of vulnerability in these settings. This theory predicts that panic attacks in these patients may be triggered by any situation which threatens to undermine already weakened defense systems. Examples of such situations may be perceived autonomic arousal suggesting loss of internal stability, perceived loss of external safety signals such as being in unfamiliar sur-

roundings, or perceived decrement in available coping strategies such as loss of a supportive partner.

At the moment, there is no convincing evidence for choosing amongst these four models. Further research, along the lines proposed above, is needed before one can decide on a definitive model.

References

American Psychiatric Association Task Force on Nomenclature and Statistics (1980, revised edn 1987) Diagnostic and statistical manual of mental disorders, 3rd edn. American Psychiatric Association, Washington, DC

Barlow D (in press) Panic, anxiety and the anxiety disorders. Guilford, New York

Barlow DH, Wolfe BE (1981) Behavioral approaches to the anxiety disorders: report of the NIMH-SUNY Albany research conference. J Consult Clin Psychol 49:448-454

Barlow DH, Cohen AS, Waddell MT, Vermilyea BB, Klosko JS, Blanchard EB, DiNardo PA (1984) Panic and generalized anxiety disorders: nature and treatment. Behav Res Ther 15:431-449

Beck AT (in press) Cognitive approaches to panic disorder: theory and therapy. In: Rachman S, Maser JD (eds) Panic: psychological perspectives. Erlbaum, Hillsdale

Beck AT, Ward CH, Mendelson M, Mock J, Erbaugh J (1961) An inventory for measuring depression. Arch Gen Psychiatry 4:561-571

Bowlby J (1973) Attachment and loss, vol 2. Separation: anxiety and anger: Basic, New York

Chambless D, Goldstein AJ (1981) Clinical treatment of agoraphobia. In: Mavissaklian H, Barlow DH (eds) Phobia: psychological and pharmacological treatment. Guilford, New York

Clark DM (1986) A cognitive approach to panic. Beh Res Ther 4:461-470

Clark DM, Salkovski PM, Chalkley AJ (1985) Respiratory control as a treatment for panic attacks. J Behav Ther Exp Psychiatry 16:22-30

Derogatis LR, Lipman RS, Covi L (1973) SCL-90: an outpatient psychiatric rating scale (preliminary report). Psychol Bull 9:13-27

Garalamo H, Zitrin CM, Klein DF (1984) Treatment of panic disorder with imipramine alone. Am J Psychiatry 141:446-448

Geer JH (1965) The development of a scale to measure fear. Behav Res Ther 345:53

Gitlin B, Martin J, Shear MK, Frances AJ, Ball G, Josephson S (1986) Behavioral therapy for panic disorder. J Nerv Dis 173:742-743

Gloger S, Grunhaus L, Birmacher B (1981) Treatment of spontaneous panic attacks with chlomipramine. Am J Psychiatry 138:1215-1217

Hamilton M (1959) The assessment of anxiety states by rating. Br J Med Psychol 32:50-55

Hand I, Angenendt J, Fischer M, Wilke C (1986) Exposure in-vivo with panic managment for agoraphobia: treatment rationale and longterm outcome. In: Hand I, Wittchen H.-U. (eds) Panic and Phobias. Springer, Heidelberg, New York

Jannoun L, Oppenheimer C, Gelder M (1982) A self-help treatment program for anxiety state patients. Behav Res Ther 13:103-111

Klein PF (1964) Delineation of two drug responsive anxiety syndromes. Psychopharmacolojia 5:397-408

Klosko J (1987) A comparison of alprazolam and cognitive-behavior therapy in treatment of panic disorder. Unpublished doctoral dissertation, State University of New York at Albany

Klosko JS, Barlow DH (1987) The treatment of panic in panic disorder and agoraphobia. A clinical replication series. Manuscript submitted for publication

Klosko JS, Barlow DH (unpublished manuscript) Behavioral treatment of panic disorder: a clinical replication series

Marks IM (1987) Behavioral aspects of panic disorder. Am J Psychiatry 144:1160-1165

Marks IM, Mathews AM (1979) Brief standard self-rating for phobic patients. Behav Res Ther 17:263-267

Marks IM, Gray S, Cohen D et al (1983) Imipramine and brief therapist-aided exposure in agorophobics having self-exposure homework. Arch Gen Psychiatry 40:153-162

Mavissakalian M, Michelson L (1983) Agoraphobia behavioral and pharmacological treatment. Psychopharmacol Bull 19:116-118

Michelson L, Mavisakalian M, Marchione K (1985) Cognitive and behavioral treatments of agoraphobia: clinical, behavioral and psychophysiological outcomes. J Consult Clin Psychol 53:913-925

Shear MK, Polan J, Harshfield G et al (1984) Ambulatory heart rate and blood pressure in panic disorder patients (abstract). Society for Behavioral Medicine, Philadelphia, October 1984

Shear MK, Kligfield P, Harshfield G, Devereux RB, Polan JJ, Mann JJ, Pickering T, Frances AJ (1987) Cardiac rate and rhythm in panic patients. Am J Psychiatry, 144:633-637

Sheehan DV, Ballenger J, Jacobsen G (1980) Treatment of endogenous anxiety with phobic,

hysterical, and hypochondriacal symptoms. Arch Gen Psychiatry 37:151–159
Spielberger CD, Gorsuch RW, Lushene RE (1970) State-trait anxiety inventory. Consulting Psychologists Press, Palo Alto
Spitzer RL, Williams JBW (1983) Structured clinical interview for DSM-III (SCID 11-1-83). Biometrics Research Department, New York State Psychiatric Institute, 722 West 168th Street, New York, New York 10032
Waddell MT, Barlow DH, O'Brien GT (1984) A preliminary investigation of cognitive and relaxation treatment of panic disorder: effects on intense anxiety vs "background" anxiety. Behav Res Ther 22:393–402
Zitrin CM, Klein DF, Woerner MG, Ross DC (1983) Treatment of phobias: I. Comparison of imipramine hydrochloride and placebo. Arch Gen Psychiatry 40:125–138

7. Cognitive Factors in the Treatment of Anxiety States

A. MATHEWS

Introduction

The apparent lack of any external focus for anxiety in generalized anxiety states or panic disorders has resulted in some lack of consensus about how such non-phobic anxiety disorders should be treated. In general such clients do not report a consistent pattern of avoidance as do phobic patients, although of course this does not mean that they never avoid anxiety-provoking situations. However, in the absence of a defined external trigger for avoidance behaviour, most therapists have abandoned straightforward exposure methods in favour of relaxation, anxiety management or cognitive therapy.

There are two important questions that need to be answered about these treatments: first, are they effective? And if so, what are the components or mechanisms responsible for their effectiveness? I think that many therapists believe that we already know the answers to these questions. Certainly it is widely believed that anxiety management and cognitive therapy are effective for non-phobic anxiety disorders, and that improvements result from the use which clients make of the specific anxiety management techniques which they have learned. Despite this optimism, I think that the answers to these two important questions remain uncertain. We do not know whether anxiety management or cognitive therapy methods are effective, in the sense of being superior to dummy or placebo treatments matched for plausibility. If the answer to this question remains in doubt, then we can hardly have much confidence in our belief that improvement results from the use of specific techniques.

By far the most popular method of assessing the effectiveness of anxiety management methods has been to use a straightforward comparison with a no-treatment condition, in which clients wait for a period before being reassessed, and then subsequently offered treatment. Published examples include the study by Jannoun et al. (1982) in which general-practice patients waited for periods varying between 4 and 8 weeks before receiving anxiety management training. Little change occurred during the waiting period, but substantial clinical improvements were obtained following treatment. The between-group comparison reported by Barlow et al. (1984) contrasted a waiting period with a complex treatment package which included relaxation, stress inoculation and cognitive therapy. Once more improvements only occurred during active treatment, although given the number of sessions (18) and the multiple techniques used, the extent of clinical improvement achieved seems relatively modest. Apparently more encouraging results were obtained in Oxford by Butler et al. (in press) in another straigthforward comparison of anxiety management and a waiting-list condition. Substantial im-

Table 1. Mean change in Spielberger trait anxiety scores

Study	AMT	WAIT	
Jannoun et al. (1982)	9.5	1.1	(Withing-subject design)
Barlow et al. (1984)	4.4	−2.1	
Butler et al. (1987)	12.1	−2.5	(Scores at follow-up only)

provements were seen in clients who were taught a variety of behavioural methods for coping with anxiety, while again little or no improvement was seen in those receiving no treatment during the waiting period (Table 1).

Needless to say, none of these studies can answer the question posed earlier: that of whether the specific techniques employed in anxiety management or cognitve therapy produce these clinical improvements, or whether these changes occur as a result of common or non-specific features inherent in the context of psychological treatment. Such common features might include the expectation of help, the reassurance provided by the therapist or by the treatment rationale, and so on. To investigate whether these common features could be responsible for the apparent effectiveness of anxiety management or cognitive therapy, requires a comparison with an alternative condition which is presented as an effective psychological treatment, but which excludes all of the specific techniques usually incorporated.

Experimental Studies

We have addressed this question in three recent studies, all of which have compared anxiety management techniques with non-directive counselling as a control condition. In non-directive counselling therapists were instructed to provide therapeutic conditions of warmth and empathy, but to avoid offering any advice about techniques for coping with anxiety, or for that matter any directive instructions at all. Instead, therapists reflected back questions and problems by rephrasing what clients said, or by asking them what they themselves thought would be best. The rationale offered to clients at the start of treatment was that specific advice could not be given because each individual needed to discover for themselves the unique causes of their own anxiety, although therapists could help and encourage the individual's own efforts towards that understanding.

In the first comparison, carried out in London and Brighton (Blowers et al., in press) trained nurse therapists treated patients referred from their general practitioner for generalized anxiety disorder. Approximately 20 patients were allocated to each of three treatment conditions: anxiety management, non-directive counselling, or a waiting-list control. Since anxiety management has in the past been used to describe such a wide range of different methods, we thought it would be useful to restrict the techniques studied here to only two: brief relaxation training and cognitive therapy based on the description given by Beck and Emery. This meant that we explicitly avoided any instructions to clients that they should expose themselves to anxiety-arousing situations, except where this was appropriate to test the validity of automatic thoughts or irrational beliefs. Since there were only eight sessions spread over 10 weeks, and the first few sessions also included relaxation training, the cognitive therapy techniques employed were necessarily rather limited. Nonetheless, we ensured that the essential core techniques were always included, such as searching for automatic anxiety-elevating thoughts, questioning their validity, and constructing rational alternatives, which could then be rehearsed in real-life situations. Typical thoughts and beliefs in this sample of generalized anxiety disorder patients were that anxiety symptoms indicated serious physical disease or insanity, that other people thought that they were stupid or incompetent in some way, or that they would fail in some catastrophic manner. All sessions were conducted by an experienced nurse therapist, and tape recordings of these sessions were discussed in supervision meetings (Table 2).

Table 2. Adjusted post-treatment ratings, CT+R better than WAIT ($P < 0.05$). (from Blowers et al. in press)

Measure	CT+R	NDC	WAIT
Tension (0–4)	1.5	1.7	2.3
Problem (0–8)			
- Cognitive	2.7	3.1	4.6
- Physical	2.8	3.2	5.1
Social impairment (0–8)	1.7	2.1	3.2

Results were assessed blind; that is, on post-treatment interviews the assessors did not know whether the patient had received treatment at all, and if so, of what type. Across a wide range of clinical ratings and self-report measures, anxiety management was generally followed by more change than the equivalent waiting period without treatment. This difference was significant on ratings of tension, intensity of the main anxiety problems, and social impairment, as well as for self-reported questionnaire scores for frequency and severity of anxiety. In striking contrast, however, there were hardly any significant differences between anxiety management and non-directive counselling. Superiority for anxiety management in this comparison was confined to peripheral measures; namely, ease of being startled, belief that panics were physically harmful, and belief that relaxation was helpful in coping with anxiety. None of these measures were central to the anxiety problem, and some (such as the helpfulness of relaxation) could clearly be attributed to the therapeutic demand implicit in the instructions given in that treatment (for example that it would be helpful to practice relaxation; Table 3).

Table 3. Adjusted post-treatment ratings, CT+R better than NDC and WAIT ($P < 0.05$). (from Blowers et al. in press)

Measure	CT+R	NDC	WAIT
Startle (0–4)	0.7	1.7	1.6
Harm from panic (0–8)	1.7	3.4	3.7
Help from relax (0–8)	5.3	3.3	3.7

No follow-up results are available for waiting-list patients, since they were subsequently given various amounts of treatment; but for the other two conditions the pattern of little or no differences persisted at 6-month follow-up. Once again, the only differences were minor, and without exception they all concerned beliefs about the cause of anxiety and methods of coping with anxiety, that were part of the rationale which they had been given in the first place. For example, patients who had earlier received cognitive therapy subsequently thought that they were better able to talk themselves out of worry. However, despite this difference the same patients did not have any lower ratings for cognitive symptoms than did those who had received non-directive therapy. It therefore appears that the different treatment approaches successfully influenced the explanations given by clients for their improvement, but these did not correspond with real improvement differences. By implication, such explanations reflect the treatment rationale which they received, rather than the actual mechanisms of change.

Unfortunately, the absolute amounts of clinical improvement seen on the central measures of clinical anxiety were relatively small, compared with other results such as those obtained by Butler et al. (in press). On the other hand, where direct comparisons between measures could be made, the amount of change was very similar to that seen in other studies, such as that reported by Barlow et al. (1984). In any event, the important point was that there were surprisingly few differences between anxiety management techniques and an equally plausible treatment condition which included no specific coping techniques at all. The superiority of anxiety management to a no-treatment waiting period was again confirmed, but there does not seem any reason to believe that this superiority can be attributed to the specific effects of relaxation and cognitive therapy.

At the same time as this trial was being carried out in England, a second study was in proggress at Pennsylvania State University, using similar treatment methods (Borkovec et al., in press). Thirty volunteers attending the University clinic were all offered training in muscular relaxation, and one-half of the total continued with additional cognitive therapy, while the remaining half continued with non-directive counselling. Thus, the question under investigation in this study was that of whether cognitive therapy added more to relaxation training than did non-directive counselling. The majority of clients were students, therapists were clinical psychologists in training, and again all sessions (12 in this case) were conducted individually, recorded and discussed in later supervision sessions.

Analysis of post-treatment data, collected in the form of self-report questionnaires and blind assessors' ratings, showed a rather different pattern to that obtained in the study presented first. Although there was no overall difference between treatments on multivariate analysis of assessors' ratings or clients' diary reports, there was a significant main effect for other self-report questionnaire data. Breaking this main effect down by individual measures revealed that cognitive therapy plus relaxation produced superior results on the Spielberger trait score, on the Marks and Mathews fear questionnaire, on a specially constructed inventory of somatic and cognitive anxiety symptoms, and on the Zung self-rating of anxiety (Table 4).

Table 4. Post-treatment change on self-report measures, CT+R better than NDC+R ($P < 0.05$). (from Borkovec et al. in press)

Measure	CT+R	NDC+R
Trait anxiety	16.0	9.9
Fear questionnaire total	12.3	2.8
Zung anxiety	10.2	6.6

Follow-up was by mail questionnaire only, and showed no significant differences between treatments for those clients who responded, although this was only one-half of the sample. In responding to questions about the reasons for their improvement, those clients who had received non-directive counselling attributed 50% of their improvement to relaxation training, compared with only 36% in those who had received cognitive therapy. Thus, clients who had cognitive therapy attributed a greater proportion of their improvement to this than the remainder did to non-directive counselling.

Reports of anxiety during relaxation training were associated with poorer outcome on some of the main clinical measures. For example, pretreatment ratings of paradoxical increases in anxiety induced by relaxation, correlated with post-treatment gains on the Hamilton anxiety scale at the −0.48 level. Learning to relax may thus have contributed some of the benefit to clients who received non-directive counselling. Despite this, a number of significant outcome differences suggest that cognitive therapy added more to relaxation than did non-directive counselling, at least as assessed by self-report. This implies that we have now established some element in cognitive therapy, or in its combination with relaxation, which has specific effects not attributable to features common to any psychotherapeutic context. There are two reservations that should be expressed, however, before accepting this conclusion. First, the significant differences found were confined to self-report measures, and did not extend to blind assessors' ratings. Second, the clients treated in this study were largely students, whose anxiety problems may be different in some important respects from those of a clinical sample. Thus, although these students met DSM-III criteria for generalized anxiety disorders, and showed substantial clinical handicaps before treatment, they may not have been representative of the population referred by general practitioners in the first study. Perhaps more verbal, younger, and less chronically disturbed clients are able to respond to some element in cognitive therapy that is not so helpful to patients referred from general practice. Certainly the response to treatment appeared greater in the second study than it was in the first, and this difference may be attributable to variations in the client sample.

In the third and final study to be reported here (Borkovec and Mathews, in press), patients with severe clinical non-phobic anxiety disorders were again seen at Pennsylvania State University clinic, and received the same treatment combinations as in the student study, but these were administered by fully qualified therapists. This trial thus allowed us to resolve the question of whether the apparent difference between treatments would again disappear when these were given to a severe and chronic clinical sample, as happened in the first study. Thirty clients referred from local mental health agencies, and with a diagnosis of either generalized anxiety disorder or panic disorder, were allocated randomly to treatment either with cognitive therapy, non-directive counselling, or coping desensitisation; the same amount of relaxation training being common to each treatment condition. In the additional treatment method, coping desensitisation, clients were required to imagine anxiety-provoking situations or to provoke related somatic sensations, and then practice eliminating anxiety using their relaxation skills, prior to using the same techniques in real life. Apart from this additional treatment, the use of more experienced therapists, and a more representative clinical client population, this study closely resembled the previous student trial (Table 5).

Table 5. Post-treatment change scores, no significant differences. (from Borkovec and Mathews, in press)

Measure	CT+R	NDC+R	CSD
Trait anxiety	8.3	8.9	10.2
Hamilton anxiety	16.1	11.0	12.3
Zung anxiety	7.0	9.6	9.6

Despite this similarity, results were strikingly different. Put simply, there were no significant differences in outcome between the three treatment conditions, either at post-treatment or at 12-month follow-up, despite trends on some measures. The main question posed by this study is thus easily answered: significant differences do indeed disappear when a more representative clinic population is studied. The apparent difference obtained with students may indeed be a reliable one, but if so, it would appear to reflect a relatively unique response of that population to cognitive therapy when assessed by self-report. Hence, when a comparison was made of the gain scores obtained on all outcome measures across all groups and conditions in these last two studies, the amount of change appeared relatively similar except for that found on self-report measures provided by students receiving cognitive therapy (Table 6).

Table 6. Comparison across studies of change in Hamilton anxiety scores (follow-up data in parentheses)

Study	AMT	WAIT	NDC
Butler et al.	9.4 (11.0)	2.0	-
Borkovec et al.	12.0	-	9.7
Borkovec and Mathews	16.1 (15.4)	-	11.0 (11.4)

Turning to the factors which appeared to have some predictive power in the preceding trail, there were again some indications that ability to relax, and the frequency of relaxation practice reported, were related to outcome. Pretreatment reports of paradoxical increases in anxiety when trying to relax were associated with poor outcome, and frequent relaxation practice during treatment was associated with good outcome. It is not clear why this should be so, given our failure to show that specific techniques make a difference, althought it seems possible that patients who are particularly sensitive to bodily sensations have a generally poorer prognosis.

Sensitivity to bodily sensations was not necessarily related to a diagnosis of panic disorder, however, and in fact there was a remarkable absence of evidence for any differences in treatment response between the two diagnostic groups. A diagnosis of panic disorder as opposed to generalized anxiety was associated with higher levels of reported worry, and (unexpectedly) with relatively higher scores for cognitive rather than somatic symptoms as assessed by questionnaire. Thus there was no evidence from our data that panic patients are relatively more somatically orientated than generalised anxiety patients, contrary to the results reported by Barlow et al. (1984). Since there was also no trend towards differences in response to any of the three treatments being associated with diagnostic group, we remain unconvinced that the distinction between panic and generalised anxiety is a useful one.

A final failure to confirm expectations arose from the lack of any interaction between treatment outcome and predominance of somatic or cognitive symptoms. For example, it might have been supposed that clients who complained more of cognitive symptoms should respond better to cognitive therapy, while those who complained more about somatic symptoms might do better with coping desensitisation. In fact, there was no evidence to support any of these expectations. There was actually only one interaction between symptom type and treatment outcome, and this suggested that among clients who received non-directive counselling, those complaining predominantly of cognitive symptoms responded relatively better. The consistent lack of any predictive power attributable to type of client or type of symptom across different treatments strongly suggests that specific anxiety management techniques do not act via changes in the symptoms or processes that form their presumed target.

Conclusions

Before discussing the implications of these negative findings, it is necessary to touch on the problem of whether the failure in two out of three trials to show outcome differences might not be interpreted as evidence of relatively weak clinical treatments, rather than evidence of the effectiveness of common or non-specific therapeutic factors. Although a difficult question to resolve, the improvements obtained in the last study were substantial, and similar in magnitude to those obtained in other well-conducted studies (for example Butler et al., in press). Thus, if our treatments are to be considered weak, then so must other related methods being employed elsewhere. Also, the equivalence of anxiety management and non-directive counselling was seen in trials where clinical effectiveness was high, as in the last study, or low, as in the first. In contrast, whenever a waiting group was included, all anxiety management conditions have proved superior to waiting. It thus appears that we must draw the following conclusions:

1. Anxiety management methods are consistently superior to no treatment.
2. None of the methods examined are clearly superior to non-directive counselling with representative clinic populations.
3. There is no convincing evidence that different anxiety management techniques act specifically on their presumed targets.

Of course these conclusions remain subject to modification as new research results are reported, and may indeed be reversed as more powerful techniques are developed. For example, one encouraging albeit insignificant trend was for improvements following cognitive therapy to persist more than following non-directive counselling, although this was again more marked for self-report measures. Nonetheless, I believe that it would be wise to grasp the nettle, and consider the implications of the present negative findings, rather than reject them on the grounds that they do not fit our preconceptions. Not all these implications can be discussed here, but there are a number which I think are particularly important.

The first, which can be dismissed fairly rapidly, is that the results of outcome trials may indeed differ across target populations. The wisdom of conducting analogue studies and drawing conclusions for clinical populations has been discussed extensively elsewhere, and there is little point in adding to that discussion. However, I think it is worth noting that student subjects, although meeting DSM-III criteria, appear to respond better to cognitive therapy than do clinical populations; while on the other hand, there is little evidence of such treatment differences in the case of severe clinical patients. Not only were there no differences overall between cognitive therapy and non-directive counselling, but there were no differences in treatment outcome between generalised anxiety or panic disorder patients. This would imply that it might be profitable to search for the underlying differences between student volunteer and clinical patients, rather than focus on perhaps less relevant differences between generalised anxiety and panic disorders.

A more fundamental implication, in my view, is the doubt that these results cast on our previous beliefs about the processes and mechanisms which we had thought were involved in anxiety management. It now seems less plausible to me that cognitive therapy acts via verbalisable thought processes, or that if it does, it cannot do so uniquely. Rather, we would have to concede that a much less structured and directed procedure, in this case non-directive counselling, has quite similar effects. This refers not just to overall outcome, but also to the type of symptom and/or the type of problem. Thus cognitive therapy was not particularly superior in the case of cognitively-orientated anxiety, or in changing specifically cognitive symptoms. This should not be taken to imply that generalized anxiety does not arise from cognitive processes, since we would still argue that it probably does. Instead, we believe that the relevant cognitive processes are not uniquely changed by existing cognitive therapy methods, perhaps because these underlying processes are not always available for conscious report. For example, we have described experimental data showing that generalised anxiety patients show an attentional bias concerned with external threat stimuli, even when they cannot report subsequently on the nature of these stimuli (Mathews and MacLeod 1986). While it may well be possible to change such an attentional bias by first changing conscious beliefs, it clearly does not follow that this is the only or even necessarily the best method of doing so.

If other features, including those which are common to coping desensitisation, cognitive therapy and non-directive counselling, may be involved in the process of change, then future research should be directed at identifying these features. If they can be identified and perhaps strengthened, then better treatments could be developed as a result. Unfortunately, our research to date has left open the nature of these factors, and only guesswork is possible. My own guess would be that all anxiety management methods redefine anxiety for clients as a problem which is soluble by his or her own efforts, rather than as a catastrophic event which is both dangerous and outside the individual's control. A related possibility is that the anxious client's problem-solving efforts are initially misdirected towards avoiding supposed physical or social dangers, leaving little or no resources available for tackling the biased cognitive processes which actually lead to their state of anxiety. By redefining anxiety as an internally generated and potentially controllable problem, cognitive resources may thus be redirected appropriately. Conceivably it makes little difference which particular technique each individual uses, whether this is relaxation, modifying automatic thoughts, or attempting to understand the underlying causes, as long as the previously exclusive focus on potential danger is modified. Clearly many other possible accounts of underlying common mechanisms are possible, and there are too many such possibilities to be fully discussed here. However, I would like to believe that by keeping an open mind about possible common treatment mechanisms, and by testing out these ideas experimentally, we should be able to improve existing methods, and make them both more specific and more effective in the future.

References

Barlow DH, Cohen AS, Waddell MT, Vermilyea BB, Klosko JS, Blanchard EB, Di Nardo PA (1984) Panic and generalized anxiety disorders: nature and treatment. Behav Res Ther 15:431–449

Blowers C, Cobb J, Mathews A Generalized anxiety: a controlled treatment study. Behav Res Ther, in press

Borkovec T, Mathews A Treatment of non-phobic anxiety disorders: a comparison of nondirective, cognitive, and coping desensitization theory. J Consult Clin Psychol, in press

Borkovec T, Mathews A, Chambers A, Ebrahimi S, Lytle R, Nelson R The effects of relaxation training with cognitive therapy or nondirective therapy and the role of relaxation-induced anxiety in the treatment of generalized anxiety. J Consult Clin Psychol, in press

Butler G, Cullington A, Hibbert G, Klimes I, Gelder M Anxiety management for persistent generalised anxiety. Br J Psychiatry, in press

Jannoun L, Oppenheimer C, Gelder M (1982) A self-help treatment program for anxiety state patients. Behav Res Ther 13:103–111

Mathews A, MacLeod C (1986) Discrimination of threat cues without awarenes in anxiety states. J Abnorm Psychol 95:131–138

8. Long-Term Efficacy of Ungraded Versus Graded Massed Exposure in Agoraphobics

W. FIEGENBAUM

Introduction

At present, exposure therapy is obviously the psychological treatment of choice for agoraphobia. About two-thirds of the patients are improved at the end of treatment, about one-third even seem to be cured. Yet, long-term efficacy of exposure therapy has not been evaluated very often, and the reported effects vary more than for the short-term evaluations (e.g., Hand et al. 1974; Mathews et al. 1977; Emmelkamp and Kuipers 1979; Goldstein 1982; McPherson et al. 1980; Munby and Johnston 1980; Burns et al. 1983; Michelson et al. 1985; Fiegenbaum 1986; Hand et al. 1986). It is possible that long-term stability of beneficial therapeutic effects varies with the type of exposure used and with the coping rationale that the patients use when confronted with agoraphobic stimuli after the end of therapy. Therefore, studies are needed that evaluate the long-term effects of different types of exposure therapy and contribute to identify those variables that favor enduring benefits.

In the present paper data are reported on a 5-year follow-up study with 127 agoraphobic patients who had been treated with one of two standardized behavioral treatment programs - either graded or ungraded massed exposure in vivo - at the universities of Münster and Marburg in the Federal Republic of Germany.

Three aspects of the long-term follow-up study will be discussed:

1. To what extent do patients who have been treated with graded vs. ungraded massed exposure in vivo differ with respect to the stability of their treatment gains 5 years after the end of therapy?
2. Will the striking long-term benefits of ungraded exposure that we had found in our first subsample of 25 patients be corroborated by the data of all 104 patients treated with ungraded massed exposure for whom 5-year follow-up data are already available?
3. What do highly successful patients of the ungraded and graded exposure groups, compared to the less successful ones, consider to be the most important basic idea of their anxiety treatment 5 years after the end of therapy?

Method

Subjects

A total of 127 patients participated in the study. All of them met DSM-III criteria for a diagnosis of agoraphobia with panic attacks. For patients treated before the publication of DSM-III, we ensured retrospectively that the criteria were met.

The average age of the patients was 34 years, with a minimum of 19 years and a maximum of 68 years; 78% of the patients were female. The mean duration of symptoms was 10.5 years. About 32% of the patients were completely housebound, a further 39% could not leave the immediate environment of their home.

Almost one-half of the patients (47%) took tranquilizers for their anxiety. Of these, 25% were dependent on medication. Most of the patients had been referred to the Psychological Department by primary-care physicians and clinics or had asked for therapy after having read reports on our agoraphobia research project. For those patients who had been able to travel at least to some extent or who lived in the region, therapies started in the areas of Marburg or Münster. For those who were housebound in other parts of the Federal Republic of Germany, or in Austria or Switzerland, therapy started in the area where they lived.

Treatment

Patients were treated with one of two fairly standardized in vivo exposure programs - namely graded massed exposure or ungraded massed exposure (Bartling et al. 1984). Each of these programs consists of the described four phases (Table 1).

Table 1. Structure of the treatment program

Diagnostic phase	4–8 hours Technical delay 7–14 days
Cognitive preparation phase	4–8 hours Decison period 7–14 days
Intensive training phase	6–10 days
Self-control phase	6–8 weeks

In the diagnostic phase, the individually relevant agoraphobic situations are specified and examples of agoraphobic experiences from the beginning of the disorder up to the present time are obtained.

In the cognitive preparation phase, the attempt is made to explain to the patients the etiology and development of their agoraphobia up to the present time in terms of an avoidance paradigm. The examples used for the explanation are taken from the patients' own reports of their experiences in agoraphobic situations. From these examples the conclusion is drawn that a massed exposure in vivo will interrupt the present vicious circle of avoidance and anxiety. After this the patients are given detailed information about the planned intensive training (graded or ungraded). They are then given a minimum of 7 days to decide whether or not they will participate.

The intensive training consists of a block of 6 to 10 consecutive days of massed in vivo exposure. The patients are not given the possibility to avoid any of the exposure situations that have been selected for therapy, neither can they themselves cut down the duration of exposure nor decide on the sequence of the situations. In the beginning of this phase the therapists accompany the patients. They train them not to distract themselves during exposure nor to fight against their anxiety, but rather to focus their attention on their symptoms and even attempt to provoke or intensify their symptoms, including their panic attacks. The patients are then progressively led to expose themselves to the agoraphobic situations.

This training is obviously more intensive and massed than is common in other exposure therapies. Table 2 shows a typical program of an ungraded massed exposure and illustrates the procedure during intensive training. The training in graded exposure is as massed as the ungraded one, but selection of agoraphobic situations follows an anxiety hierarchy, i.e., patients start with the less anxiety-provoking situations and step by step move to the top of the hierarchy.

During the subsequent self-control phase, the patients continue the training by themselves. They observe carefully in which situations of their everyday life they might still profit from prolonged exposure. In the first part of our project 25 of the patients had been assigned to ungraded and 23 to graded massed exposure. Groups were matched with respect to age, sex, duration of agoraphobia, and educational status. The next 79 patients were uniformly assigned to ungraded massed exposure.

Table 2. Example of a typical intensive therapy program: ungraded massed exposure

First day:
- Collection from home town and journey by car (2-door, patient sitting in the back) to Marburg
- Confinement in narrow, dark room (approx. 1 m^2, 1–2 h)
- Walk in unfamiliar area (1–2 h)
- Flight in sporting plane (approx. 45 min, ideally 2–3 take-offs/landings)
- Meal in overcrowded canteen
- Train to Frankfurt (approx. 1 h)
- Travel by underground in Frankfurt (approx. 2–4 h, evening rush hour, first trips without therapist)
- Sleeper journey Frankfurt–Milan (approx. 10 h)

Second day:
- Approx. 7 a.m. arrival in Milan; then underground, bus, tram, specified paths through town, top of cathedral, department stores, cinema, eat in overcrowded restaurants (approx. 11–12 h)
- Flight Milan–Munich
- Night in hotel

Third day:
- Munich: Morning – Subway, Olympic Tower, department stores. Afternoon – Journey by train, rack-railway (approx. 40 min in tunnel), cablecar to “Zugspitze“ (highest mountain in germany). Evening – Night train home

Other days:
- Exercises in home town of patient

Therapists

Therapies were conducted by senior graduated students or psychologists who had completed their university training (Dipl.-Psych. or Master's level). They received a thorough special training in massed exposure therapies and were supervised by experienced behavioral therapists during the whole course of therapy.

Assessment

Follow-up assessments were carried out by specially trained psychologists who did not know which type of exposure therapy the former patients had received. Assessment consisted of a set of rating scales, symptom checklists, personality questionnaires, and a behavioral test (exposure to the individual top agoraphobic situation).

Results

Comparison of Graded and Ungraded Massed Exposure (Subsample of 48 Patients)

The data of our first subsample are shown in Table 3. Patients of the graded and

Table 3. Patients' self-evaluation 5 years after therapy

	Ungraded exposure ($n = 25$)		Graded exposure ($n = 23$)	
	(n)	(%)	(n)	(%)
Symptom-free	19	76.0	8	34.8
Higly improved	1	4.0	5	21.7
Moderately improved	4	16.0	3	13.0
Unchanged	0	0.0	4	17.4
Deteriorated	1	4.0	3	13.0

Chi-square = 12.2, $P < 0.05$

ungraded exposure groups differ significantly in their *subjective evaluations of their symptom status.* The ungraded treatment is superior to the graded one in that 76% vs. 35% are in their own view completely free of symptoms 5 years after therapy.

The same is found with regard to the anxiety scores obtained on *fear questionnaires,* e.g., FSS-III (Wolpe and Lang 1964) and STAI (Spielberger et al. 1970). Patients also had to *rate* their *anxiety levels* with regard to their three individual top agoraphobic situations as assessed prior to therapy using a 100-point rating scale (Table 4).

Table 4. Mean anxiety ratings (0–100) for the three individual top agoraphobic situations prior to therapy and at 5-year follow-up

	Prior to therapy ($\bar{x}$)	At follow-up ($\bar{x}$)
Ungraded exposure ($n = 25$)	89.1	15.9
Graded exposure ($n = 23$)	86.4	56.7

$t = -7.6$, $P < 0.001$

We again found pronounced superiority of the ungraded massed exposure treatment.

Finally, patients underwent a behavioral test. They were asked to *expose themselves* to their formerly most anxiety-provoking situation and stay in this situation for an individually defined period of time (Table 5).

Striking differences between groups were found. Again, results clearly favor ungraded massed exposure. Eighty percent of the patients in this group were able to complete exposure compared to only 22% of the other group.

It should be mentioned that we had also evaluated the short-term effects of both therapeutic procedures for the above sample. At the end of treatment and 8 months later both procedures showed equally good outcomes on almost all of the variables assessed. Yet, contrary to our expectations, patients participating in the graded procedure showed objectively, and subjectively, significantly higher levels of stress during training. Therefore, we decided to discontinue the graded approach and to treat all further patients with ungraded massed exposure.

Table 5. Behavioral tests at 5-year follow-up (%)

	Ungraded exposure ($n = 25$)		Graded exposure ($n = 23$)	
	(n)	(%)	(n)	(%)
Exposure completed	20	80.0	5	21.7
Exposure terminated prematurely	0	0.0	0	0.0
Exposure refused	5	20.0	18	78.3

Chi-square = 14.0, $P < 0.001$

Follow-Up Data for the Total Sample of Patients Treated with Ungraded Massed Exposure

Table 6 shows the results for all 104 patients with ungraded massed exposure that we have now followed up for 5 years. Again data show that almost 78% of the sample consider themselves to be completely symptom-free.

The mean anxiety rating for the three individual top agoraphobic situations decreased from about 85 on a 100-point rating scale prior to therapy to 20.5 at 5-year follow up. Most importantly, in the behavioral test, about 80% of the subjects were able to complete exposure to their top agoraphobic situation.

Table 6. Outcome of ungraded massed exposure at 5-year follow-up (total sample, $n = 104$)

Patients' self-evaluation	*(n)*	(%)
Symptom-free	81	77.9
Highly improved	7	6.7
Moderately improved	13	12.5
Unchanged	1	1.0
Deteriorated	2	1.9

Mean anxiety ratings (0–100) for the three individual agoraphobic situations: $\bar{x} = 20.5$

Behavioral tests	*(n)*	(%)
Exposure completed	83	79.8
Exposure terminated prematurely	1	1.0
Exposure refused	20	19.2

Relationship Between Exposure, Success of Treatment, and Therapeutic Rationale in the View of the Patient

We wanted to get an idea of the therapeutic rationale that might have guided the patients over the 5-year period. We therefore asked them, what they considered to be the most important basic idea of their anxiety therapy (Table 7).

Interestingly, about 75% of the subjects from the ungraded exposure group but only 13% from the graded exposure group said that they had learned the rule "Expose yourself to the situation until anxiety has gone." In contrast, 52% of the graded, but only about 2% of the ungraded patients said they had learned: "Cope with your anxiety step by step."

It may be that the cognition "Expose yourself..." leads to a behavioral strategy that is incompatible with avoidance or escape behavior, whereas the cognition "Cope stepwise" might imply that total avoidance is replaced by partial avoidance.

There should be a higher probability for the "Expose yourself" patients to profit from treatment than for patients using rationales that give room to avoidance behavior. Data from our behavioral test clearly support this hypothesis (Table 8). Of those 83 patients who completed the exposure test, 74 had the rationale "Expose yourself until anxiety has gone," only 9 had other rationales. Of those 20 subjects who refused exposure 15 had not the rationale "Exposure yourself..."

Table 8. Outcome of exposure test for patients with vs. without the rationale "Expose yourself to the situation until the anxiety has gone" (ungraded exposure group only, $n = 104$)

	"Expose yourself until anxiety has gone" *(n)*	Other rationales *(n)*
Exposure completed	74	9
Exposure terminated prematurely	0	1
Exposure refused	5	15

Chi-square= 38.7, $P < 0.001$

Table 7. "What do you consider the most important basic idea of your anxiety therapy?"

	Group 1: ungraded exposure *(n)*	(%)	Group 2: ungraded exposure *(n)*	(%)	Group 3: graded exposure *(n)*	(%)
"Expose yourself to the situation until the anxiety has gone"	18	72.0	79	76.0	3	13.0
"Cope with your anxiety step by step"	0	0.0	2	1.9	12	52.2

Chi-square: Group 1 vs. 3: 22.7, $P < 0.001$; group 2 vs. 3: 55.9, $P < 0.001$

As a consequence of this study, we suggest that the probability of long-term benefits in agoraphobics with panic attacks may be increased by taking two guidelines into consideration:

a) Perform exposure therapies in a way that definitely gives no room to avoidance behavior.
b) Make sure that the patients internalize the rationale "Expose yourself until anxiety has gone."

References

Bartling G, Fiegenbaum W, Krause R (1984) Reizüberflutung. Kohlhammer, Stuttgart

Burns LE, Thorpe GL, Cavallero A, Gosling J (1983) Agoraphobia eight years after behavioral treatment: a follow-up study with interview, questionnaire and behavioral data. 17th Congress of AABT/World Congress for Behavior Therapy, Washington, DC

Emmelkamp PMG, Kuipers ACM (1979) Agoraphobia: a follow-up study four years after treatment. Br J Psychiatry 134:352-355

Fiegenbaum W (1986) Longterm efficacy of exposure therapy in cardiac phobia. In: Hand I, Wittchen H-U (eds) Panic and phobias. Springer, Berlin Heidelberg New York

Goldstein AJ (1982) Agoraphobia: treatment successes, treatment failures and theoretical implications. In: Chambless DL, Goldstein AJ (eds) Agoraphobia: multiple perspectives on theory and treatment. Wiley, New York

Hand I, Lamontagne Y, Marks I (1974) Group exposure (flooding) in vivo for agoraphobics. Br J Psychiatry 124:588-602

Hand I, Angenendt J, Fischer M, Wilke C (1986) Exposure in vivo with panic management: treatment rationale and longterm outcome. In: Hand I, Wittchen H-U (eds) Panic and phobias. Springer, Berlin Heidelberg New York, p 104-128

Mathews AM, Teasdale J, Munby M, Johnston DW, Shaw P (1977) A homebased treatment program for agoraphobia. Behav Res Ther 8:915-924

McPherson FM, Brougham I, McLaren S (1980) Maintenance of improvement of agoraphobic patients treated by behavioural methods - four year follow-up. Behav Res Ther 18:150-152

Michelson L, Mavissakalian M, Marchione K (1985) Cognitive and behavioral treatments of agoraphobia: clinical, behavioral, and psychophysiological outcomes. J Consult Clin Psychol 53:913-925

Munby M, Johnston DW (1980) Agoraphobia: the long-term follow-up of behavioural treatment. Br J Psychiatry 137:418-427

Spielberger CD, Gorsuch RL, Lushene RE (1970) Manual for the state-trait anxiety inventory. Consulting Psychologists Press, Palo Alto

Wolpe J, Lang P (1984) A fear survey schedule for use in behaviour therapy. Behav Res Ther 2:27-30

9. Exposure Treatment of Agoraphobia with Panic Attacks: Are Drugs Essential?

G. Andrews and C. Moran

Introduction

There is a body of opinion that holds that panic disorder and agoraphobia are different to the other anxiety disorders. This opinion is based on three sets of observations:

a) panic disorder and agoraphobia seem to be influenced by specific genetic factors;
b) the attacks of panic can be precipitated by the administration of lactate and other substances; and
c) treatment with antidepressants is "uniquely effective" (Sheehan 1982).

As these disorders afflict some 5% of the population (Robins et al. 1984), a specific remedy that blocked panic without producing side-effects, sedation, or dependence, would be of value. New drugs are being produced for panic, but before we embark on their use it might be prudent to consider three questions. First, is there satisfactory evidence that these disorders are under some type of specific genetic control, or is the evidence more consistent with the general genetic diathesis that has been shown to contribute to all the anxiety disorders? We have already drawn attention to the incompatibility with genetic hypotheses of the familial risks observed in agoraphobia (Moran and Andrews 1985), and recently produced data to support the general genetic diathesis hypothesis (Andrews et al. 1987). The second question, which concerns the specificity of certain chemical stimuli in producing panic in susceptible subjects, has been recently reviewed (Holt and Andrews 1987). There seems little doubt that many persons who regularly experience panic attacks can be induced to panic if placed in a laboratory situation, surrounded by resuscitation equipment, and given chemicals that cause perturbations of the autonomic system, not unlike the early symptoms of panic; but no panic will occur in nonanxious people. It had been hoped that some evidence of some underlying biochemical vulnerability to panic might be the link between these chemicals and the resultant panic attacks, but no such evidence has yet emerged (Holt and Andrews 1987).

This paper is concerned with the third question. Are drugs essential in the treatment for agoraphobia with panic attacks? The results of 50 patients treated with a very structured cognitive behavior therapy program will be presented. This program was specifically aimed at teaching control of panic through slow breathing and relaxation and elimination of avoidance behavior by graded exposure. Therapy was also aimed at reducing the general propensity to anxiety and the externalized locus of control shown by many of these patients. In the discussion we shall review the benefits that can be expected from both drug and nondrug therapies for these disorders.

Method

There were three considerations in doing this study. First, to ensure that all subjects suffered from an agoraphobia with panic attacks that was consistent with DSM-III criteria. Second, as ensuring quality of treatment in the psychotherapies is difficult (Andrews 1984), we developed a highly structured treatment protocol, fully described in a treatment manual that each patient, under supervision, read in detail as treatment proceeded. Third, we sought to use well-established measures so that the results could be easily compared with those from other studies.

Subjects and Measures

The subjects were 50 consecutive patients referred by their family physician or psychiatrist for treatment of agoraphobia. Forty-four were female and six were male. Their ages ranged from 18 to 59, mean age was 34.6 years. They had had agoraphobia for a mean of 8 years (range 1–30 years). All subjects completed the symptom and vulnerability measures at the time of the first diagnostic interview, and this diagnosis was confirmed in the week prior to treatment by the diagnostic interview schedule (Robins et al. 1981). They completed the symptom and vulnerability measures again at this interview, at the end of treatment, and at 6 months and 12 months after treatment had concluded.

The following measures were used. Symptoms were measured with the Symptom Check List (SCL-90R Derogatis et al. 1974) and the global anxiety and phobic avoidance subscales will be reported. Panic, for which there is as yet no generally accepted method of assessment, was assessed from responses to question 72 of the SCL 90R scale: "In the last two weeks how much were you distressed by spells of terror or panic?" Scores ranged from 0 (not at all) to 4 (extremely). The behavioral avoidance test was a measure of the distance subjects could travel on their own from the clinic to a shopping center 5 miles distant. It was scored on a 9-point logarithmic type scale so that 9 meant only able to go to the door of the clinic office, 5 able to reach the hospital gate 500 yards away on one's own, and a score of 1 able to travel alone to a shopping center 5 miles away.

The vulnerability measures analysed were the Eysenck personality inventory neuroticism scale (Eysenck and Eysenck 1964), a trait measure of emotionality, strongly correlated with other trait measures of anxiety that has been found to predict the emergence of general neurotic symptoms in a general population and to predict relapse after psychotherapy (Henderson 1981; Weissman et al. 1978). The second vulnerability measure, the locus of control of behavior scale (Craig et al. 1984), was developed in this laboratory as a measure of the locus of personal control in respect to chronic conditions like stuttering and agoraphobia. It has been shown to be a powerful predictor of relapse in stutterers (Craig and Andrews 1985).

Results are presented in terms of means and standard deviations, and in effect size units (ES), a measure of the number of standard deviations of improvement that follows therapy. Data were analysed using planned contrasts analysis of variance on repeated measures with the critical alpha set in advance as $P < 0.05$.

Treatment Program

The patients were treated as in-patients, in groups of six, over a period of ten working days. Treatment was full-time, with didactic sessions and practice outings continuing from 9 a.m. to 5 p.m. each day. Patients were expected to review the day's material each evening. When each patient was initially offered treatment the program was described as "like going to college. You will learn about anxiety, panic, and agoraphobia. You will learn how to control your anxiety and panic attacks, and how to overcome your fears of situations. We will also teach you some ways of controlling worrying thoughts and some ways to assert yourself more effectively."

The agoraphobic patients seemed surprisingly naive in their approach to understanding anxiety. For the purposes of this program, anxiety was held to be the result of an external stressor being identified as threatening to the individual, and resulting in prolonged arousal, hypervigilance, and various autonomic symptoms associated with anxiety. Prior adversive experience with similar stressors, the presence of high trait anxiety, and poor coping skills were given as the principal determinants of one's proneness to anxiety. Coping with anxiety was described as a two-stage process. First, the use of the relaxation response to prevent anxiety becoming debilitating, and, second, the use of mature coping strategies like anticipation and rehearsal of possible solutions to the threat, suppression until such strategies could be used, and stoic acceptance if the situation appeared chronic, intractable, and unavoidable.

Panic was defined as an acute attack of anxiety in which the physiological concomitants of anxiety themselves became a primary cause of concern, either because they were unpleasant or because they were thought to herald some calamity like loss of control, insanity, or fatal heart attack. Agoraphobia was described as avoidance of situations for fear of panic, particularly situations in which escape would be difficult or help not available if a severe panic occurred. Patients were told that proper anxiety management would lessen the likelihood of panic attacks occurring, specific panic control procedures would stop panic attacks escalating, and that avoidance behavior could then be overcome by confronting the feared situations.

Panic control was achieved by training patients in a specifically designed slow breathing technique (Andrews and Moran 1986), whereby they learned to reduce their respiration rates to 10 breaths per minute if required. By doing this they would be able to reverse the physiological effects of hyperventilation, induce a relaxation response, and distract themselves from debilitating self-statements about the imminence of panic. Although the slow-breathing concept is simple: "when you feel yourself begin to panic hold your breath for 10 seconds then breathe in and out on a 6 second cycle, saying relax as you breathe out"; in practice the steps involved in such training are more complex. Patients learn to identify the phases of inspiration and expiration; monitor their natural respiration rate at rest, during activity, and in phobic situations; and practice regulating their respiration rates in all situations. This training and practice takes some 6 h of the 80-h program.

Isometric relaxation was also taught as a technique to be used to control panic. Situational panics were quite effectively dealt with in these ways for the anticipatory anxiety warns the patient to use these techniques before the anxiety becomes debilitating. Once these techniques became practised and indeed overlearned, spontaneous panic attacks could be aborted in the same fashion.

Training in deep muscle relaxation was offered to all patients and even those who initially become distressed by the threatened loss of control that can accompany the relaxation response were encouraged to persist, for both mastery and regular practice of the relaxation response were considered to be the groundwork necessary if isometric relaxation was to be effective, and essential if a reduction in trait anxiety was to occur in the longer term.

Patients were instructed in the theory and application of graded exposure. Two sets of hierarchies were constructed, one, a standard set of tasks that ranged from walking alone in the hospital grounds, to travelling on one's own to the city 9 miles distant by bus and while there using the subway and taking an elevator to a 7th-floor boutique. The steps on this hierarchy were first completed in the company of the therapist and then performed alone. Successful completion of each step was rewarded by a combination of therapist and group acclaim and a cash reward. The second hierarchy was a set of personal assignments which patients constructed to apply to their own home and work environs.

Many patients who can control their panic attacks and who have learned to confront previously feared situations still are troubled by anticipatory fears of the type "What if next time I can't control the panic?". We therefore provided instruction and practice in replacing such negative and self-defeating thoughts with more positive thoughts which, together with practice in thought stopping and distraction, gave patients control over their anticipatory anxieties. Most of our patients had been agoraphobic for years, and had gradually become dependent on others and unprepared to take the initiative and cope with their own real world or other agoraphobia-related anxieties. Accordingly, the last 10h of the program were spent on restructuring irrational thinking and in assertiveness training.

Thus, in summary, during the 2-week intensive treatment period patients received some 40 h therapy covering the nature of their illness, the control of panic, techniques for entering feared situations, and the steps required if they were to habitually use mor mature coping mechanisms to deal with anxiety. In addition they spent a further 40h completing a hierarchy of graded exposure assignments, one-half under the supervision of the therapist and one-half on their own. The program has been developed from a number of sources (Jacobsen 1938; Marks 1975; Ellis 1962; Jakubowski and Lange 1976) and from our own clinical experience over a 7 year period.

Results

The results for the 50 agoraphobic subjects treated with this intensive and structured treatment program, and measured on two occasions prior to treatment, at the end of treatment, and 6 and 12 months later are presented in Table 1. The scores on all four symptom measures were stable during the baseline pretreatment period (mean effect size, −0.01). All the symptom scores improved significantly during the 2-week treatment period ($P < 0.05$, mean ES = 1.98). Follow-up data were available for 46 of the 50 subjects and these data showed that this improvement was not reduced over the 12-months follow-up period (mean ES at 6 months = 2.42; mean ES at 12 months = 2.12). None were retreated for their agoraphobia during this period. The improvement was similar on all four symptom measures, general anxiety, phobic anxiety, the panic question, and the behavioral avoidance test. These results are displayed in Fig. 1 in effect size units. In regard to the panic question at 12 months, 50% scored 0 or 1, while 38% still scored 3 or 4 on the SCL-90R question.

The two measures chosen to assess vulnerability to neurosis, the Eysenck Personality Inventory Neuroticism Scale and the Locus of Control of Behaviour Scale, changed with treatment and remained significantly improved throughout the 12-month follow-up period. The means, standard deviations, and numbers of subjects measured are also displayed in Table 1, and the improvement in effect size units is shown in Fig. 1. To what extent does improvement in these factors repre-

Table 1. Agoraphobia treatment outcome: Symptom measures (SCL 90 general anxiety and phobic anxiety scales, the panic question, and a test of behavioral avoidance) and vulnerability measures (EPI neuroticism and locus of control) given as means, with standard deviations and number of subjects measured in parentheses

	Symptom outcome measure				Vulnerability factors	
Measurement occasion	SCL 90 Anxiety	SCL 90 Phobic anxiety	SCL 90 Panic question	Behavioral avoidance	EPI Neuroticism	Locus of control
1. Initial interview	2.76 (0.65; 50)	3.28 (0.67; 50)	3.36 (0.85; 50)	4.58 (2.10; 36)	18.60 (3.97; 42)	37.23 (7.21; 39)
2. Pretreatment	2.77 (0.62; 50)	3.22 (0.68; 50)	3.48 (0.85; 50)	4.74 (1.44; 49)	18.40 (3.63; 50)	35.94 (9.33; 48)
3. Posttreatment	1.68* (0.93; 50)	1.86* (1.04; 50)	2.08* (1.54; 50)	1.20* (0.54;50)	16.64* (4.94; 50)	26.29* (11.31; 48)
4. 6 months post-treatment	1.27* (0.82; 31)	1.48* (0.97; 31)	1.61* (1.39; 21)	2.10*+ (1.52; 30)	14.26* (6.07; 31)	25.68* (8.82; 31)
5. 12 months post-treatment	1.39* (0.97; 42)	1.66* (1.11; 42)	1.76* (1.56; 42)	2.36*+ (1.98; 39)	14.91* (5.95; 42)	29.52* (13.35; 42)

* Significantly different to pretreatment measure (2);
\+ significantly different to posttreatment measure (3)

sent a lessening in vulnerability as distinct from merely being evidence of some general improvement? Both vulnerability measures are intercorrelated with symptom measures, but because of the reduction in symptoms due to treatment it was impossible to decide if there was any evidence of an independent reduction in vulnerability during the treatment period. Symptom scores were stable between the 6- and 12-months follow-up assessments and so using data from the 42 subjects who had been treated to criterion (defined as at the end of treatment being able to travel at least 5 miles by public transport on their own), we performed a hierarchical multiple regression to examine the influence of the two vulnerability factors and symptoms at the 6-months point on symptoms of anxiety at the 12-months point. The two vulnerability factors at 6 months accounted for 35% of the variance in symptom scores at 12 months ($P < 0.05$; $n = 24$), while symptoms of anxiety at 6 months, entered into the regression last, accounted for 30% of the variance in symptoms observed at 12 months ($P < 0.05$; $n = 24$). We concluded that vulnerability factors measured at 6 months were contributing to the stable posttreatment outcome at 12 months.

Discussion

A very structured and very detailed behavioral treatment program delivered in 80 h over 2 weeks produced a significant change in symptoms in a group of 50 agoraphobic patients and this improvement was sustained over the next 12 months. The improvement in symptoms included reductions in anxiety, phobic avoidance, and panic, and an improvement in the ability to travel alone. Prior to treatment these patients were severely

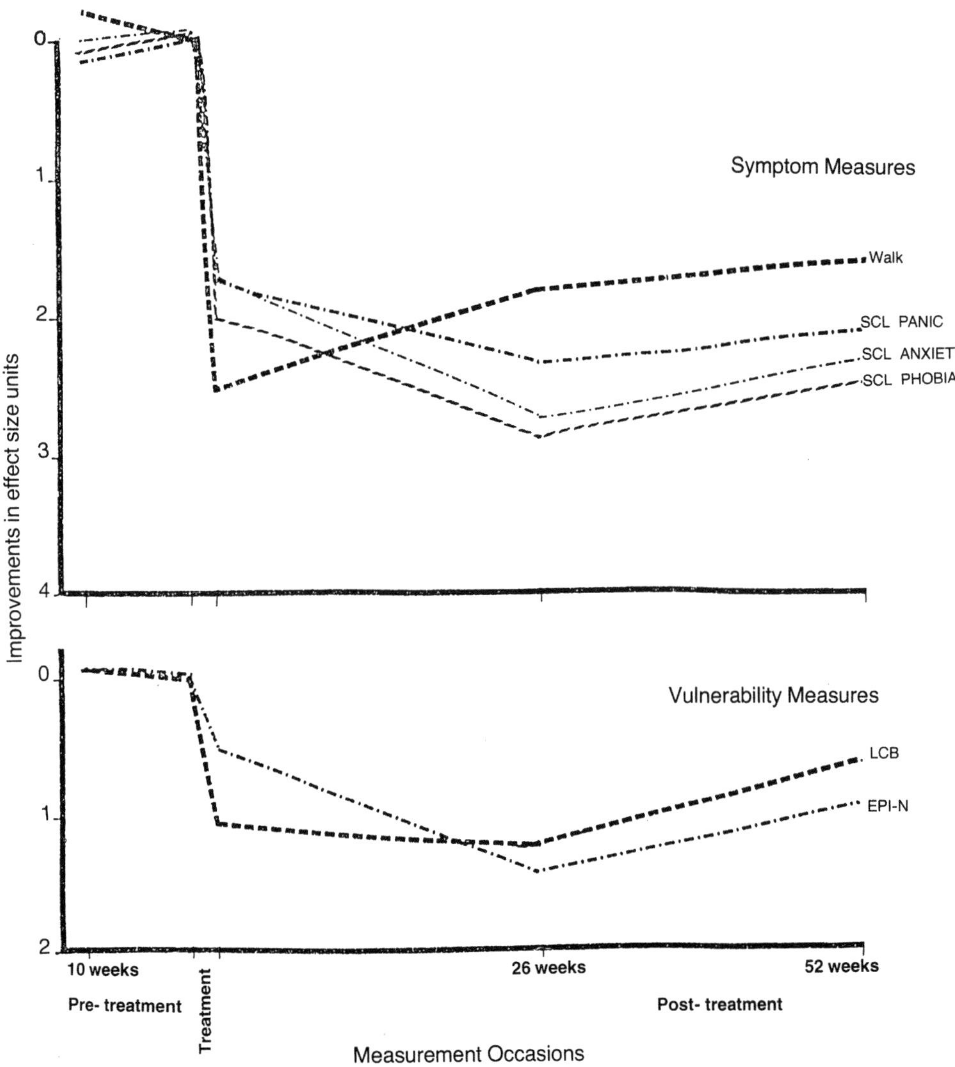

Fig. 1. Results of the cognitive behavioral treatment of agoraphobia with panic attacks in a base line pre-post design and with follow-up for 52 weeks after treatment had concluded. Symptoms measured included a behavioral avoidance test (walk), and three measures derived from the SCL 90. Vulnerability measures include the locus of control of behavior scale and the Eysenck personality inventory neuroticism scale

handicapped by avoidance, the average patient being unable to reach the hospital gate unaccompanied. There was also evidence that despite initially abnormal neuroticism and locus of control scores, this treatment program had resulted in a reduction of neuroticism and an internalization of locus of control to the extend that the probability of relapse in the future should be reduced.

The 50 patients were a large unselected consecutive series of patients referred for behavioral treatment, whose age, sex, and illness characteristics were similar to those of other groups of agoraphobics reported in the literature. At the time of referral many were taking drugs, but all had ceased taking benzodiazepines and had reduced all other drugs by the end of therapy. The assessment of outcome was based on a baseline pre-post design, a design which is justified in view of the chronic nature of the disorder and because neither regression to the mean, spontaneous remission, nor response to nonspecific factors have been shown to affect outcome. Pre-post designs have also been found to be of value in other chronic disorders such as stuttering (Andrews et al. 1980), hypertension (Andrews et al. 1982), and obsessive-compulsive disorder (Christensen et al. 1987).

Many studies of nondrug therapies suffer in comparison with drug therapies be-because they do not ensure the standardization and quality of the intervention (Andrews 1984). In this study, standardization was ensured because all patients read and discussed a 20 000-word manual with the therapist, and quality was ensured by having both authors closely involved in either the therapy or supervision of the treatment program. Compliance was therefore maximized and multiple-choice questionnaires given during treatment showed that patients were absorbing the material satisfactorily. The measures used werd standard, and have been used in other studies of agoraphobia (Sheehan et al. 1980; Noyes et al. 1984).

Symptom measures were available for all patients at the end of treatment, and for 92% of patients at either the 6- or 12-month follow-up. Thus, dropouts were minimal.

The present results compare well with other reports of cognitive behavioral interventions in agoraphobia with panic. Five studies reported on a combination of instructions to confront feared situations and cognitive restructuring techniques to reduce anxiety in the feared situation, and their results for measures of phobia were broadly comparable with the present study (mean ES = 1.37; SD = 0.27) (Emmelkamp et al. 1978; Emmelkamp and Mersch 1982; Emmelkamp et al. 1983; Williams and Rappoport 1983).

The present results also compare well with drug treatment in agoraphobia with panic attacks. Five studies have explored the utility of monoamine oxidase inhibitors in agoraphobia. The first was a retrospective study of 196 patients most of whom had agoraphobia (Kelly et al. 1970). It reported that phobic behavior was improved and panic attacks ceased in one-half the patients treated with a monoamine oxidase inhibitor, usually phenelzine. As some patients also received benzodiazepines and others also were taking tricyclic antidepressants, this report can only be regarded as suggestive. Three other studies (Sheehan et al. 1980; Lipsedge et al. 1973; Solyom et al. 1973) of patients treated with such drugs showed improvement in phobias but did not measure panic. The one study that did measure panic attacks found phenelzine to be no more effective than placebo (Tyrer et al. 1973).

We have recently reviewed the treatment of the anxiety disorders (Christensen et al. 1987; The Quality Assurance Project 1985) and used the metaanalytic technique to allow the results of the various studies to be compared. The technique is a cross-over design with propanolol, and so may be imprecise. The one study of alprazolam (5.4 mg/day) on 16 patients which measured panic (Sheehan et al. 1984) did not produce results suggesting that this drug was to be preferred on the grounds of greater efficacy. Data after treatment had ended were available for all treatments involving in vivo exposure and it was clear that improvement had been maintained over the follow-up period. There were not data on outcome after drug treatment without exposure had ceased.

Table 2. A metaanalysis of the 24 studies of agoraphobia which have measured panic attacks. Results by treatment type given for each measure (in terms of mean effect size, standard deviation and number of studies) for improvement pre- to posttreatment and pretreatment to follow-up, a median of 6 months after treatment ended

	Pre- to posttreatment					Pretreatment to follow-up				
Treatment type (*n* subjects)	Panic	Phobia	Anxiety	Beh Av Test	Depression	Panic	Phobia	Anxiety	Beh Av Test	Depression
Imipramine and in vivo exposure ($n = 70$)	1.06 (0.51; 6)	2.37 (0.86; 6)	1.78 (0.60; 5)	1.53 (0.82; 2)	1.41 (0.64; 6)	0.99 (0.38; 3)	2.86 (0.74; 3)	1.82 (0.55; 3)		1.54 (0.31; 3)
Placebo and in vivo exposure ($n = 67$)	0.92 (0.56; 5)	2.02 (0.78; 5)	1.30 (1.24; 4)		0.92 (0.25; 5)	1.03 (0.68; 3)	2.24 (1.14; 3)	1.77 (1.68; 3)		1.02 (0.35; 3)
Imipramine alone ($n = 17$)	0.85 (0.79; 2)	1.35 (0.72; 2)	1.20 (NA; 1)	0.42 (0.20; 2	1.15 (0.08; 2)					
In vivo exposure ($n = 191$)	0.95 (0.60; 9)	2.15 (0.99; 9)	0.90 (0.53; 7)	3.05 (0.91; 2)	0.49 (0.24; 7)	1.30 (0.70; 4)	2.19 (1.22; 4)	1.14 (0.92; 4)	1.68 (NA; 1)	0.39 (0.25; 2)
Diazepam ($n = 17$)	0.81 (NA; 1)	1.86 (NA; 1)	1.32 (NA; 1)							
Triazolam ($n = 16$)	0.52 (NA; 1)	0.73 (NA; 1)	0.70 (NA; 1)		0.23 (NA; 1)					

NA, not applicable

There appears to be little published evidence that imipramine, phenelzine, diazepam, or alprazolam are "uniquely effective" (Sheehan 1982) in the control of panic in agoraphobia. Given the absence of evidence that patients remain improved after drugs have been ceased, it is probable that treatment with in vivo exposure programs is to be preferred in both the short and the long term. The present treatment program comprised 80 h of education about the disorder, training in techniques to control panic, practice in rational thinking, and considerable supervised experience in confronting feared situations. It appears to us that the highly structured format of the treatment program was very important for thereby were we able to ensure that all patients, having read and discussed and practised the instructions in the protocol in painstaking detail, clearly understood the path to sustained recovery.

The patients in the present study were improved after 2 weeks of intensive, full-time therapy and were still improved 1 year later without further therapy. It therefore seems important to ask whether drugs are essential in the treatment of agoraphobia with panic attacks, for these patients had already finished treatment by the time patients placed on imipramine would still have been building up to a described in those papers. For this present paper we were able to find 23 studies (reported in 12 papers) that gave accounts of treatment outcome that included a measure of panic and from which an effect sice could be calculated. Effect sizes were calculated from the difference between measures before and after treatment, divided by the standard deviation of the pretreatment scores. If subject were allocated to more than one treatment group then the pretreatment standard deviations were pooled. The results are presented in Table 2. Changes in panic, phobic anxiety or avoidance, and in behavioral avoidance tests are presented along with changes in measures of general anxiety or depression taken immediately after treatment and at a median 6 months after treatment had ended. There were five studies of imipramine and in vivo exposure (Telch 1983; Zitrin et al. 1983; Marks et al. 1983; Mavissakalian and Michelson 1982; Mavissakalian and Michelson 1983) four studies of placebo and in vivo exposure (Telch 1983; Zitrin et al. 1983; Marks et al. 1983; Mavissakalian and Michelson 1982), only two studies of imipramine uncomplicated by instructions to expose (Telch 1983; Mavissakalian and Michelson 1982), and six studies (including the present study) of in vivo exposure uncomplicated by drugs or placebo (Ost et al. 1984; Emmelkamp and Emmelkamp 1975; Emmelkamp and Wessels 1975; Hafner and Marks 1976; Mavissakalian et al. 1983). Like imipramine, in vivo exposure was given in varying doses, from simple advice to confront feared situations, through directed programs of exposure, to therapist-accompanied assignments.

These treatments, whether imipramine and/or in vivo exposure, produced about a one standard deviation improvement in panic, and a two standard deviation improvement in the phobias. Few of the studies included data on performance as measured by some form of a behavioral avoidance test. All treatments resulted in improvement in general anxiety, but the treatments containing imipramine (median dose 125 mg/day) resulted in a significantly greater reduction in depression. There was one study of diazepam (30 mg/day) (Noyes et al. 1984), which measured panic in 17 patients but the effect-size calculation was confounded by the crosstherapeutic dose of that drug (Mavissakalian and Penel 1985), and would then have been faced with months of drug taking ahead. Programs similar to that described in this report will result in faster and greater improvement in panic, phobias, and disability than those offered by any drug for which evidence is presently available.

Why then are such behavioral psychotherapies so rarely used outside specialist clinics? First, because in vivo exposure is often understood to mean the therapist leaving the office to accompany the patient into the feared situation. There is evidence that shows that detailed planning of a hierarchy of tasks, dispatching the patient to do the task, and reviewing progress with the patient when the task is done is as effective, and considerably more convenient, than accompanying the patient (The Quality Assurance Project 1985). The second problem concerns the lack of acceptance of standardized therapy programs. While all psychiatrists are happy, and indeed grateful, to be able to prescribe doses of standard drugs, few are content to give standard psychotherapy programs. Most have been trained in the importance of an individualized formulation and individualized therapy for each patient. But in some disorders a simple diagnosis accounts for most of the decisions about treatment, and the personal predicament of each patient is redundant, at least until the disorder has been treated. Schizophrenia and melancholia are two disorders in which the diagnosis is paramount. It is therefore not surprising that psychatrists agree on the standard treatments necessary for these conditions (Andrews et al. 1988, in press). Agoraphobia with panic attacks is another condition which responds well to standardized treatments. Perhaps it would help if training in the behavioral psychotherapies, so useful in this condition, were available to psychiatrists, for as a profession we must take care to promote effective nondrug remedies with the same thoroughness with which the pharmaceutical remedies are promoted.

References

Andrews G (1984) On the promotion of non-drug treatments. Br Med J 289:994–995

Andrews G, Moran C (1986) The control of hyperventilation. Videotape. Audio Visual Unit, University of New South Wale, Sydney

Andrews G, Guitar B, Howie P (1980) Meta-analysis of the effects of stuttering treatment. J Speech Hear Disord 45:289–307

Andrews G, MacMahon SW, Austin A et al (1982) Hypertension: a comparison of drug and non-drug treatments. Br Med J 284:1523–1526

Andrews G, Allen R, Henderson AS (1987) The genetics of four anxiety disorders: a twin study. J Affective Disord (in press)

Andrews G, Hadzi-Pavlovic D, Christensen H et al. (1988) The treatment of anxiety and somatoform disorders: views of practising psychiatrists. Am J Psychiatry (in press)

Christensen H, Hadzi-Pavlovic D, Andrews G (1987) Behavior therapy and tricyclic medication in the treatment of obsessive compulsive disorder: a quantitative review. J Consult Clin Psychol 55:000–000

Craig A, Franklin J, Andrews G (1984) A scale to measure locus of control of behaviour. Br J Med Psychol 57:173–180

Craig A, Andrews G (1985) The prediction and prevention of relapse in stuttering: the value of self-control techniques and locus of control measures. Behav Modif 9:427–442

Derogatis LR, Lipman RS, Rickels K et al (1974) The Hopkins Symptoms Check List (HSCL): a self-report symptom inventory. Behav Sci 19:1–15

Emmelkamp PM, Emmelkamp-Benner A (1975) Effects of historically portrayed modeling and group treatment on self observation: a comparison with agoraphobics. Behav Res Ther 13:135–139

Emmelkamp PM, Mersch PP (1982) Cognition and exposure in vivo in the treatment of agoraphobia: short-term and delayed effects. Cogn Ther Res 6:77–89

Emmelkamp PM, Wessels H (1975) Flooding in imagination versus flooding in vivo: a comparison with agoraphobics. Behav Res Ther 13:7–15

Emmelkamp PM, Kuipers AC, Eggeraat JB (1978) Cognitive modification versus prolonged exposure in vivo: a comparison with agoraphobics as subjects. Behav Res Ther 16:33–41

Emmelkamp PM, van der Hout A, Devries K (1983) Assertive training for agoraphobia. Behav Res Ther 21:63–68

Ellis A (1962) Reason and emotion in psychotherapy. Lyle-Stuart, New York

Eysenck HJ, Eysenck SBG (1964) Manual of the Eysenck personality inventory. University of London Press, London
Hafner J, Marks I (1976) Exposure in vivo of agoraphobics: contributions of diazepam, group exposure, and anxiety evocation. Psychol Med 6:71-88
Henderson AS (1981) Neurosis and the social environment. Academic, Sydney
Holt PE, Andrews G (in press) Provocation of panic: a comparison on three elements of the panic reaction in four anxiety disorders. J Abnorm Psychol
Jacobsen E (1938) Progressive relaxation. University of Chicago Press, Chicago
Jakubowski P, Lange AJ (1976) Responsible assertive behavior: assertive option. Research Press, Champaign
Kelly D, Guirguis W, Frommer E et al (1970) Treatment of phobic states with anti-depressants: a retrospective study of 246 patients. Br J Psychiatry 116:387-398
Lipsedge MJ, Hajioff J, Huggins P et al (1973) The management of severe agoraphobia: a comparison of iproniazid and systematic desensitisation. Psychopharmacologia 32:67-80
Marks I (1975) Behavioral treatments of phobic and obsessive-compulsive disorders: a critical apparaisal. In: Herson M, Eisler R, Miller P (eds) Progress in behavior modification, vol 1. Academic, New York
Marks IM, Gray S, Cohen D et al (1983) Imipramine and brief therapist-aided exposure in agoraphobics having self-exposure homework. Arch Gen Psychiatry 40:153-162
Mavissakalian M, Michelson L (1982) Agoraphobia: behavioral and pharmacological treatments, preliminary outcome, and process findings. Psychopharmacol Bull 18:91-103
Mavissakalian M, Penel J (1985) Imipramine in the treatment of agoraphobia: dose-response relationships. Am J Psychiatry 142:1032-1036
Mavissakalian M, Michelson L, Pealy RS (1983) Pharmacological treatment of agoraphobia: imipramine versus imipramine with programmed practice. Br J Psychiatry 143:348-355
Mavissakalian M, Michelson L, Greenwald D et al (1983) Cognitive-behavioural treatment of agoraphobia: paradoxical intention versus self-statement training. Behav Res Ther 21:75-86
Moran C, Andrews G (1985) The familial occurrence of agoraphobia. Br J Psychiatry 146:262-267
Noyes R, Anderson D, Clancy J et al (1984) Diazepam and propranolol in panic disorder and agoraphobia. Arch Gen Psychiatry 41:287-292
Ost LG, Jerramalm A, Jansson L (1984) Individual response patterns and the effects of different behavioural methods in the treatment of agoraphobia. Behav Res Ther 22:697-707
Robins LN, Helzer JG, Croughan J et al (1981) National Institutes of Mental Health Diagnostic Interview Schedule. Its history, characteristics and validity. Arch Gen Psychiatry 38:381-389
Robins LN, Helzer JE, Weissman MM et al (1984) Lifetime prevalence of specific psychiatric disorders in three sites. Arch Gen Psychiatry 41:949-958
Sheehan DV (1982) Panic attacks and phobias. N Engl J Med 307:156-158
Sheehan DV, Ballinger J, Jacobsen G (1980) Treatment of endogenous anxiety with phobic, hysterical and hypochondrical symptoms. Arch Gen Psychiatry 37:51-59
Sheehan DV, Coleman JH, Greenblatt DJ et al (1984) Some biochemical correlates of panic attacks with agoraphobia and their response to a new treatment. J Clin Psychopharmacol 42:66-75
Solyom L, Heseltine GFD, McClure DJ et al (1973) Behavior therapy versus drug therapy in the treatment of phobic neurosis. Can J Psychiatry 18:25-32
Telch MJ (1983) A comparison of behavioral and pharmacological approaches to the treatment of agoraphobia. Doctoral dissertation, Stanford University, University Microfilms International
The Quality Assurance Project (1985) Treatment outlines for the management of anxiety states. Aust NZ J Psychiatry 19:138-151
Tyrer P, Candy J, Kelly D (1973) A study of the clinical effects of phenelzine and placebo in the treatment of phobic anxiety. Psychopharmacologia 32:237-254
Weissman MM, Prusoff BA, Klerman GL (1978) Personality as a predictor of long-term outcome of depression Am J Psychiatry 137:797-800
Williams SL, Rappoport A (1983) Cognitive treatment in the natural environment for agoraphobics. Behav Res Ther 14:299-313
Zitrin CM, Klein DF, Woerner MG et al (1983) Treatment of phobias I: comparison of imipramine hydrochloride and placebo. Arch Gen Psychiatry 40:125-138

Part III

Specific Variables Affecting Mode of Treatment: Experimental Studies on Physiology and Cognition

10. Panic Attacks in Nonclinical Subjects

J. Margraf and A. Ehlers

Introduction

Sudden episodes of intense anxiety accompanied by a number of predominantly somatic symptoms (now usually called panic attacks) are the primary feature of the psychological disturbance termed panic disorder in DSM-IIIR (APA 1987). This diagnosis was introduced based on the idea that panic attacks are a distinct type of anxiety in need of their own diagnostic entity. However, recent research has shown that panic attacks are not specific to panic disorder since they also occur across a wide range of other psychological disorders and even in nonclinical populations. Barlow et al. (1985) studied 108 patients with the DSM-III diagnoses simple phobia, social phobia, generalized anxiety disorder, panic disorder, agoraphobia with panic attacks, obsessive-compulsive disorder, and major depressive episodes. The great majority of patients in each of these categories (at least 83%) reported having experienced panic attacks. Although the frequency of attacks varied across diagnoses, there were only few differences in terms of the symptom pattern associated with the attacks. Furthermore, symptom severity was similar for patients with situational (predictable, expected) and spontaneous (unpredictable, unexpected) attacks. These results are in line with those of the Munich Follow-Up Study (MFS, Wittchen 1986) in which panic attacks were observed in 9.3% of a representative community sample, a percentage higher than the combined frequencies of panic disorder and agoraphobia with panic attacks.

If it is established that panic attacks are not specific to people suffering from a specific disorder, it is important to study the distribution of the phenomenon in the general population. There have been a first few attempts to approach this question using questionnaire screening methods. Norton et al. (1985, 1986) initiated this line of research. They found surprisingly high prevalences of panic attacks in nonclinical subjects. About one-third of their two samples of undergraduate students reported having experienced at least one panic attack in the past year. They concluded that panic attacks often occur in presumably normal people and that these panic attacks share many similarities with those of patients who have well-defined panic disorders (Norton et al. 1985).

Aside from the question of the distribution of panic attacks in the population, there are at least two other important reasons to study panic attacks in nonclinical subjects. The first reason concerns sampling bias. With the exception of large epidemiological studies such as the Epidemiological Catchment Area Program (ECA, Regier et al. 1984) or the MFS (Wittchen 1986) previous studies of panic attacks have exclusively investigated clinical populations. There are a number of reasons to expect that these samples represent a biased selection of the total population of persons with panic attacks. Highly symptomatic individuals are more likely to seek treatment or to be detected in clinical screenings, an effect Motulsky (1978) termed "ascertainment bias." This bias increases the probability of persons with two disorders to be part of clinical samples and thus may lead to mistaken assumptions about the relationship between such disorders. For example, almost all agoraphobic patients seen in clinical settings have panic attacks (cf. Mendel and Klein 1969; Thyer and Himle 1985). In nonclinical community samples, however, the picture looks quite different. Weissman et al. (1986) and Wittchen (1986) found that only a small percentage of all subjects meeting criteria for agoraphobia also exhibited panic disorder (ranging from 6% to 16% in the various ECA and MFS sites) and only another 17% to 50% showed limited panic symptoms in addition to agoraphobia.

Another example for sampling bias is the postulated relationship between panic disorder and mitral valve prolapse (MVP). We have argued elsewhere (Margraf et al., 1988) that the higher prevalence of MVP observed in some studies of panic disorder patients represents a problem of comorbidity rather than a true functional relationship. If the sampling bias inherent in studying clinical samples is eliminated, the association between panic attacks and MVP vanishes. This was shown by Hartman et al. (1982) and Devereux et al. (1986), who studied MVP patients and their family members who had not sought treatment themselves. Family members with and without MVP were not different from each other with respect to number of panic attacks and other symptoms; both groups were far less symptomatic than the original sample of MVP patients who had been referred to the clinic. Thus, sampling bias may strongly influence the results of research on clinical samples. It is therefore important to complement such research by studies of the characteristics of nonclinical subjects with the same disturbance.

A second important reason to study nonclinical panickers is related to the fact that many of these people are infrequent panickers. They experience fewer attacks than patients who seek treatment for the full-blown syndrome. Infrequent panickers may form the basic population out of which some people will continue to develop the full clinical syndrome. If this is the case, infrequent panickers offer a unique opportunity to study possible vulnerability factors for panic attacks. Most of our current etiological research on panic attacks is correlational in the sense that groups of panic patients and controls are compared in cross-sectional designs. True experimental designs would for instance involve attempts to produce panic disorder in previously "normal" subjects. For obvious reasons such studies cannot be conducted. Thus, we cannot make firm statements about causal antecedents of the disorder. If infrequent panickers are the basic population for panic disorder they should show whatever diathesis for panic exists. In this case we can assume that characteristics of patients that are not found in infrequent panickers are consequences rather than causes of the disorder. On the other hand, infrequent panickers may represent a different basic population than frequent panickers (panic disorder patients). It is possible that even though both groups show identical manifest symptoms (panic attacks) they suffer from different underlying disturbances. In this case, infrequent panickers should be studied to gain insight into such a heterogeneity of the panic attack phenomenon.

Questionnaire Studies

The first studies of panic attacks in presumably normal populations were reported by Norton et al. (1985, 1986). In their initial study, 186 students were screened using the Hopkins Symptom Checklist (HSCL-90, Derogatis et al. 1973) and a specially designed anxiety questionnaire asking for current levels of anxiety as well as frequency and symptoms of panic attacks. A striking 34.4% of the subjects reported having had one or more panic attacks in the past year, and 2.2% reported having had at least three attacks in the past 3 weeks. The symptoms reported to occur during these attacks were similar to the ones described by clinical samples of panic attack patients (Barlow et al. 1985; Margraf et al. 1987). The most severe symptoms were heart pounding, trembling, sweating, flushing, and dizziness. Subjects describing at least one panic attack in the anxiety questionnaire scored significantly higher than those without attacks on the HSCL-90 subscales anxiety, phobic anxiety, depression, interpersonal sensitivity, somatization, and anger/hostility. There were no significant differences with respect to obsessive-compulsiveness, psychoticism, paranoid ideation, or sleep difficulties.

In a second study, Norton et al. (1986) screened 256 students with a refined version of their questionnaire, now termed the Panic Attack Questionnaire (PAQ). Subjects also completed the State-Trait Anxiety Inventory (STAI, Spielberger et al. 1970), the Beck Depression Inventory (BDI, Beck et al. 1961), and the Profile of Mood States (POMS, McNair et al. 1981). In addition, subjects were either given the Fear Survey Schedule (FSS-III, Arrindell 1980) or the Fear Questionnaire (FQ, Marks and Mathews 1979). Very similarly to the first study, 35.9% of the sample reported having experienced at least one panic attack in the past year, and 3.1% reported having had at least three attacks in the past 3 weeks. Panickers scored significantly higher on state and trait anxiety (STAI, anxiety scale of the POMS), depression (BDI, depression scale of the POMS), fatigue (POMS), and anger (POMS). In contrast, there were no differences compared to nonpanickers on any of the FSS-III or FQ subscales (agoraphobia, social phobia, blood/injury phobia, aggression, animal phobia) or the POMS scales activity and confusion. Panickers and nonpanickers were similar in the frequency of reported previous treatments for any mental or physical disorder. Similarly, the two groups were comparable with respect to age, sex, or socioeconomic status. Panickers reported significantly more first-degree relatives who had panic attacks.

As in the first study, the most severe symptoms of panic attacks were palpitations, trembling, sweating, dizziness, and hot/cold flashes. Other characteristics of panic attacks included a sudden onset in the majority of cases (59% under 10 min), an average of eight DSM-III symptoms, and a wide variety of situational contexts in which attacks occurred, especially social situations. The great majority of panickers reported having experienced at least one life stressor at the onset of their panic attacks. Most frequently mentioned were difficulties at work, family crises, and loss of a significant other. Subjects who experienced some unpredictable attacks were different from those who experienced only predictable attacks on 9 out of 40 comparisons. Those subjects with unpredictable attacks reported more attacks in more different situations, as well as more severe feelings of unreality and tachycardia.

Together, these studies show that panic attacks may occur in more persons than previously assumed and that subjects who have panic attacks report more psychopathology than do nonpanickers. In addition, the panic attacks experienced by nonclinical panickers and patients with anxiety disorders are very similar. While these studies have yielded some fascinating data and initiated an important line of research, they also pose some new challenges. A first problem is to establish the reliability and validity of the PAQ as compared to standard structured interview diagnoses. Norton et al. (1986) reported that 22 out of 24 cases, previously identified as nonclinical panickers by the PAQ, also met DSM-III criteria for panic attacks in a structured interview. However, they did not give information as to what interview was used, whether interviewers were blind to the questionnaire results, and the reliability of their interview and questionnaire methods. A second challenge is to go beyond mere questionnaire assessment of psychopathology and to compare nonclinical panickers, clinical panickers, and normal controls on psychophysiological variables or the response to stressors. More recent studies have attempted to address these issues.

Laboratory studies

Beck and Scott (1987) compared ten subjects who had panic disorder with ten infrequent panickers. All subjects were recruited from the community using media announcements. Infrequent panickers were defined as subjects reporting four of the 12 DSM-III symptoms during typical attacks, but never having experienced three attacks in 3 consecutive weeks. The screening instrument was the Anxiety Disorder Interview Schedule (ADIS-R, DiNardo et al. 1983). Laboratory paradigms were four 2-min tasks (neutral imagery, hospitalization imagery, signal detection, paced arithmetic). Assessments included continuous measurement of trapezious electromyogram (EMG), skin conductance level (SCL), and heart rate, as well as thought-listing and ratings of the DSM-III panic symptoms immediately following each task. Overall, there were relatively few differences between panic disorder subjects' and infrequent panickers' responses to the test paradigms. Panic disorder subjects showed more EMG and SCL reactivity to the two imagery tasks, infrequent panickers more EMG and SCL reactivity to paced arithmetic. There were no differences in heart rate reactivity or on the thought-listing measure. With respect to panic symptoms, panic disorder subjects scored significantly higher on four and infrequent panickers scored higher on six out of 52 comparisons.

Sandler et al. (1987) reported a comparison of nonclinical panickers and control subjects without panic attacks. Eighty subjects were recruited through screening of college students with a panic attack questionnaire. Subsamples included frequent panickers, infrequent panickers, and panic-free controls. Cardiovascular reactivity to a psychological (challenge reaction time task) and a physical (cycling) stress task was assessed by measuring heart rate and blood pressure at intervals before, during, and after the tasks. All of the measures showed progressive declines during the pretask baseline periods, increases during the stress tests, and declines during the post-task recovery phases. There were no differences between groups with respect to cardiovascular reactivity. This is similar to what is seen in most so-called panic induction studies of clinical samples (cf. Ehlers et al. 1986a, 1986b, 1988; Margraf et al. 1986a). In contrast to these studies, however, differences in baseline heart rate levels were lacking. The only apparent difference was some modest evidence for slower recovery from exercise in those subjects reporting the most frequent occurrence of panic attacks.

It is interesting to note that neither Sandler et al. (1987) nor Beck and Scott (1987) found differences in cardiovascular reactivity. There were few reactivity differences between frequent and infrequent panickers in Beck and Scott's study and no reactivity differences between panickers and nonpanickers in Sandler et al.'s study. This is in contrast to the consistent and strong differences on several of the questionnaire measures in the two Norton studies. We have recently conducted two studies trying to combine questionnaire and laboratory measures in a comparison of nonclinical panickers and controls.

The Marburg and Tübingen Studies

During late 1986 and early 1987 we conducted two independent studies of nonclinical panickers. The first study (Ehlers and Meisner, in preparation) involved a sample of 170 undergraduate students at Philipps University in Marburg in the central part of West Germany. The second study (Margraf, Wrobel, and Jakschik, in preparation) involved a sample of 136 undergraduate students at the university of Tübingen in southern Germany. These studies pursued three specific goals:

1. To replicate the Norton et al. (1985, 1986) findings using a German translation of their PAQ
2. To determine the reliability and validity of the questionnaire screening method as compared to a standard structured interview approach
3. To compare nonclinical panickers and controls on a questionnaire battery and a psychophysiological laboratory assessment

Table 1. Definition of a panic attack given in the version of the panic attack questionnaire used in the German studies

A **panic attack** (anxiety attack) is a discrete period of **sudden onset of intense apprehension, fear, or terror,** often associated with feelings of impending doom. The following symptoms may be experienced:

Racing, pounding, or irregular heart beat
Dizziness or lightheadedness
Shortness of breath
Sweating
Chest pain or discomfort
Trembling or shaking
Hot and cold flashes
Choking or smothering sensations
Numbness or tingling in parts of the body
Fear of dying
Faintness
Nausea or abdominal distress
Feelings of unreality or being detached
Fear of losing control or going crazy

The questions on the following pages refer to panic attacks in situations that were **not life-threatening.** The attacks have to be accompanied by **at least four** of the symptoms listed above.

Figure 1 gives an overview of the studies. Each study consisted of three phases. First, a large group of undergraduate students was screened using our German translation of the PAQ. The definition of a panic attack given to the subjects is shown in Table 1.

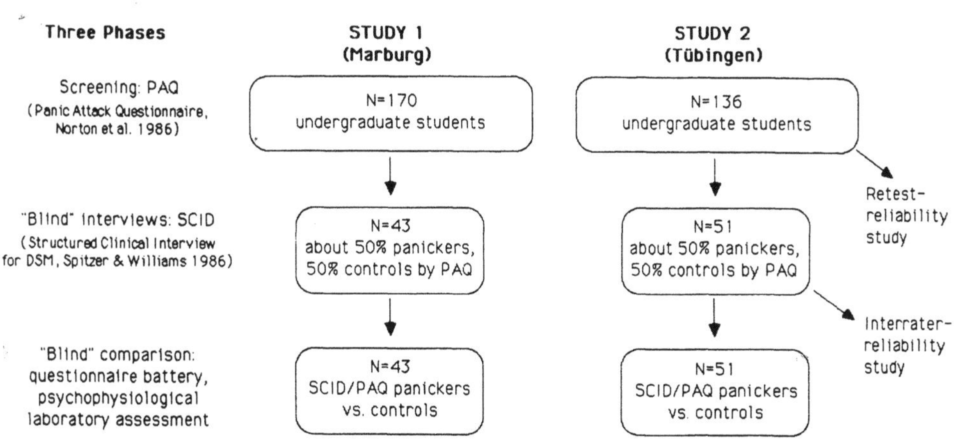

Fig. 1. Overview of the Marburg and Tübingen studies of panic attacks in nonclinical subjects

In phase two, we selected subsamples of PAQ determined panickers and nonpanickers or "controls" (about 50% each) using strict criteria (panickers: reporting at least one spontaneous attack, at least four symptoms, attacks not only in social situations; controls: no attacks or anxiety symptoms). We then conducted blind diagnostic interviews to determine the agreement between the interview and questionnaire methods. The interview was a German translation of the Structured Clinical Interview for DSM (SCID) by Spitzer and Williams (1986). In the third phase, subjects meeting both PAQ and SCID criteria for panic attacks ("nonclinical panickers") and controls were compared using an extensive questionnaire battery and a psychophysiological laboratory assessment involving a baseline and a hyperventilation task. In addition, two substudies assessed the retest reliability of the PAQ and the interrater reliability of the SCID in our hands. In the following, we will present the results of the preliminary analyses conducted so far.

The retest reliability of the PAQ proved to be generally good. Similarly, the interrater reliability of the SCID in our hands was good. Table 2 summarizes the results of the retest reliability study.

Information about the occurrence, number, and intensity of attacks as well as stress at the onset of panic, avoidance behavior, and family history was given reliably. In contrast, subjects were not able to give reliable information about whether they had ever experienced unexpected ("spontaneous") attacks, panicked only in social situations, or experienced most of their symptoms within 10 min.

Table 3 compares the number of subjects reporting panic attacks on the PAQ in our two studies with the numbers reported by Norton et al. (1985, 1986). The mean ages of our samples were 24 (study 1) and 25 years (study 2), while 69% (study 1) and 65% (study 2) of all subjects were female.

While we found a somewhat higher percentage of panickers for the past year, results for the past 3 weeks closely resemble those of Norton et al. (1985, 1986). Thus, their finding of a high percentage of nonclinical panickers is replicated using the questionnaire method. However, when using the structured interview approach, a different picture emerge. We found that only 12 out of 23 (study 1, Marburg) and 15 out of 29 (study 2, Tübingen) PAQ-determined panickers also met SCID criteria for panic attacks. While we thus had a high rate of false positives, there were only a few false negatives:

Table 2. Retest-reliability of the Panic Attack Questionnaire (sample size: $n = 39$, retest interval 14-28 days with a mean of 20 days)

Item (or groups of items)	Reliability coefficient	Statistic
Ever had panic attack	0.80	Kappa
Ever had 3 attacks in 3 weeks	0.80	Kappa
Ever worried for 4 weeks about attack	0.82	Kappa
Number of attacks past year	0.85	Spearman
Most symptoms within 10 min	0.33	Kappa
Ever had unexpected panic	0.53	Kappa
Panics only in social situations	0.43	Kappa
Stress at onset of panic (8 items)	0.67-1.0	Kappa
Age of onset, treatment, self-medication, familiy history, avoidance behavior (14 items)	0.65-0.72	Kappa, Spearman
Average duration, anxiety, number of symptoms	0.70-0.76	Spearman, Pearson

Table 3. Frequency of panic attacks determined by the Panic Attack Questionnaire (percent of all subjects)

	Study 1: Marburg ($n = 170$)	Study 2: Tübingen ($n = 136$)	Norton et al. 1985 ($n = 186$)	1986 ($n = 256$)
Panickers (last year)	46	59	34	36
Panickers (last 3 weeks)	21	29	24	23
Three attacks in 3 weeks (lifetime)	12	15.5	*	*
Three attacks in last 3 weeks	2	1	2	3

* These results were not reported by Norton et al.

pooled across both studies only 4 out of 42 PAQ nonpanickers met SCID criteria for panic. Overall rates of agreement were as low as 74% and 65% (kappa: 0.50 and 0.32, studies 1 and 2, respectively). A post hoc analysis of those subjects who indicated panic attacks on the PAQ, but did not meet SCID criteria, revealed that disagreement was not of a pure "chance" nature. Rather, it seemed that these false positives reported milder variants of the same phenomenon (cf. the concept of limited symptom attacks in DSM-IIIR) and that the interview had a more conservative cut-off between panic and nonpanic.

The comparison of nonclinical panickers (PAQ and SCID criteria) and controls on the questionnaire battery yielded a number of pronounced differences. Since study 2 (Tübingen) used a more comprehensive battery, the pattern of its results is shown in Fig. 2. The results of study 1 were generally similar. The questionnaires used in study 2 were the Panic and Agoraphobia Profile (PAP, cf. Margraf and Ehlers 1987), Fear Survey Schedule (FSS, Arrindell 1980), Symptom Checklist-90 (SCL, Derogatis 1977), Self-report Inventory of somatic symptoms (SISS, King et al. 1986), state-trait anxiety inventory (STAI, Spielberger et al. 1970, trait form), Beck Depression Inventory (BDI, Beck et al. 1981), and the Mobility Inventory (MI, Chambless et al. 1985).

The different questionnaires use very different scales. For a standardized presentation, we computed the difference between the means of panickers and controls divided by the standard deviation of the control group. The bars in Fig. 2 thus indicate the difference between the two groups in units of the standard deviation of the controls. The upper part of Fig. 2 shows those scales on which the two groups differed significantly ($P < 0.05$), the lower part scales without significant differences. It is important to note that questionnaires measuring similar constructs also yielded similar results. Therefore, such scales were grouped together.

Nonclinical panickers reported considerably higher levels of phobophobia, agoraphobic fears (but not avoidance behavior), somatization, anxiousness, depressiveness, and injury phobia than nonpanickers of comparable age, sex, and socioeconomic background. Of the two depression scales, the BDI that focusses more on

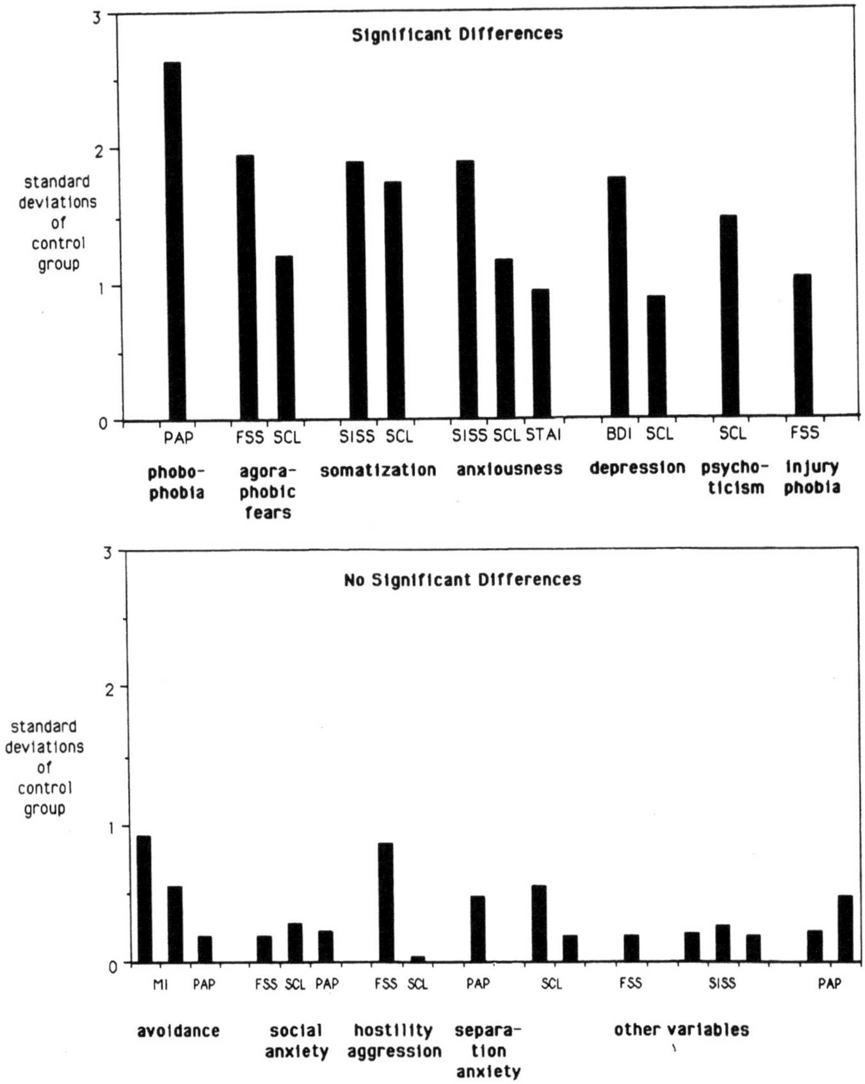

Fig. 2. Comparison of panickers and controls using a questionnaire battery (study 2, Tübingen). The *bars* represent the difference between the scores of the two groups divided by the standard deviation of the control group. Scales measuring similar constructs are grouped together. The abbreviations referring to the questionnaires containing the scales are explained in the text. The *upper half* of the figure shows scales yielding significant differences between panickers and controls: phobophobia (PAP), agoraphobia (FSS), phobic anxiety (SCL), total somatization disorder score (SISS), somatization (SCL), neurotic symptoms (SISS), anxiety (SCL), trait anxiety (STAI), depression (BDI), depression (SCL), psychoticism (SCL), and blood/injury phobia (FSS). The scales listed in the *lower half* of the figure yielded no significant differences between panickers and controls: mobility alone and mobility accompanied (MI), general avoidance (PAP), social fears (FSS), interpersonal sensitivity (SCL), fear of social embarrassment (PAP), aggression (FSS), hostility (SCL), separation anxiety (PAP), obsessive-compulsiveness and paranoid ideation (SCL), animal phobia (FSS), cardiovascular, gastrointestinal, and muscular awareness (SISS), fear of loss of control and fear of somatic distress (PAP)

the cognitive concomitants of depression yielded a stronger difference than the depression scale of the SCL-90 that contains more vegetative symptoms. The difference on the SCL-90 psychoticism scale is probably due to several ambiguous items that can be interpreted as signs of psychotic ideation as well as indicating typical panic symptoms (e.g., a fear of going crazy, losing control over one's body, derealization). Somewhat surprisingly, there were no differences in terms of self-reported avoidance behavior, social anxiety, hostility, or aggression. Separation anxiety, which has been linked causally to the development of panic attacks (Klein 1980; cf. Margraf et al. 1986b for a critique), was not heightened in nonclinical panickers. It should be noted that the separation anxiety scale used here has been shown to be highly sensitive to the separation anxiety found in clinical panickers as well as in agoraphobics (Margraf and Ehlers 1987).

The results for the baseline and hyperventilation tasks of the psychophysiological laboratory assessment are summarized in Fig. 3 (study 1) and 4 (study 2). We chose hyperventilation (60 cycles/min, 2 min) as the stress task because it has frequently been associated with panic attacks. Separate repeated measures ANOVA's (using the Greenhouse-Geisser correction when appropriate) for the different dependent variables showed significant baseline differences between panickers and controls in self-reported anxiety and panic symptoms, but not control symptoms which are not usually associated with anxiety, heart rate, systolic blood pressure, and diastolic blood pressure. Blood pressure results are not included in the figures. The responses to the hyperventilation task were similar in both groups with the exception of a greater increase in self-rated anxiety in panickers. In study 2 (Tübingen) the EKG was monitored continuously throughout the different paradigms and a rather strong heart rate increase in response to hyperventilation was observed. This was not the case in study 1 (Marburg) because heart rate could not be measured during but only before and after paradigms.

Overall, the results of the Marburg and Tübingen studies replicate earlier findings: There is a high number of persons with panic attacks in nonclinical samples. These persons also show more self-reported psychopathology, but not the cardiovascular differences typical for clinical cases of panic disorder. These replications are complemented by data on the reliability and validity of the questionnaire screening method and results from a more comprehensive battery of questionnaires. In addition, hyperventilation was again shown to produce increases in anxiety, panic symptoms, and heart rate. Nonclinical panickers showed higher baseline anxiety and a greater response to hyperventilation on the anxiety rating scale than nonpanickers.

Conclusions

Taken together, published studies of nonclinical or infrequent panickers and our own preliminary results suggest that Norton et al. (1985, 1986) identified a valid phenomenon. Panic attacks occur relatively frequently in nonclinical subjects. As in clinical studies, the exact proportion depends in part on the measures or criteria we use to determine panic attacks. In our studies, at least 50% of questionnaire-determined panickers did not meet SCID criteria for panic attacks. This occurred in spite of the fact that the subjects invited for the interview had not only indicated a panic attack but also reported on the PAQ at least one spontaneous attack, at least four symptoms during attacks, and panic attacks not only in social situations. Thus, the proportions of panickers given in Table 3 are probably upper limits of the prevalence of panic

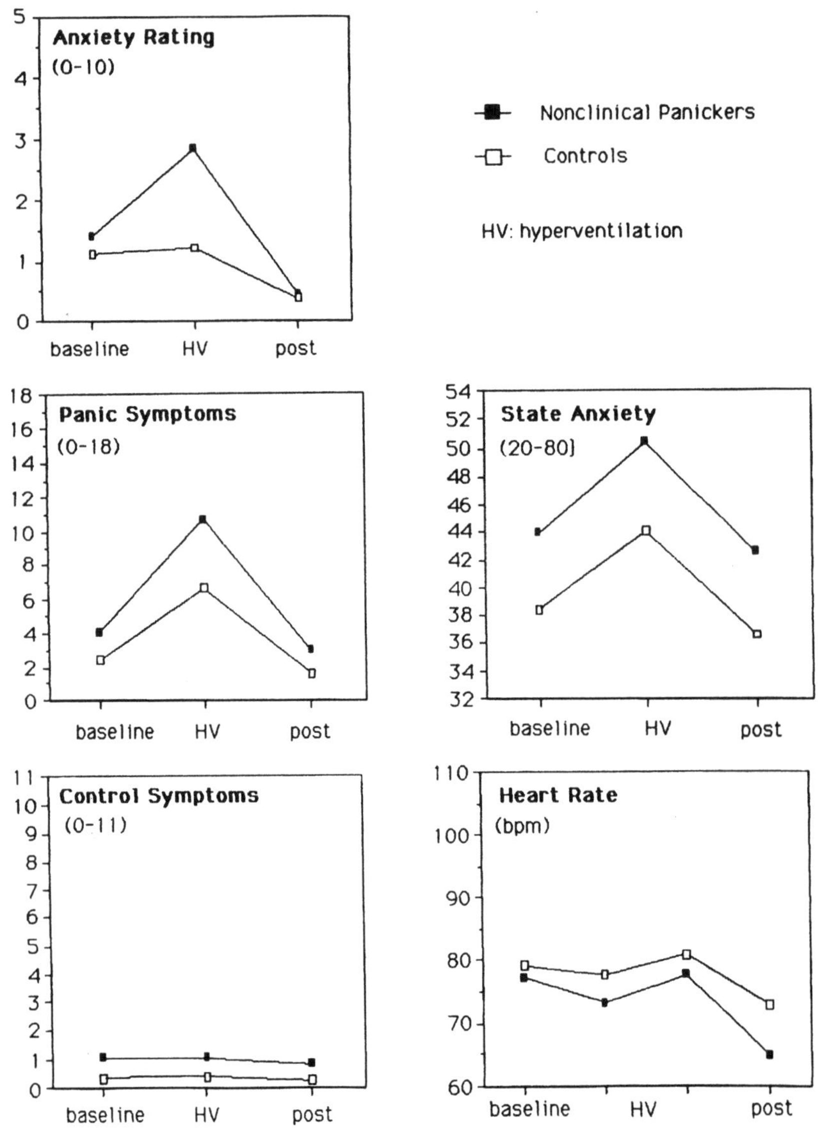

Fig. 3. Selected results of the psychophysiological laboratory assessment in study 1 (Marburg). Shown are self-rated anxiety (on a 0–10 scale), number of panic symptoms (on a list of 18 symptoms), state anxiety (STAI, 20–80 scale, Spielberger et al. 1970), number of control symptoms (on a list of 11 symptoms), and heart rate (in beats per min) at baseline, during hyperventilation (2 min, 60 cycles per min), and at the end of the laboratory session. Heart rate was measured at baseline, immediately before and *after* hyperventilation, and at the end of the session. *Black squares* represent panickers, *open squares* represent controls

attacks in nonclinical subjects. In spite of the high number of "false positive" results, the low proportion of "false negative" results and its good retest reliability make the PAQ a valid screening device. However, if one wants to assure compatibility with the diagnostic standards in clinical studies, a structured interview has to complement the questionnaire in its present form. Nevertheless, it may be

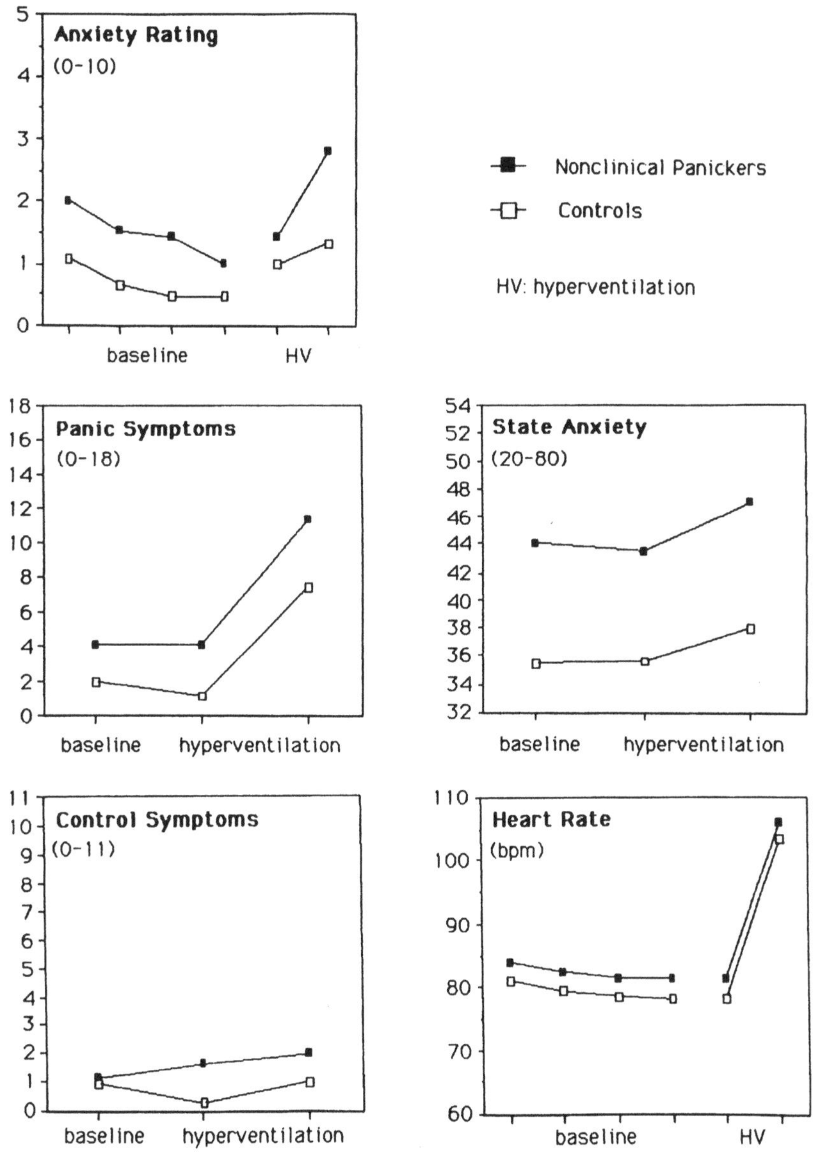

Fig. 4. Selected results of the psychophysiological laboratory assessment in study 2 (Tübingen). Shown are the same variables as in Fig. 3 during a 12-min baseline and a 2-min hyperventilation test (60 cycles per min). For the hyperventilation paradigm, self-report measures were taken immediately before and after hyperventilation, heart rates were calculated from the EKG immediately before and *during* the last 20 s of hyperventilation. *Black squares* represent panickers, *open squares* represent controls

possible to develop future forms of the PAQ that agree better with instruments such as the SCID. It is also possible that the low agreement was due to the lack of reliability of certain criteria for the diagnosis of panic in DSM-IIIR. The fact that information about the "spontaneity" and the rapidity of onset of panic attacks was not given reliably raises doubt as to the usefulness of these criteria.

What are nonclinical panickers like? There are a number of variables in the self-report domain that differentiate nonclinical panickers from controls. These are primarily measures of phobophobia, agoraphobic fears, somatization, anxiousness, and depression. The physiological variables assessed so far as well as reactivity to laboratory stressors differentiate much less well or not at all between panickers and controls in nonclinical samples. The most consistent difference found in our laboratory assessments were tonically elevated levels of self-reported anxiety and symptoms. Reactivity to stress tasks differentiated only poorly and cardiovascular measures differentiated not at all in our studies and in that of Sandler et al. (1987). Even the significant differences on laboratory parameters reach a magnitude of only about one standard deviation (of the control group) and are thus much smaller than some of the questionnaire differences.

Several of the features of nonclinical panickers have previously been found in clinical panic disorder patients (e.g., phobophobia, somatization, general anxiousness, depression). However, further studies are needed that directly compare nonclinical and clinical samples. It is an open question whether the infrequent panickers studied by Beck and Scott (1987) represent a clinical or a nonclinical population since all subjects were recruited through media announcements for people with panic attacks. In our experience, infrequent panickers who respond to such advertisements are more similar to self-selected clinical cases than to nonclinical subjects recruited from community screenings. This could be one reason for the lack of differences between the two samples reported by Beck and Scott (1987).

The results of studies of nonclinical panickers are consistent with the psychophysiological, cognitive, or psychological models of panic proposed by several researchers (e.g., Barlow 1986; Clark 1986; Margraf et al. 1986a, 1986b; van den Hout, 1988) in showing a number of postulated causal factors for the development of panic (e.g., fear of anxiety symptoms, anxiety response to hyperventilation) to be present in this population. They are not consistent with views that assume separation anxiety or active avoidance behavior as necessary antecedents of panic attacks.

If we want to use these results to make more causal statements about the development of panic attacks, we need prospective longitudinal studies. These studies have to determine whether infrequent panickers are the basic population out of which some subjects go on to develop the full-blown clinical picture of panic disorder or even agoraphobia with panic attacks or whether the phenomenon of panic is heterogeneous, representing different subgroups of underlying causes. Either possibility is of high scientific and clinical interest. In the first case, we have a fascinating opportunity to study possible vulnerability factors in subjects at a high risk to develop panic disorder. In the second case, we may gain insights into differential etiologies of panic attacks possibly connected to clinical outcome in the long run. In addition, the longitudinal study of nonclinical panickers may give us information about possible factors protecting most of them from becoming clinical "cases". We have recently started such a prospective longitudinal follow-up study of infrequent panickers at the Clinical Research Unit of the Department of Psychology at Philipps University. On the whole, the studies presented in this chapter illustrate the usefulness of supplementing the usual study of clinical samples by investigating of panic attacks in nonclinical subjects.

Acknowledgements: Preparation of this chapter was supported in part by German Research Foundation grant Eh 97/1-1.

Additional financial support by the Department of Psychology of Philipps University and the help of I. Florin, G. Jakschik, W. Lutzenberger, K. Meisner, B. Rockstroh, F. Schneider, and F. Wrobel is gratefully acknowledged.

References

American Psychiatric Association (1987) Diagnostic and statistical manual of mental disorders, Third edition-revised. American Psychiatric Press, Washington, DC

Arrindell WA (1980) Dimensional structure and psychopathology correlates of the Fear Survey Schedule (FSS-III) in a phobic population: a factorial definition of agoraphobia. Behav Res Ther 18:229-242

Barlow DH (1986) A psychological model of panic. In: Shaw BF, Cashman F, Segal ZV, Vallis Tm (eds) Anxiety disorders: theory, diagnosis, and treatment, Plenum, New York

Barlow DH, Vermilvea J, Blanchard EB, Vermilyea BB, Di Nardo PA, Cerny JA (1985) The phenomenon of panic. J Abnorm Psychol 94:320-328

Beck JG, Scott SK (1987) Frequent and infrequent panic: a comparison of cognitive and autonomic reactivity. J Anx Disord 1:47-58

Beck AT, Ward CH, Mendelson M, Mock J, Erbaugh J (1961) An inventory for measuring depression. Arch Gen Psychiatry 4:561-571

Chambless DL, Caputo GC, Jasin SE, Gracely EJ, Williams C (1985) The mobility inventory for agoraphobia. Behav Res Ther 23:35-44

Clark DM (1986) A cognitive approach to panic. Behav Res Ther 24:461-470

Derogatis LR (1977) SCL-90. Administration, scoring and procedures. Manual-I for the r(evised) version and other instruments of the psychopathology rating scale series. Johns Hopkins University School of Medicine, Baltimore

Derogatis LR, Lipman RS, Covi L (1973) HSCL-90. An outpatient psychiatric rating scale: preliminary report. Psychopharmacol Bull 9:13-25

Devereux RB, Kramer-Fox R, Brown WT, Shear MK, Hartman N, Kligfield P, Lutas EM, Spitzer MC, Litwin SD (1986) Relation between clinical features of the mitral valve prolapse syndrome and echocardiographically documented mitral valve prolapse. J Am Coll Cardiol 8:763-772

DiNardo PA, O'Brien GT, Barlow DH, Waddell MT, Blanchard EB (1983) Reliability of DSM-III anxiety disorder categories using a new structure interview. Arch Gen Psychiatry 40:1070-1075

Ehlers A, Margraf J, Roth WT (1986a) Experimental induction of panic attacks. In: Hand I, Wittchen H-U (eds) Panic and phobias. Springer, Berlin Heidelberg New York

Ehlers A, Margraf J, Roth WT, Taylor CB, Maddock RJ, Sheikh J, Gossard D, Blowers GH, Agras WS, Kopell BS (1986b) Lactate infusions and panic attacks: do patients and controls respond differently? Psychiatry Res 17:295-308

Ehlers A, Margraf J, Roth WT (1988) Interaction of expectancy and physiological stressors in a laboratory model of panic. In: Hellhammer D, Florin I, Weiner H (eds) Neurobiological approaches to human disease. Huber, Toronto

Hartman N, Kramer R, Brown WT, Devereux RB (1982) Panic disorder in patients with mitral valve prolapse. Am J Psychiatry 139:669-670

King R, Margraf J, Ehlers A, Maddock RJ (1986) Panic disorder - overlap with symptoms of somatization disorder. In: Hand I, Wittchen H-U (eds) Panic and phobias. Springer, Berlin Heidelberg New York

Klein DF (1980) Anxiety reconceptualized. Compr Psychiatry 21:411-427

Margraf J, Ehlers A (1987) Fear of fear in panic disorder and agoraphobia: the Panic and Agoraphobia Profile (PAP). 17th Annual meeting of the European Association for Behaviour Therapy, Amsterdam, August 1987

Margraf J, Ehlers A, Roth WT (1988) Mitral valve prolapse and panic disorder: a review of their relationship. Psychosom Med in press

Margraf J, Ehlers A, Roth WT (1986a) Sodium lactate infusions and panic attacks: a review and critique. Psychosom Med 48:23-51

Margraf J, Ehlers A, Roth WT (1986b) Biological models of panic disorder and agoraphobia: a review. Behav Res Ther 24:553-567

Margraf J, Taylor CB, Ehlers A, Roth WT, Agras WS (1987) Panic attacks in the natural environment. J Nerv Ment Dis 175:558-565

Marks IM, Mathews AM (1979) Brief standard self-rating for phobic patients. Behav Res Ther 17:263-267

McNair DM, Lorr M, Droppleman LF (1981) Profile of Mood States. Edits, San Diego

Mendel JGC, Klein DF (1969) Anxiety attacks with subsequent agoraphobia. Compr Psychiatry 10:190-195

Motulsky AG (1978) Biased ascertainment and the natural history of diseases. N Engl J Med 298:1196-1196

Norton GR, Harrison B, Hauch J, Rhodes L (1985) Characteristics of people with infrequent panic attacks. J Abnorm Psychol 94:216-221

Norton GR, Dorward J, Cox BJ (1986) Factors associated with panic attacks in nonclinical subjects. Behav Ther 17:239-252

Regier DA, Myers JK, Kramer M, Robins LN, Blazer DG, Hough RL, Eaton WW, Locke BZ (1984) The NIMH epidemiologic catchment area program - historical context, major objectives, and study population characteristics. Arch Gen Psychiatry 41:934-941

Sandler L, Wilson KG, Ramsum D, Asmundson G, Ashton G, Larsen D, Schumacher B (1987) Psychophysiological characteristics of individuals with frequent panic attacks (Abstract). Psychophysiology 24:609

Spielberger CD, Gorsuch RL, Lushene RE (1970) State-Trait Anxiety Inventory. Consulting Psychologists Press, Palo Alto

Spitzer RL, Williams JB (1986) Structured Clinical Interview for DSM (SCID). New York State Psychiatric Institute, New York

Thyer BA, Himle J (1985) Temporal relationship between panic attack onset and phobic avoidance in agoraphobia. Behav Res Ther 23:607-608

van den Hout MA (1988) The explanation of experimental panic. In: Maser J, Rachman S (eds) Panic and cognition. Plenum, New York

Weissman MM, Leaf PJ, Blazer DG, Boyd JH, Florio L (1986) The relationship between panic disorder and agoraphobia: an epidemiologic perspective. Psychopharmacol Bull 22:787-791

Wittchen H-U (1986) Epidemiology of panic attacks and panic disorders. In: Hand I, Wittchen H-U (eds) Panic and phobias. Springer, Berlin Heidelberg New York

11. Panic, Perception, and pCO_2

M. A. VAN DEN HOUT

Introduction

Explanations of panic disorder (PD) refer to underlying pathogenic processes that are assumed to be specific to PDs. There are various ways to test the validity of such theories on the dynamics of panic. Particularly important, if not decisive, are tests aimed at triggering and neutralizing the hypothetical underlying process. Triggering the pathogenic mechanism should arouse panic, preferably only in PD, while neutralizing the process should reduce pathology.

As for panic reduction, considerable investments in pharmacological research have shown that some drugs - most notably the tricyclics and alprazolam - lead to a decrease in complaints of PD's (Charney et al. 1986; Chouinard et al. 1982; Alexander and Alexander 1986). Side-effects and withdrawal problems seem to be common (Monteiro et al. 1987; Lydiard et al. 1987; Fyer et al. 1987). Though there is a strong body of evidence pointing to the beneficial effects of exposure-based treatments for agoraphobia (Emmelkamp 1982), there is a paucity of psychological treatment studies aimed specifically at PD. The few data that are available suggest that PD responds very well to cognitive/behavioral interventions, with no side-effects or withdrawal problems (Rapee 1987). To the author's knowledge, only one study has been completed in which a direct comparison was made between alprazolam and psychological treatment of panic. Psychological treatment proved to be superior in eliminating panic attacks (Barlow, this volume). What is badly needed here are more tightly controlled replications from different centers. Many psychological treatment studies are at this very moment being prepared or carried out.

In this paper, the focus will not be on panic-reduction studies and their implications; excellent summaries are included elsewhere in this book. Attention will be focused instead, upon the opposite of panic reduction. That is, on deliberate attempts to provoke panic or panic-like phenomena by experimental means. In the course of this discussion, the explanatory and predictive power of psychological accounts will be highlighted. This is not because I feel that, in the final analysis, biology vs psychology will prove a useful dichotomy, but because the final analysis still lies rather far ahead. For the time being, we may be better off taking a pragmatic stance and asking ourselves how far we can get if we use psychological theories to explain, infer, and predict relevant phenomena.

Psychological Notes on Panic and Panic Disorder

Several authors have noted that although panics in PD may be nonsituational, this does not imply that they are uncued.

More specifically, one has reasoned that panics in PDs may be triggered by distinct interoceptive sensations. Thus, the physical symptoms that are characteristic of panic may not be neutral interoceptive stimuli, but sufficient to cause panic. From this perspective, those who suffer from nonsituational panic are a subgroup of phobics; they are said to represent those phobics for whom the fear-eliciting cues stem from the perceived internal, rather than external, milieu. Particular sensations, once felt, trigger anxiety and typically increase the saliency of the feared symptom comples. The patient might thus be trapped in a positive feedback loop (Clark 1986; van den Hout 1987).

Considering the fact that, in general, the psychological processing of internal stimuli is not fundamentally different from the processing of external cues (Pennebaker 1982), the mere existence of interoceptive phobias would not be surprising. Plausibility aside, the idea that interoceptive fear maintains PD is only as good as the hypothesis to which it gives rise.

A first straightforward deduction is that panics are preceded by the perception of bodily sensations. Two studies addressed and confirmed this hypothesis. Ley (1985) and Hibbert (1984) found that 80% and 53%, respectively, of their PDs said that a bodily sensation was the first thing they noted when having an attack. In Hibbert's study, only zero percent of non-PD neurotic controls mentioned perceiving bodily sensation before subjective anxiety.

A second prediction from the interoceptive fear hypothesis of PD is that interoceptive fears are not merely a symptom of neurosis in general, but rather that they are specific to PDs. A self-report study again corroborates this idea: 29 PDs, 29 nonpanicking neurotic controls, and 30 normal controls indicated their fear of 14 distinct somatic symptoms. On none of the 14 items did normals score significantly lower than nonpanicking neurotics. For 13 of the 14 symptoms, PDs did express higher anxiety than the two other groups; the exception was feeling paralyzed, a prospect as frightening to PDs as to the others (van den Hout et al. 1987a). Data are given in Fig. 1.

The findings are in line with data from other centers (Reiss et al. 1986; Cambless et al. 1984).

With regard to the important question of why PDs become so frightened by interoceptive sensations that happen to be part of the anxiety response, Clark and Salkovskis (this volume) offered thought-provoking data. In a paper-and-pencil task, PDs were found to catastrophically misinterpret ambiguous bodily sensations that are associated with panic. In several respects, this phenomenon was highly specific: PDs did not misinterpret ambiguous social situations or nonpanic related bodily changes any more than normals or nonpanicking neurotics. The misinterpreation of bodily feelings of the PDs occurred significantly less in the two control groups.

Given that PDs are likely to become anxious when perceiving certain bodily states, one wonders what physiological processes produce the symptoms that are so frightening to PDs. Do PDs merely overreact to sensations that are commonly felt, or do identifiable physiological peculiarities underlie the disorder?

Several authors believe that the latter is true and maintain that acute changes in acid-base status and, more specifically, hyperventilation are responsible.

Psychological Reactions to Change in pH and pCO_2

To assess whether pH/pCO_2 changes are involved in panic, direct measurements during attacks should be made. Only rarely is there an opportunity to do so; however, the few casuistic observations

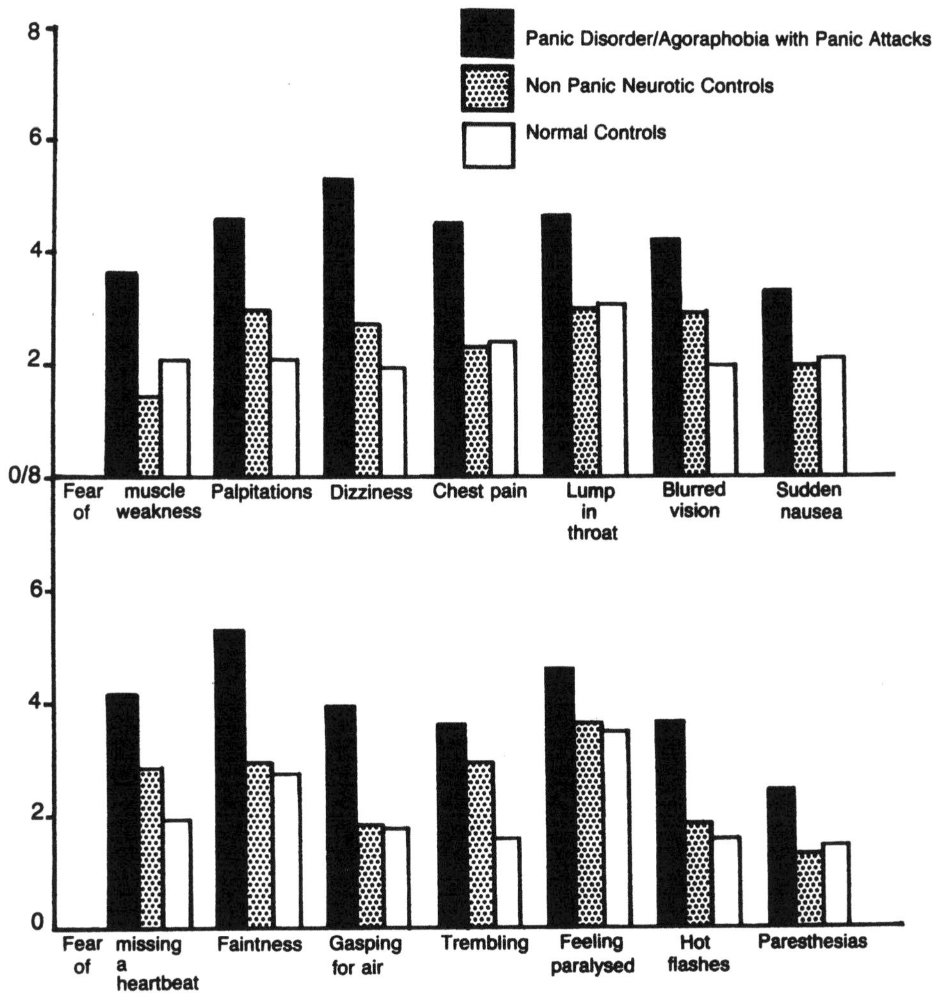

Fig. 1. Fears of interoceptive sensations in panic patients, nonpanic neurotic controls, and normal controls. (From van den Hout et al. 1987a)

that have been made have shown massive plasma pCO_2 drops/pH rises during full-blown panics (Salkovskis et al. 1986; Griez et al. 1987). Similarly, Hibbert's data on ambulatory CO_2 monitoring, though hampered by technical problems, indicated that pCO_2 drops coincided with anxiety (Hibbert 1985).

To check whether pCO_2 changes are not just associated with panic but are causes of panic, data from experimental manipulation of acid-base status are relevant. There is a large body of evidence indicating that changing pH by lactate infusion, a single inhalation of 35% CO_2/65% O_2, or continuous 5% CO_2 breathing does, indeed, produce high anxiety in PDs; interestingly, normal controls and nonpanicking neurotics typically do not become highly anxious (van den Hout 1987; Shear 1986).

Garssen et al. observed that approximately two out of every three agoraphobics recognize the symptoms produced by hyperventilation provocation as being similar to panic symptoms (Garssen et al. 1983), while Margraf et al. (1987) documented that PDs show steeper increases in anxiety after hyperventilating than do normal controls.

The question remains of how hyperventilation (provocation)-induced, lactate-induced, 35% CO_2-induced, or 5% CO_2-induced acid-base changes are related to panic symptoms. Do these interventions trigger pathophysiological abnormalities in PDs, and is this why they induce anxiety in PDs? Or do these acid-base changes induce panic because the bodily sensations that ensue are frightening to PDs?

A series of recent studies has addressed the hypothesis that pCO_2/pH change-induced anxiety is psychologically mediated. The results are consistent. First it should be noted that hyperventilation, lactate, and or CO_2 inhalation all induce – in everybody – salient physical symptoms feared by PDs. Thus, the fact that PDs specifically react anxiously is fully consistent with the interoceptive fear hypothesis. Second, though hyperventilation, lactate, and CO_2 all affect the acid-base balance, they do so in an *opposite* direction: 5% CO_2 increases plasma CO_2 and decreases pH, while lactate decreases CO_2 and increases pH. Both, however, produce *comparable* interoceptions in all subjects and *comparable* affective reactions in PDs. This favors a psychological account of pH/pCO_2 changes inducing anxiogenesis.

Particularly relevant are data from experiments in which attempts were made to manipulate the affective responses to CO_2 or lactate challenges by experimentally influencing the psychological state of the subjects. Rapee et al. (1986) gave a single inhalation of 50% CO_2/50% O_2 to 16 PDs and 16 social-phobics. One-half of the subjects from both groups were told beforehand what symptoms to expect and that the occurrence of symptoms was perfectly normal after CO_2 inhalation. The other subjects were not prepared in this fashion. In both conditions, social-phobics mentioned little, if any, anxiety. Panic patients who had previously been informed and reassured reported significantly less anxiety, fewer cognitions about impending catastrophes, and less similarity between CO_2-induced anxiety and natural panic.

These data are not unlike recent preliminary results from two experiments by Margraf et al. (1987) showing that affective and cardiovascular effects of voluntary overbreathing are strongly influenced by expectational variables.

Repeated and prolonged exposure to phobic cues reduces phobic fears. From the idea that PD represents a form of interoceptive phobia and that it is precisely this feature that explains the anxiogenic power of lactate and CO_2 challenges, it follows that repeated and prolonged administrations of lactate or carbon dioxide to vulnerable individuals will produce less anxiety as the number and duration of administrations increase. Bonn et al. (1973), using lactate infusion to induce maximum anxiety in 33 anxiety neurotics during six 20-min sessions, found that "the phobophobic element which was so frequently elicited from these patients was substantially reduced." This study, however, was uncontrolled in that it did not use challenge-by-challenge ratings, did not use a placebo control condition, and did not include a normal control sample.

The authors carried out a carbon dioxide experiment under all of these necessary conditions which provided a robust confirmation of this hypothesis (van den Hout et al. 1987b). In this study, 14 panic patients and 8 controls received a series of 35% CO_2/65% O_2 inhalations (6 sessions; 10 inhalations per session), as well as air inhalations (3 sessions; 10 inhalations per session). The order was: carbon dioxide (3 sessions), air (3 sessions), carbon dioxide (3 sessions) or air (3 sessions), carbon dioxide (3 sessions), carbon dioxide (3

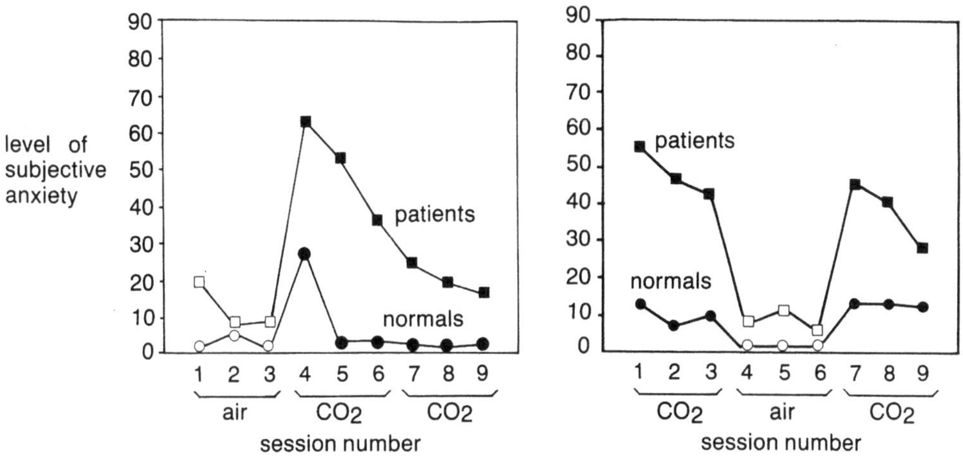

Fig. 2. Reduction of CO_2-induced anxiety after repeated exposure to CO_2 challenge. (From van den Hout et al. 1987b)

sessions). Subjects reported anxiety on a 100-point scale after each inhalation and all scores for a given session were averaged. There was a clear habituation effect in the patient groups. Normals did not report any distress after air and only very little, transient anxiety after carbon dioxide inhalation. The data are presented in Figure 2.

These studies demonstrate that by manipulating psychological variables, pCO_2/pH challenge responders can be turned into nonresponders. Of course, the hypothesis would gain explanatory power if it could be shown, the other way around, that *challenge nonresponders become responders* by prechallenge psychological interventions. In a recent study (van der Molen et al. 1986), 13 normal volunteers were given sodium lactate and glucose in a randomized order. Seven of the subjects were told that the infusions would be anxiogenic and the other six were told to expect pleasant excitement, as when watching a movie. Affective changes were indicated on a scale ranging from +100 (a very high level of pleasant excitement) to −100 (extreme, subjective anxiety), with 0 indicating the mood before the infusion. The results of the double-blind study are presented in Fig. 3. The induced expectation did not affect mood in the placebo conditions, but had a powerful effect on the lactate challenges: The subjects in group A expected to experience anxiety and reported sharp increases in subjective anxiety, but the subjects in group B showed no systematic change. The average subjective anxiety indicated on the 100-point scale by the group A subjects was 65. This figure closely matches the level of subjective anxiety reported by PDs after 35% CO_2 inhalation (van den Hout et al. 1987b), 5% CO_2 inhalation (Ehlers et al. 1986), and lactate challenge (Ehlers et al. 1986). The findings strongly suggest that lactate is panicogenic because it triggers interoceptive fears: When normals without any psychiatric history become fearful of interoceptive changes, their lactate responses become indistinguishable from those of PDs. The studies cited above suggest that it is not specific physiological effects of pH/CO_2 changes that produce anxiety.

As mentioned, increasing pCO_2 by 5% CO_2 inhalation may be as anxiogenic as

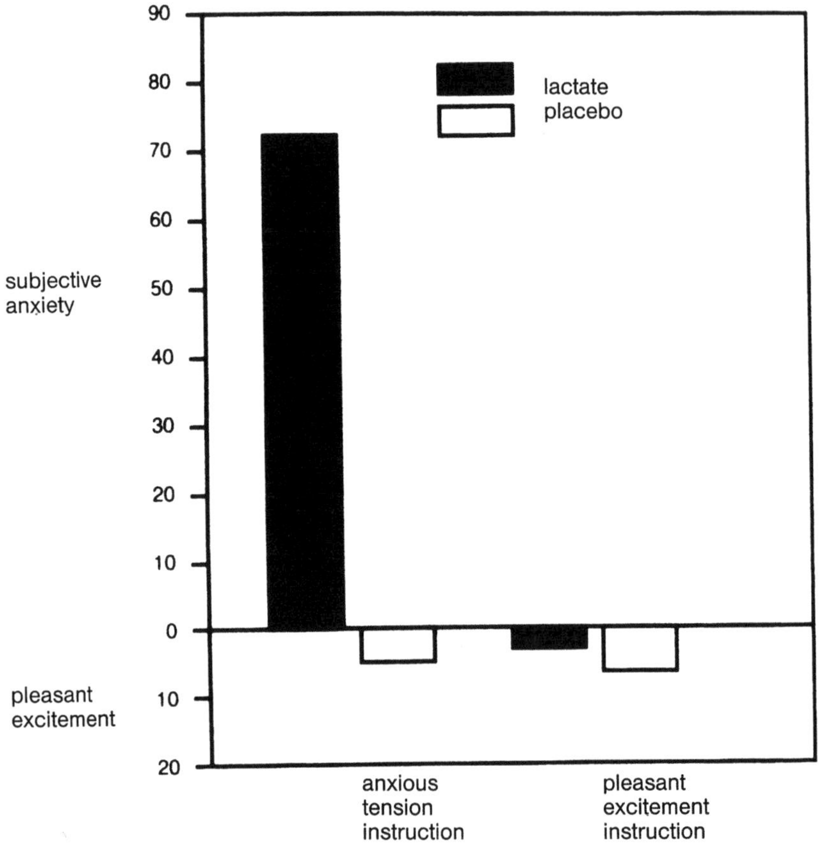

Fig. 3. Healthy subjects reporting high anxiety after lactate/anxiety instruction and no anxiety after lactate/pleasant instruction. (Data from a double-blind, placebo-controlled study; van der Molen et al. 1986)

decreasing CO_2 by lactate, and hyperventilation in one study seemed less anxiogenic than 5% CO_2 (Gorman et al. 1984). The authors of this study reasoned that possible beneficial effects of paper bag rebreathing might not be attributable to physiological reasons, but rather to distraction.

The idea that effects of the commonly used paper bag rebreathing depend on psychological factors was tested in two related experiments (van den Hout et al. 1987c). In experiment 1, a group of 12 healthy volunteers were told that we were investigating how quickly hyperventilation-induced symptoms disappear when the paper bag is used and when it is not used. Each subject participated twice in a randomized, balanced, cross-over study. On both occasions, subjects overbreathed. After 2 min, they either started to ventilate normally or to rebreathe into a paper bag. As expected, paper bag rebreathing resulted in a much quicker pCO_2 restoration and a much quicker disappearance of physical symptoms.

To check whether the quicker disappearance of symptoms was affected by expectational factors, the procedure used in experiment 2 was identical in all but two

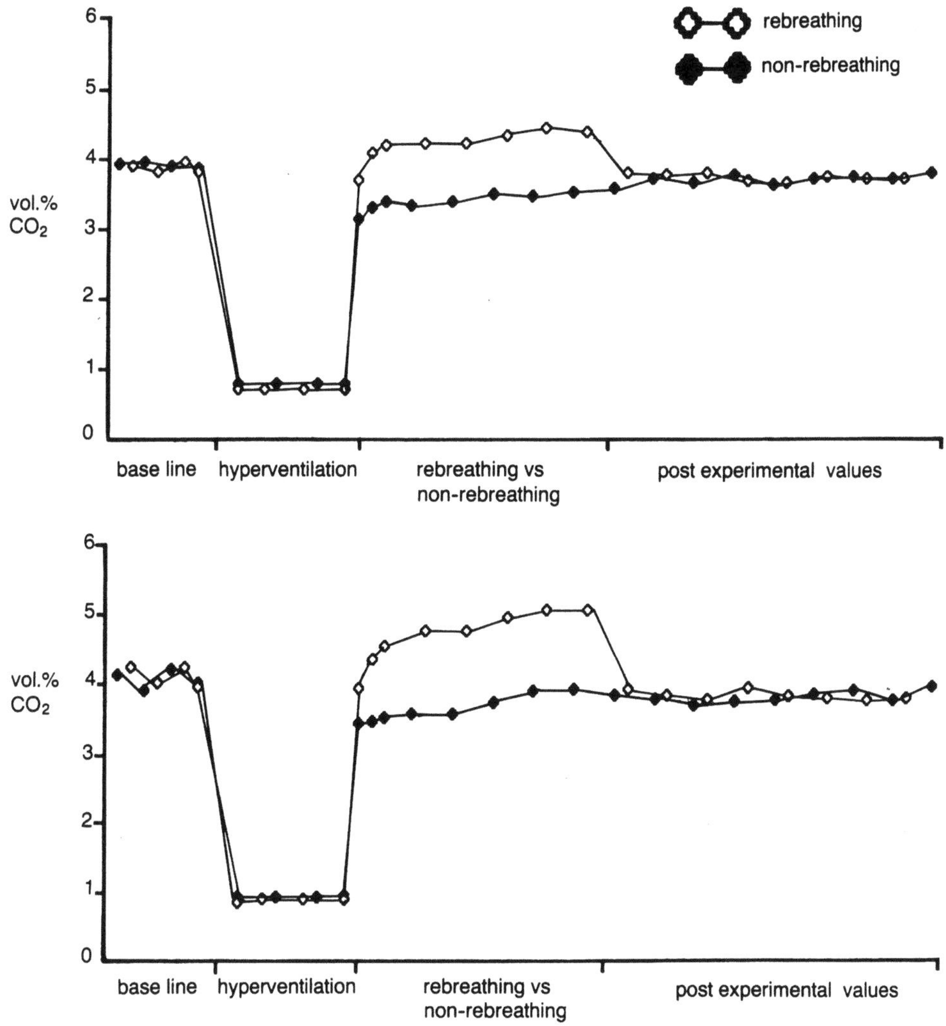

Fig. 4. Effects of voluntarily hyperventilating and subsequent rebrething on alveolar CO_2. (Results from two experiments; van den Hout et al. 1987c)

ways. Rebreathing was not done into a paper bag but into a semiclosed tube system. Normal post-hyperventilation breathing was done in the same way except that this time its valves were open. On both occasions subjects believed they were breathing into a closed system Again, of course, pCO_2 restoration was quicker in the rebreathing condition. A graphic representation showing the identical pCO_2 curves in both experiments is given in Fig. 4.

In this second experiment, however, there was no between-condition difference in the time interval between stopping hyperventilation and disappearance of symptoms. These results indicate that possible beneficial effects of rebreathing to cope with hyperventilation are highly dependent upon expectations.

In sum, the experiments described above support the idea that interoceptive fear is an important underlying and maintaining factor in PD.

Biological Peculiarities Possibly Predisposing One to Interoceptive Fears and Panic Disorder

Hyperventilation is a common component of stress (Garssen 1986), and the literature suggests that excessive hyperventilation takes place during panic attacks.

In an early pilot study, Drury found that patients suffering from "soldiers heart syndrome" (a syndrome similar to PD) displayed intolerable hyperpnea at lower CO_2 levels than did normals. Alveolar ventilation is mainly controlled by the CO_2 stimulation of the respiratory centers of the brain, located near the central surface of the medulla. It may be speculated that PDs characteristically have hypersensitive chemoreceptors, implying a tendency for them to overbreathe. Woods et al. (1986) challenged 14 PDs with a CO_2 rebreathing test in order to see whether PDs - as compared to normals - show greater increases in ventilation as a function of increased CO_2 pressure. No significant differences were found between patients and controls. Yet, in a recent study by members of our research group, 19 PDs showed a considerably steeper increase in ventilation during CO_2 rebreathing than in 14 matched normals (Lousberg et al. 1987). Data are given in Fig. 5)

One could, of course, argue that the patients' ventilatory overreaction was not due to the CO_2 challenge per se, but rather that it resulted from anxiety due to CO_2-induced interoceptions. Two observations argue against this interpretation, however. First, PD/control differences emerged very quickly, that is, when interoceptive changes were still absent or only very minor. More important, just like normals, PDs displayed a strictly linear ventilatory response to the increasing CO_2. Interoceptive fear mediation would have predicted a nonlinear, exponential increase as a manifestation of the proposed positive feedback loop. Recently, comparable findings on chemoreceptor oversensitivity were reported by Gorman and co-workers. The authors are inclined to believe that the chemoreceptory system of PDs is more sensitive to CSF pCO_2.

A second line of evidence concerns the regulation of noradrenaline turnover. The hypothesis that PDs are noradrenergically overreactive is corroborated by evidence from two sources. First, 20 mg of the alpha 2 autoreceptor antagonist Yohimbine produces significantly higher plasma levels of MHPG - an NA metabolite - in frequently panicking PDs than it does in normals (Charney et al. 1984). Patients also report sharper increases in anxiety with such dosage, than do normals

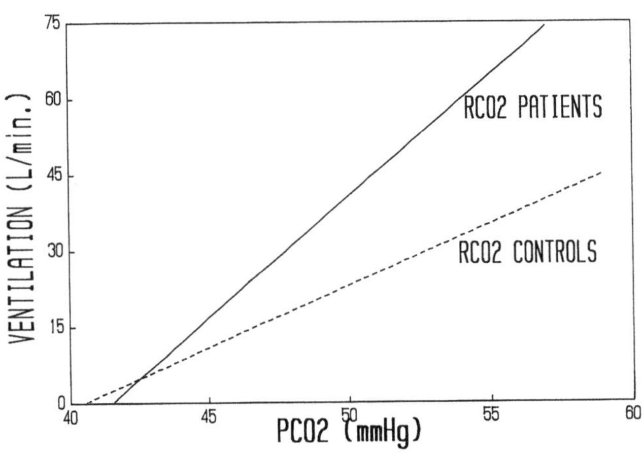

Fig. 5. Chemoreceptor sensitivity in panic patients and matched controls. $RCO_2 = CO_2$ responsivity. (From Lousberg et al., in press)

(Woods et al. 1986). It does not seem likely that interoceptive cueing gives an exhaustive explanation of Yohimbine anxiogenesis. Ten healthy subjects received 20 mg Yohimbine and placebo in a randomized, balanced order, double-blind crossover study. Subjects were told that they might get a placebo twice, or an "active substance" followed by placebo, or placebo followed by an "active substance," or twice an "active substance". During the trials subjects were asked 30, 60, 90, and 120 min after drug intake if they had had placebo or an "active substance." Of the 4 × 10 guesses in the Yohombine conditions, 36 were wrong; 32 of the 40 guesses in the placebo condition were right. Interestingly, when guessing on what active substance was given, subjects were fairly uncertain, regardless of whether the guess was right or wrong. On the contrary, when thinking a placebo was given, subjects were significantly more certain, no matter whether they in fact had had Yohimbine or placebo. Findings are represented in Fig. 6.

The straightforward conclusion from the data seems that healthy subjects cannot tell Yohombine from placebo (van den Hout 1987; unpublished data). Comparable results were observed by Albus (1987; unpublished data), who not only found that controls do not discriminate Yohimbine from placebo any better than chance, but that PDs are able to do so. Thus, unlike lactate and CO_2, Yohimbine challenge produces in controls no salient bodily feelings of the type that produces anxiety in PDs. Another strong argument in favor of an NA hypothesis of PD is provided by the observation that clonidine, an alpha 2 agonist, produces greater heart rate reduction and hypotensive effects in PDs than it does in normals (Nutt 1986).

The data on CO_2 and NA hypersensitivity meanwhile do not at all indicate that such biological constituents are necessary or sufficient to produce PD. One reason is that there is considerable variance in CO_2 sensitivity among PDs and controls, while there is considerable overlap between the two groups. There are even tentative indications that some PDs habitually hypoventilate and are chemoreptorally hyposensitive (Gorman et al. 1985; Pearson et al. 1985). As for the NA hypothesis, Yohimbine challenge only produced higher plasma MHPG in high-frequency panickers and not in PDs as a group (Charney et al. 1984).

At present, considering the robustness of the interoceptive fear findings, the most parsimonious formulation would be that

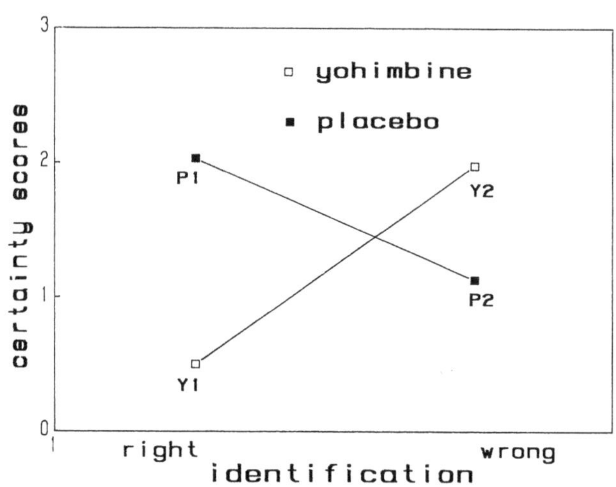

Fig. 6. Healthy subjects being uncertain whether they believe they have had Yohimbine when the guess is right (*y1;* 4 observations) or wrong (*y2;* 36 observations); certainly scores were significantly higher when they rightly (*p1;* 32 observations) or wrongly (*p2;* 8 observations) guessed they had had placebo

CO_2 and NA sensitivity represent continua. PDs might have a greater chance of being located in the right tail of this assumed distribution. While this might be a benign deviation from the mean, it might still imply a greater risk for the development of PD. Prospective studies can be conceived and should be welcomed.

Concluding Remarks

In the first part of this chapter, evidence was presented indicating: that the perception of bodily sensations precedes panic attacks in PDs, that PDs are likely to catastrophically misinterpret these feelings which they greatly fear, that hyperventilation may often take place during panics, that provoking the relevant sensations in PDs by giving lactate or CO_2 and, thereby, changing the acid-base balance induces anxiety in PDs, that challenge responders can be turned into nonresponders by behavioral and cognitive interventions, that nonresponders can become responders by changing their cognitive set, and that expectations may play a crucial role in blocking hyperventilation by rebreathing. Considering the robustness of the data and recalling that various panic challenges have opposing acid-base effects, it may be concluded that there is substantial evidence to support the idea that interoceptive fear plays a causal role in PD. I also discussed a number of studies that show that chemoreceptor and locus coerelleus NA hypersensitivity may be a characteristic of many PDs.

Just *how* chemoreceptor hypersensitivity, noradrenergic hypersensitivity, hyperventilation, and interoceptive fears *interact* is unclear, but hypotheses can be formulated. To illustrate the empirical and potentially fruitful nature of such biopsychological speculating, this chapters finishes with a conjecture.

As for the association between CO_2 and NA hypersensitivity, it was observed that increased pCO_2 produces increased NA turnover (Elam et al. 1981). Thus, CO_2 challenges may produce NA surges, especially in vulnerable individuals. It can be speculated that, considering the findings on CO_2-induced NA stimulation, the system works the other way around as well, namely that decreasing PCO_2 produces decreases in NA turnover. If this were true, it would mean that an often efficient way of limiting the degree of NA discharge would be to hyperventilate. During nonpanic episodes, mild NA overactivity could be counteracted by overbreathing. This would be a highly reinforcing type of self-medication, for those subjects who are fearful of bodily feelings associated with increased NA discharge. Central NA turnover is controlled by many more factors than just CSF pCO_2, and it would be expected that NA discharge could only be limited by overbreathing to a certain extent. Hyperventilating during panic attacks might prove to be a vigorous, but unsuccessful, way of reducing relatively large NA discharges. Thus, during nonpanic episodes, hyperventilation might be sufficient to reduce feared NA discharge related interoceptions to an acceptable degree. During panics, the hyperventilation strategy may be insufficient to combat the occurring NA discharge.

Hyperventilation might even become counterproductive in that it may start to produce the type of sensations that it aimed to reduce. This theory is, of course, highly speculative and may turn out to be false altogether. It may demonstrate, however, that in principle, biological and psychological notions are not mutually exclusive and that testable theories can be formulated that incorporate crucial finding from both areas.

References

Alexander PE, Alexander DD (1985) Alprazolam treatment for panic disorders. J Clin Psychiatry 47:301-304

Bonn JA, Harrison J, Rees L (1973) Lactate infusion in the treatment of "free-floating" anxiety. Can HJ Psychiatry 18:41-46

Chambless DL, Caputo GG, Bright P, Gallagher R (1984) Assessment of fear of fear in agoraphobics: the body sensations questionnaire and the agoraphobic cognitions questionnaire. J Consult Clin Psychol 52:1090-1097

Charney DS et al (1984) Noradrenergic function in panic anxiety. Arch Gen Psychiatry 41:751

Charney DS, Woods SW, Goodman WK, Rifkin B, Kind MRN, Aiken B, Quadrino MS, Heninger GR (1986) Drug treatment of panic disorder; the comparative efficacy of imipramine, alprazolam and trazodone. J Clin Psychiatry 47:580-586

Chouinard G, Annable L, Fontaine R, Solyom L (1982) Alprazolam in the treatment of generalized anxiety and panic disorders: a double blind placebo controlled study. Psychopharmacology 77:229-233

Clark DM (1986) A cognitive approach to panic. Behav Res Ther 24:461-470

Ehlers A, Margraf J, Roth WT (1986) Experimental induction of panic attacks. In: Hand J, Wittchen HU (eds) Panic and phobias. Empirical evidence of theoretical models and long-term effects of behavioral treatments. Springer, Berlin Heidelberg New York

Elam M, Yao T, Thoren T, Svensson TH (1981) Hypercapnia and hyperoxia: chemoreceptor mediated control of locus coereleus neurons and splanchnic sympathetic nerves. Brain Res 222:373-381

Emmelkamp PMG (1982) Phobic and obsessive compulsive disorders: theory, research and practice. Plenum, New York

Fyer AJ, Liebowitz MR, Gorman JM, Campeas R, Levin A, Davies SO, Goetz D, Klein DF (1987) Discontinuation of Alprazolam treatment in panic patients. Am J Psychiatry 144:303-308

Garssen B, van Veenendaal W, Bloemink R (1983) Agoraphobia and the hyperventilation syndrome. Behav Res Ther 21:643-649

Garssen B (1986) Psychofysiologie van de ademhaling en het hyperventilatiesyndroom; psychophysiology of respiration and the hyperventilation syndrome (with a summary in English). Doctoral thesis, Utrecht, Holland

Gorman JM; Askanazi J, Liebowitz MR, Fyer AJ, Stein J, Kinney JM, Klein DF (1984) Response to hyperventilation in a group of patients with panic disorder. Am J Psychiatry 141:857-861

Gorman JM, Fyer AJ, Ross DC, Cohen S, Martinez JM, Liebowitz MR, Klein DF (1985) Normalization of veneus pH, pCO_2 and bicarbonate levels after blockade of panic attacks. Psychiatry Res 14:57-65

Griez E, Pols H, van den Hout MA (1987) Acid base balance in real life panic. J Affective Disord 12:263-266

Hibbert GA (1984) Ideational components of anxiety: their origin and content. Br J Psychiatry 144:618-624

Hibbert GA (1985) Ambulatory monitoring of transcutaneous pCO_2. In: Lacey J, Sturgeon J (eds) Proceedings of the 15th European conference on psychosomatic medicine. Libby, London

Hout MA van den (1987) The explanation of experimental panic. In: Rachman S, Maser JD (eds) Panic: psychological perspectives. Erlbaum, Hillsdale, pp 237-258

Hout MA van den, van der Molen GM, Griez E, Lousberg H (1987a) Specificity of interoceptive fear to panic disorders. J Psychopathol Behav Assess 9:99-109

Hout MA van den, van der Molen GM, Griez E, Lousberg H, Jansen A (1987b) Reduction of CO_2-induced anxiety in patients with panic attacks after repeated CO_2 exposure. Am J Psychiatry 144:788-791

Hout MA van den, Boek C, van der Molen GM, Jansen A, Griez E (1987c) Rebreathing to cope with hyperventilation. Experimental tests of the paper bag method. J Behav Med (in press)

Ley R (1985) Agoraphobia, the panic attack and the hyperventilation syndrome. Behav Res Ther 23:79-81

Lousberg H, Griez E, van den Hout MA (to be published) Carbon dioxide chemosensitivity in panic disorder. Acta Psychiatr Scand

Lydiard RB, Laraia MT, Ballenger JC, Howell EF (1987) Emergence of depressive symptoms in patients receiving alprazolam for panic disorder. Am J Psychiatry 5:664-665

Margraf J, Ehlers A, Roth WT (1987) Expectancy effects and hyperventilation as laboratory stressors. In: Hellhamer D, Florin I, Weiner H (eds) New frontiers in stress research. Huber, Toronto

Molen GM van der, van den Hout MA, Vroemen J, Lousberg H, Griez E (1986) Cognitive determinants of lactate induced anxiety. Behav Res Ther 24:677-680

Monteiro WO, Noshirvani HF, Marks IM, Lelliot PP (1987) Anorganismic from clomipramine in obsessive compulsive disorder. A controlled trial. Br J Psychiatry 151:107-112

Nutt DJ (1986) Increased central $alpha_2$ adrenoceptor sensitivity in panic disorder. Psychopharmacology. 90:268-269

Pearson MG, Peattie B, Quadiri MR, Finn R (1985) Abnormalities of respiratory centre function and pottasium homeostasis in the chronic hyperventilation syndrome. Paper presented at the 5th international symposium on respiratory psychophysiology. Nijmegen, The Netherlands

Pennebaker JW (1982) The psychology of physical Symptoms. Springer, Berlin Heidelberg New York

Rapee R (1987) Psychological treatment of panic attacks: theoretical conceptualization and review of evidence. Clin Psychol Rev 7:427-438

Rapee R, Matlich R, Murrell E (1986) Cognitive mediation in the affective component of spontaneous panic attacks. J Behav Ther Exp Psychiatry 17:245-253

Reiss S, Peterson RA, Garsky DM, McNally RJ (1986) Anxiety sensitivity, anxiety frequency and the prediction of fearfulness. Behav Res Ther 24:1-8

Salkovskis PM, Warwich HMC, Clark DM, Wessels DJ (1986) A demonstration of acute hyperventilation during naturally occurring panic attacks. Behav Res Ther 24:91-94

Shear MK (1986) Pathophysiology of panic: a review of pharmacologic provocative tests and naturalistic monitoring data. J Clin Psychiatry [Suppl] 47:18-26

Woods SW, Charney DS, Loke J, Goodman WK, Redmond DE, Henninger GR (1986) Carbon dioxide sensitivity in panic anxiety. Arch Gen Psychiatry 43:900-909

12. Selective Information Processing, Interoception, and Panic Attacks

A. Ehlers, J. Margraf, and W. T. Roth

Introduction

Panic attacks have recently been given a central role in the classification of anxiety disorders (DSM-IIIR, *Diagnostic and Statistical Manual of Mental Disorders* of the American Psychiatric Association, third edition-revised, APA 1987). The etiology of these anxiety attacks is controversial. One of their most puzzling and fascinating features for clinicians and researchers is that panic attacks often occur in the absence of any perceived situational triggers. This apparent spontaneity has led researchers to search for possible causes of panic attacks "within" the patient.

Many biologically oriented researchers believe that panic attacks represent an "endogenous" form of anxiety resulting from metabolic dysfunction. Detailed critical reviews of these medical models of panic disorder are found in Margraf et al. (1986a) and Margraf and Ehlers (in press). While medical models presume that yet unknown metabolic dysfunctions of the central nervous system cause spontaneous panic attacks, psychophysiological models assume that internal anxiety triggers can be identified and that panic attacks are a fear response to these internal stimuli.

The present paper will focus on these alternative models of panic attacks that have recently received increasing attention and empirical support. After a description of the psychophysiological models, some recent evidence will be reviewed. The need for further specification of the models will be discussed. We will focus on two aspects of possible specifications: the role of selective information processing and the role of interoception in panic attacks. Preliminary results from our laboratories will be presented.

Psychophysiological Models of Panic Attacks

Patients report that many panic attacks occur without any situational triggers. In contrast to medical models, psychophysiological models do not take these reports at face value. It is assumed that anxiety triggers can be identified even for "spontaneous" panic attacks. The role of *internal* triggers is emphasized. These include body sensations like palpitations or dyspnea, thoughts related to danger, and other cognitive changes such as inability to concentrate or feelings of derealization. Since bodily symptoms are most prominent in panic attacks, most researchers have concentrated on body sensations as possible triggers for panic. We will follow this tradition in the present paper. Note, however, that for individual patients cognitive events such as derealization may be more important than bodily cues in triggering panic attacks.

In the past few years, a number of researchers have presented models that explain panic attacks as the result of a positive feedback loop between internal stimuli (body sensations or cognitive events) and anxiety responses. To emphasize the close interaction between psychological and physiological responses, we use the term "psychophysiological models" (Margraf et al. 1986a, b). However, other groups have used the terms "cognitive" (Beck et al. 1985; Clark 1986; Rapee, in press) or "psychological" (Barlow 1986; van den Hout and Griez 1983; Rapee, in press) models. The idea that positive feedback can lead to panic attacks had already been presented by Lader and Mathews in 1968. These authors assumed that panic was on a continuum with orienting and defense reactions. They argued that panic attacks result from lack of habituation due to a high level of activation and repeated stimulation. However, they emphasized internal anxiety cues to a lesser extent than current models and did not explain why anxiety attacks are less likely when the patient is accompanied by a friend or spouse.

Psychophysiological models of panic are related to the old concept of "fear of fear" often mentioned in the literature on agoraphobia (Evans 1972; Fenichel 1945; Frankl 1975; Freud 1895; Shands and Schor 1982; Westphal 1871; see Goldstein and Chambless 1978 for the most developed "fear of fear" model and for further references). The concept of "fear of fear" explains the large variety of situations that agoraphobic patients fear: They are not afraid of the situation itself, but they are afraid of having a panic attack. Therefore, they start to avoid situations in which a panic attack is likely or would have severe social or physical consequences. Since the "fear of fear" hypothesis was developed in relation to agoraphobia, the authors were mostly interested in panic attacks occurring in feared situations and avoidance behavior. Thus, they elaborated less on what factors lead to "spontaneous" panic. Current psychophysiological models which were developed to explain spontaneous as well as situational attacks take into account that some anxiety attacks occur without preceding anxiety and explicitly address fluctuations in symptomatology (e.g., "good" and "bad" days). Thus, they avoid some of the problems of overprediction of the "fear of fear" hypothesis (see also Clark 1988).

Psychophysiological models of panic attacks are characterized as follows:

1. In contrast to current medical models (for a review see Margraf et al. 1986a), it is generally not assumed that panic attacks are a distinct form of anxiety qualitatively different from fear or anticipatory anxiety.
2. Panic attacks are seen as the result of a positive feedback loop between certain internal cues (body sensations or cognitive events) that the person associates with immediate threat or danger, and the resulting anxiety reaction.
3. It is assumed that psychological interventions that change the person's responses to anxiety symptoms by habituation or reinterpretation are effective in the treatment of panic attacks. This is again in contrast to current medical models that assume that medication is necessary to treat the postulated biological malfunction underlying panic attacks.

Figure 1 shows a schematic presentation of our current understanding of the psychophysiological model. The central part of the schema shows a positive feedback loop (illustrated by black arrows in Fig. 1) leading to a panic attack. Its components are physiological, cognitive, and emotional responses of the panicking person. Note that the positive feedback may start with any of its following components.

- Physiological or cognitive changes occur as a consequence of various causes such as physical effort, drug intake (e. g., caffeine), situational stressors (for example, heat), or emotional responses (e. g., anger or anxiety).
- The person perceives such changes. Note that patients may feel changes in their body sensations even in the absence of physiological changes. For example, patients might feel that their

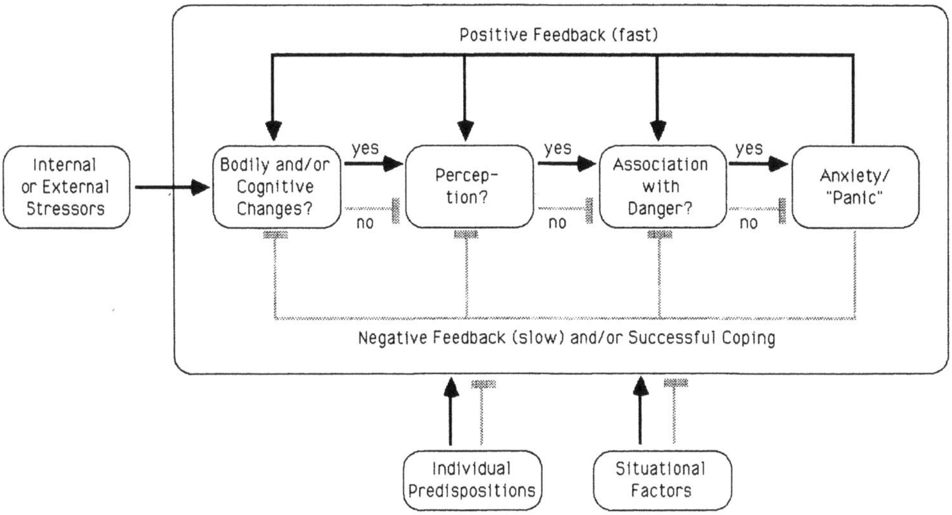

Fig. 1. Schematic presentation of the psychophysiological model of panic attacks. *Black arrows* represent facilitatory, *grey arrows* inhibitory influences. For further explanations see text

heart rate has accelerated after going to bed because changes in body posture have increased their cardiac awareness.

- The bodily changes or cognitive symptoms are associated with threat or danger. Clark (1986) emphasizes the immediate nature of the anticipated threat. Note that this association can take various forms ranging from conditioning (Goldstein and Chambless 1978; van den Hout and Griez 1983; Barlow 1986; Margraf et al. 1986b) to catastrophic misinterpretations in conscious thoughts (Ottaviani and Beck 1987; Clark 1986; Goldstein and Chambless 1978; Margraf et al. 1986b). The positive feedback may start at this level when situational variables are associated with immediate threat (see below). For example, simple phobics may experience a panic attack when confronted with their phobic stimulus. In agoraphobic patients, the phobic situations are probably only indirectly associated with danger through the association with body sensations (Foa and Kozak 1986).
- The person responds to the perceived threat with anxiety that in turn leads to physiological changes, body sensations, and/or cognitive symptoms (positive feedback).
- If these symptoms are again perceived and associated with danger, further anxiety increases occur. The patient's anxiety influences these processes. Thus, positive feedback operates at all the stages discussed above.
- The positive feedback may escalate into a panic attack. Note that is a fast process. It is unclear, at what point anxiety should be called panic. We think that this is a question of severity. We have argued elsewhere that from our laboratory and ambulatory monitoring data, panic attacks do not seem to be an all-or-none phenomenon (Ehlers et al. 1987). Again, the patients' perception and appraisal of their body sensations and of situational variables influence whether they call their anxiety panic (see below).

Panic attacks are time-limited phenomena. The positive feedback model does not explain what terminates a panic attack. Therefore, we have to assume parallel processes that counterbalance the effects of positive feedback. Two kinds of processes seem relevant: negative feedback mechanisms and the patient's coping strategies.

- Negative feedback mechanisms are a well-known phenomenon in physiology. We assume that such mechanisms operate during panic attacks and counterbalance the positive feedback (grey arrows in Fig. 1). Physiological and psychological negative feedback influences all of the components involved in the positive feedback loop and leads to a reduction in anxiety. The negative feedback operates more slowly than the positive feedback. Thus, a panic attack may rapidly develop, but anxiety will decrease with time. Examples for negative feedback processes are habituation and fatigue both of which decrease physiological responses. An example for negative feedback influencing the association with danger is that patients may notice after a while that no catastrophic consequence of their palpitations has occurred.

  Parallel to negative feedback mechanisms, successful coping strategies will decrease anxiety (grey arrows in Fig. 1). Again, coping attempts may influence any of the components of the positive feedback loop. An example for coping strategies influencing physiological symptoms is paced breathing. Distraction strategies, for example, focusing the attention on external cues, operate at the perceptual level. Cognitive strategies such as reattribution of bodily sensations affect the association with danger. A very common coping strategy is avoidance of help-seeking behavior that changes the situational context in which anxiety occurred.
- Note that failure of coping may, on the other hand, increase anxiety. When the patients notice that they experience dizziness or palpitations or feel anxious in spite of attempts to control these sensations, this may feed into the positive feedback cycle.

A number of variables determine the probability of a person experiencing a panic attack:

Internal or external stressors: Their presence will increase the probability of physiological or cognitive events that may trigger the positive feedback loop.

Individual predispositions: These include *biological* predispositions that will influence the likelihood of body sensations like disturbances of noradrenergic function (Charney and Heninger 1986); physical fitness (Taylor et al., in press); specific organic dysfunctions like vestibular dysfunction (Jacob et al. 1985); drug tolerance or intolerance (e. g., caffeine; Boulenger et al. 1984); and genetic factors (Marks 1986). *Psychological* predispositions such as anxious expectations (e.g., Lazarus and Averill 1972; Epstein 1972), selective attention to threat cues (see below), attributional styles, lack of assertiveness (Goldstein and Chambless 1978), learned associations (e.g., Breggin 1964), and coping strategies (e.g., Lazarus and Averill 1972; Epstein 1972) also influence whether body sensations occur and whether they are perceived and associated with threat. Psychological predispositions like the patients' learning history (reinforcement and modeling) with respect to somatic symptoms and emotional experiences influence whether they report panic attacks and seek help for them (cf. cross-cultural studies on report of pain; Melzack and Wall 1973).

Situational factors: Various situational variables determine whether body sensations are perceived (e.g., body posture, complexity of concurrent external stimulation). Furthermore, situational variables influence whether body sensations are associated with danger (e.g., the presence of a spouse or therapist, being in a situation where escape is difficult like driving on a freeway or standing in line in a crowded supermarket, the availability of explanations for the body sensations like physical exercise, and availability of coping resources such as medication or relaxation). Finally situational variables can in themselves be associated with danger and trigger a panic attack (see above).

Empirical Support for the Psychophysiological Models

Evidence from Interview and Questionnaire Studies

Psychophysiological models would predict that patients usually experience unpleasant body sensations *before* the full-blown panic attack. Studies using structured interviews support this hypothesis. Hibbert (1984) found that the most frequently reported sequence of events in panic attacks was the perception of an unpleasant body sensation (e.g., dyspnea, palpitations, or sweaty hands) followed by anxious catastrophizing cognitions and the full-blown picture of a panic attack. An unpublished study from our laboratory replicated this result (Zucker et al.). Similarly, Ley (1985) found that somatic symptoms preceded fear in the majority of patients interviewed. Ottaviani and Beck (1987) could identify specific misattributions of physical sensations as panic triggers in each of 30 patients.

The latter finding leads us to a second prediction from psychophysiological models: Panic patients are more likely than controls to associate body sensations with danger. Questionnaire studies by Clark et al., Foa and coworkers, and van den Hout et al. (see their chapter in this book), support this hypothesis. Similarly, Chambless et al. (1984) and McNally and Lorenz (1987) found that agoraphobics with panic attacks report more fear of body sensations than controls. McNally and Foa (1987) and Clark et al. (see their chapter in this book) demonstrated that agoraphobics and panic patients tend to misinterpret ambiguous scenes (McNally and Foa) or body symptoms (Clark) in a catastrophic fashion when chosing from a series of alternatives.

Thus, cognitive distortions may be involved in the association between anxiety, body sensations, and danger during panic attacks. There is evidence that catastrophic misinterpretations do indeed occur during panic attacks. In the studies of Beck et al. (1974), Hibbert (1984), Ottaviani and Beck (1987), Rapee (1985b), Rachman et al. (1987), and Zucker et al. (unpublished), patients reported catastrophic ideation during panic attacks that centered around physical (e.g., death, heart attack) or mental (e.g., losing control, going crazy) catastrophes. Patients with generalized anxiety disorder (Hibbert, Rapee) or nonclinical subjects (Zucker et al.) reported different thought patterns for their anxiety episodes. In the Zucker et al. study, 20 panic disorder patients were compared with 10 controls who were free of any history of psychiatric disorders. Patients reported thoughts that centered around physical or mental crises, loss of control, and need to escape. In contrast, thoughts of controls were more focused on external events like time constraints. The studies of the Beck group found that the majority of panic patients also described imagery that was closely related to the catastrophic ideation. Evidence for imagery was less clear in the Hibbert and Zucker studies. Questionnaire studies are in line with the interview results. Agoraphobics with panic attacks reported having more catastrophic ideation when being anxious than controls (Chambless et al. 1984; McNally and Lorenz 1987). Rachman et al. (1987) found that the cluster of bodily sensations and cognitions that patients reported during panic attacks induced by exposure to feared situations was meaningfully linked.

Thus, the interview and questionnaire data collected so far support the psychophysiological models of panic attacks. However, without further support from experimental studies, the evidence is not conclusive because it depends on the patients' recollections of their panic attacks. In addition, questionnaire and interview studies assess conscious processes while the reported "spontaneity" demonstrates that patients have only limited insight into what triggers panic. Thus, at least some of the processes involved in panic might not be accessible by introspection.

Evidence from Experiments

Recent experimental data support the validity of the questionnaire findings described above. Consistent with the psychophysiological model, the anticipation of anxiety in itself induces anxiety and its physiological concomitants in panic disorder patients to a larger degree than in controls (Ehlers et al. 1988b). Patients and controls had to breathe room air through a gask mask on two different occasions. On the 2nd test day they were informed that they would receive carbon dioxide at some point of the inhalation period that could induce anxiety and bodily symptoms. In contrast, they knew that they would only receive room air on the 1st day. Patients showed larger increases in self-reported anxiety and cardiovascular measures only on the 2nd test day, i.e., in anticipation of the anxiety induction procedure.

In another study, panic patients and controls were given false feedback of an abrupt heart rate increase. Only the patients responded with increases in anxiety and physiological arousal (Ehlers et al. 1988a). One patient even experienced a severe panic attack in response to the false feedback (Margraf et al. 1987a). These studies show that a positive feedback loop can be triggered when patients believe that bodily changes have occurred or when they expect to become anxious. Patients were more prone to respond in the direction of positive feedback than controls.

These results are in line with those of Clark et al. and Foa (see their chapter in this book) who found that panic patients show larger anxiety responses than controls when reading word pairs of bodily symptoms and catastrophes (Clark) or during imagery of panic symptoms (Foa). In addition, Clark et al. used a contextual priming task and found that patients reacted faster to catastrophic misinterpretations of bodily sensations than to neutral interpretations suggesting a bias to interpret bodily symptoms as dangerous.

Further support for the psychophysiological models comes from a research area that used to be primarily associated with medical models of panic. The results from so-called panic induction studies that attempt to provoke anxiety by application of biochemical substances such as sodium lactate or carbon dioxide are consistent with the psychophysiological models (Margraf et al. 1986b; Clark 1986; van den Hout 1988). As all of these procedures induce various unpleasant physical sensations, they can be interpreted as a powerful way to trigger the positive feedback loop described above. Thus, it is not necessary to assume a direct biochemical effect on anxiety to explain the anxiety-inducing effects of pharmacologic panic-provocation. The psychophysiological model has the advantage that it explains the variety of procedures that induce panic and, in some cases, have opposite physiological effects (e. g., hyperventilation and lactate infusion induce alkalosis, whereas inhalation of 5% CO_2 induces mild acidosis; Ehlers et al. 1986a).

In addition, there are results from panic induction studies that cannot be accounted for by a pure biological interpretation. For example, response to panic induction methods is modified by the subject's expectations. This was demonstrated by manipulating the experimental instructions in healthy subjects (van den Hout and Griez 1982; van der Molen et al. 1986) as well as in panic patients (Margraf et al., in press; Rapee et al., in press). In the study of Margraf et al., patients were more affected by the expectancy manipulation than controls. A recent study from Barlow's laboratory (Sanderson et al; submitted) demonstrated that the patients' response to carbon dioxide depends on their sense of control. When panic patients thought they had control over CO_2 delivery, few of them panicked - although they never used the control mechanism. In contrast, when they knew that they had no control the majority reported a panic attack. Furthermore, medical models cannot explain the case reports of Guttmacher and Nelles (1984) and Shear and Fyer (1987) that patients who had "panicked" during sodium lactate infusion before treatment did not "panic" in response to lactate after successful behavior therapy. Furthermore, they do not explain the efficacy of repeated lactate infusion or CO_2 inhalation in the treatment of panic attacks or other anxiety states (Bonn et al. 1973; Griez and van den Hout 1986).

Overall, experimental evidence presented here supports psychophysiological models of panic attacks. In addition, there is a large literature on the relationship of hyperventilation and panic attacks that is in line with a psychophysiological perspective. This literature is reviewed in detail elsewhere (Bass et al., in press; Ley 1987; Rapee, in press).

Evidence from Treatment Studies

There has been controversy between proponents of medical and psychophysiological models whether panic attacks can be successfully treated without giving medication. This question has only recently been addressed by systematic treatment studies. In the large literature on treatment of agoraphobia, for a long time, little emphasis was placed on panic attacks. While the efficacy of exposure therapy in the reduction of agoraphobic avoidance behavior was clearly demonstrated - with follow-ups of up to 9 years (e.g., Burns 1983; Emmelkamp and Kuipers 1979; Fiegenbaum 1986; Goldstein 1982; Hand et al. 1974, 1986; Mathews et al. 1977; McPherson et al. 1980; Michelson et al. 1985; Munby and Johnston 1980), few studies have assessed the effect of the treatment procedures on panic attacks. In their 1984 review, Jacob and Rapport identified only eight studies that reported results on panic attacks. Six of these studies found improvement in panic frequency and/or severity after exposure treatment. Since the focus was agoraphobic avoidance behavior, measures of panic attacks were often unsatisfactory and the results should only be considered preliminary. More recent studies that used better assessment of panic attacks usually found positive effects of exposure to anxiety-provoking situations on panic frequency and intensity (Telch et al. 1985; Michelson et al. 1985; Lelliott et al. 1987; Marchione et al. 1987). No effect was found in the study by Arnow et al. (1985).

In the last few years a number of single-case (Griez and van den Hout 1983; Rapee 1985a; Waddell et al. 1984) and group studies (Barlow et al. 1984; Bonn et al. 1984; Clark et al. 1985; Gitlin et al. 1985; Griez and van den Hout 1986; Öst 1988; Salkovskis et al. 1986; Sartory 1985; Sokol-Kessler and Beck, cited from Ottavani and Beck 1987) have been presented that demonstrated the efficacy of cognitive-behavioral treatments of panic attacks. Treatment components included education about panic attacks and treatment rationale, exposure to feared internal and external stimuli, cognitive therapy, controlled respiration, methods to increase vagal tone, and relaxation techniques. The most common outcome criteria were diary reports of panic frequency and intensity. All studies found marked and stable improvement or complete remission. Follow-ups ranged from 3 months to 2 years. Interestingly, most studies found further gains during follow-up. For further evidence from more recent treatment studies see the chapters by Barlow, Clark et al., Fiegenbaum, and Shear et al. in this book.

Although some of the studies used very small samples, the consistency of the results is impressive. Thus, there is sufficient evidence to conclude that cognitive-behavioral treatments are effective in the treatment of panic attacks. However, treatment effectiveness can only be seen as an indirect support of the psychophysiological models. First, the treatment mechanism remains unclear. Second, even with a purely metabolic etiology of panic attacks psychological treatments could be effective. However, the efficacy of psychological treatments clearly contradicts the assumption of proponents of medical models that medication is necessary to treat panic attacks.

Possible Specification 1: Role of Interoception

In the psychological literature on panic attacks we often read that panic patients suffer from interoceptive fears. Psychophysiological models usually start with explaining what happens *after* the patient has perceived certain changes in his body or cognitive functioning. Thus, little is said about the perceptual process itself. As we will outline here, we think that it is worthwhile to study the process of perception of bodily changes in this population.

There are several reasons to study interoception in persons with panic attacks: First, individual differences in interoception may be one factor involved in the *etiology* of panic disorder. One problem with the psychophysiological model is that usually people have only limited awareness of their bodily functions like cardiac or gastrointestinal activity, especially if these processes are within their normal range of functioning. We therefore have to specify conditions that influence whether a panic patient experiences body sensations. It is conceivable that panic patients differ from other people in their ability to detect changes in their bodily functions like heart rate increases or arrhythmias. Individual differences in interoception could influence the probability of people developing concerns about their heart as well as the probability of positive feedback in the sense of the psychophysiological model. It is also possible that persons who have experienced spontaneous panic attacks will begin to monitor their internal state more closely (e. g., by taking their pulse repeatedly or by shifting their attentional focus). Again, this could increase the probability of positive feedback. Thus, interoception could be involved in the etiology and/or maintenance of panic attacks.

Second, interoception is important for the *treatment* of panic disorder. Several of the psychological interventions include self-control techniques such as controlled breathing (Salkovskis et al. 1986), stimulation of vagal tone (Sartory 1985), or relaxation (Barlow et al. 1984; Gitlin et al. 1985; Öst 1988). These techniques require the patients' ability to monitor their bodily state and to decide when to use the techniques. The same applies to medication prescribed on a p.r.n. basis. Third, interoception may be a *prognostic* factor in panic disorder. Little is known about predictors of long-term outcome in panic patients or persons with infrequent panic attacks. The ability of a person to detect changes in bodily functions may be one factor influencing prognosis.

In the following, we will discuss cardiac awareness as an example of the possible role of interoception in panic disorder. Cardiac awareness is especially relevant since palpitations are the most commonly reported symptom of panic attacks. In a recent diary study, palpitations were reported in 68% of 175 recorded attacks (Margraf et al. 1987b). Do patients with panic disorder differ from controls in their cardiac awareness? If we look at the patients' self-reports, the answer is yes. Panic patients report to be much more aware of sensations from their heart than nonanxious control subjects (King et al. 1986).

There is a lack of studies corroborating self-reports by objective tests of cardiac perception. The literature on interoception shows that untrained subjects show generally poor cardiac perception (Katkin 1985). There is some, although inconsistent, evidence that persons with high state anxiety show better heart beat perception (Schandry 1981) and that persons with good cardiac perception are emotionally more responsive than poor perceivers (Schandry 1983; Katkin 1985). However, it was generally found that correlations between self-reported awareness of bodily function and objectively measured visceral sensitivity are very small (for example, McFarland 1975; Whitehead et al. 1977). It is unclear whether these results in nonclinical populations also apply to panic disorder patients.

Studies of cardiac awareness in patients with anxiety disorders are sparse. Tyrer et al. (1980) compared 23 patients with anxiety neurosis, 19 patients with phobias (including agoraphobia), and 18 patients with hypochondriasis. Subjects rated their perception of heart rate ten times after exposure to short film segments showing either driving through the city at different speeds or a swan on a river. Their ten ratings were individually correlated with their objective heart rates. Patients with anxiety neurosis and hypochondriasis showed higher correlations than phobic patients. Patients whose primary somatic symptoms were cardiac sensations reached the highest correlations. Despite some methodological weaknesses (small number of assessments, unclear diagnostic criteria), the study supports the idea that there might be systematic differences in cardiac perception between diagnostic groups. However, we cannot draw conclusions from this study unequivocally about cardiac awareness in panic patients because both anxiety neurotics and agoraphobics experience panic attacks.

A recent study by Harbauer-Raum (1987) is more definitive. She assessed 27 patients with cardiac neurosis, a diagnosis that probably represents a subgroup of panic disorder (Buller et al. 1987). In the laboratory, these patients performed better in a heart beat perception task (counting their heart beats without taking their pulse) than 16 normal controls. They were also better than controls and patients with mitral valve prolapse ($n = 27$) in detecting cardiac arrythmias occurring during 24-h ECG monitoring. The latter result was subsequently refined by Stalmann et al. (1987) who found that patients with cardiac neurosis ($n = 25$) noticed cardiac arrhythmias better than control subjects ($n = 14$) and patients with hyperthyreosis ($n = 5$) or autonomic neuropathy ($n = 12$). Cardiac neurotics detected ventricular extrasystoles but not tachycardias better than patients with mitral-valve prolapse ($n = 23$).

It is uncertain whether these results can be generalized to the entire population of panic disorder patients. The diagnosis of cardiac neurosis is given to a patient group much more homogeneous with respect to their interpretation of cardiac sensations. Furthermore, not all panic patients are primarily concerned about their cardiac function. There are other reasons to believe that such a generalization may not be valid. Most importantly, we found a discrepancy between patients' reports of palpitations in the majority of panic attacks and concurrent heart rate recordings. Based on the patients' descriptions of panic attacks, we usually assume that panic attacks are accompanied by abrupt and large increases in heart rate as observed in single cases (Cohen et al. 1985; Lader and Mathews 1970; Margraf et al. 1987a). Taylor et al. (1986), however, found that this only applies to a subgroup of panic attacks. More recently, we recorded heart rates and levels of physical activity in a larger sample of 44 naturally occuring panic attacks using a portable microcomputer (Margraf et al. 1987b). We found that, on the average, spontaneous panic attacks were not accompanied by heart rate increases. During panic attacks occurring in feared situations, mild heart rate elevations were observed compared to a matched period 24 h later, but these elevations were already present during the 15 min preceding the attacks and may be accounted for by increased levels of physical activity.

In addition, results from other studies cast doubt on a high visceral awareness of panic disorder patients. In our studies, patients tended to report physical symptoms indiscriminately (Ehlers et al. 1986b). Other studies have shown that there is a substantial overlap between hyperventilation and panic disorder (see reviews of Bass et al. in press; Ley 1987; and Rapee, in press). In this literature, it is usually assumed that the patients are unaware of their hyperventilation, i.e., show poor interoception in this respect.

Thus, previous research on interoception in disorders related to panic attacks has shown inconsistent if not contradictory findings. We have therefore started a research program designed to study cardiac awareness in carefully diagnosed patients with panic disorder and persons with infrequent panic attacks. We combine a cross-sectional with a longitudinal study. Preliminary results of the cross-sectional part are presented below.

The first two studies conducted at Stanford University compared patients with panic disorder and normal controls that were free of any history of psychiatric disorders. Subjects were asked to do a heart-rate perception test at the beginning and end of a psychophysiological laboratory assessment. Subjects were instructed to match the rate of a train of tone pips to their heart rate without actually taking their pulse. The task was similar to a procedure developed by Porges and Raskin (1969). Subjects were given 1 min to complete the test using a dial with a range from 1 to 10. In the first study, the dial was set at 5 (equalling 60 bpm) before the subject started. Between the first and second test, subjects received 6 min of true and 2 min of false heart rate feedback as described in Ehlers et al. (1988a). The results from this study (based on 24 patients and 24 controls) are shown in Fig. 2 (study 1). Performance in the heart rate perception test was assessed by the absolute difference between the real and the estimated heart rate (in beats per minute, bpm).

In study 1, there was no overall difference in accuracy between the groups. However, controls but not patients improved their estimations after receiving heart rate feedback. The vast majority of subjects in both the patient and control groups, underestimated their heart rates. We were concerned that the setting of the dial might have biased the subjects' estimations. Therefore, we repeated the experiment starting with a dial setting of 120 bpm. In this study, no heart rate feedback was given. The preliminary analysis of 22 patients and 16 controls is shown in Fig. 2 (study 2). There were no significant group or time effects or interactions in the ANOVA. As in study 1, the majority of subjects underestimated their heart rates.

Thus, the studies showed that both patients and controls are generally inaccurate in their heart rate estimations. If we compare the results of studies 1 and 2,

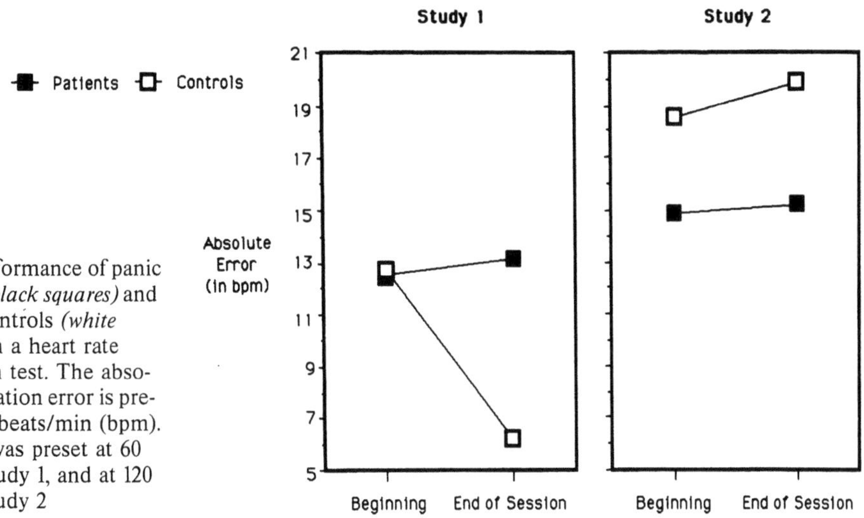

Fig. 2. Performance of panic patients *(black squares)* and normal controls *(white squares)* in a heart rate perception test. The absolute estimation error is presented in beats/min (bpm). The dial was preset at 60 bpm in study 1, and at 120 bpm in study 2

however, it appears that patients were more stable in their judgements than controls. Controls were more influenced by the heart rate feedback and by the setting of the dial. When the two protocols were compared in an overall ANOVA, a significant group × protocol interaction was found. Thus, although patients are inaccurate in their heart rate estimations, they seem to be less influenced by external information in making these judgements. One reason for this may be that they rely more on internal information than controls.

Before final conclusions are drawn from these studies we have to bear in mind, however, that the test of cardiac perception has a number of disadvantages. First, it involves matching of an external and an internal signal. Thus, the task is more complex and requires further stages of information processing beyond accurate interoception (for example, the subject's abilities to monitor two signals at the same time, to compare two rhythms, to compare between two modes of perception, and/or to remember rhythms). Second, the task involves motor activity that in itself has an impact on the subject's heart rate.

We have started a new study at Philipps University (Marburg) using different methods to assess heart rate perception. One of the tests we use is the "heart rate tracking" method described by Schandry (1981). Subjects are asked to count their heart beats repeatedly during signalled intervals of 35, 25, and 45 s without taking their pulse and without knowledge of the number of seconds in these intervals. This task was used by Harbauer-Raum (1987), who found superior heart rate perception in patients with cardiac neurosis as described above. Preliminary analyses of this test showed a trend towards a higher percentage of panic patients classified as good cardiac perceivers compared to infrequent panickers and normal controls. There was no indication of better cardiac perception in infrequent panickers.

Thus, while panic patients insist that they are very aware of cardiac sensations, it is unclear whether these sensations reflect objectively measurable changes in cardiac function. The evidence collected so far suggests that good cardiac perception is only found in a subgroup of panic patients. In these patients, however, excessive awareness of cardiac sensations may be one of the factors contributing to the maintenance of the disorder.

Possible Specification 2: Role of Selective Information Processing

Several studies using methods developed in experimental cognitive psychology have demonstrated that anxiety patients show an attentional bias towards threat cues related to their respective disorders. Burgess et al. (1981) used a dichotic listening task and found that six patients with social phobia or agoraphobia detected fear-relevant words (like "public speaking" or "shopping alone") in the unattended channel better than control groups of six nonanxious subjects and 12 psychology students with high scores on phobia scales. Similarly, in a study of Foa and McNally (1986), 11 obsessive-compulsive patients detected fear-relevant words like "feces" in the unattended channel better than control words and also showed larger skin conductance responses to these words. These differences disappeared after successul behavior therapy, indicating that the effects were not due to differences in familiarity with the stimulus material.

The pattern of results is in line with those of Watts et al. (1986a), who assessed reaction times of spider phobics and normal controls in a modified Stroop color-naming task. Before, but not after treatment, spider phobics showed a larger interference when color-naming words related to spiders such as "creepy" or "crawl." In contrast, interference was similar in both groups for the standard Stroop test (color words) or other control words. Deficits in the patients' recognition memory were less clear (Watts et al. 1986b). The subjects were shown dead spiders and had to recognize them later. Patients gave fewer correct answers for big spiders only. In a second experiment, this result was only partly replicated.

In a study of Streblow et al. (1985), phobic inpatients (type of phobia was not specified) and matched controls were presented slides showing three objects. Their task was to focus their attention on the central item and decide whether this object belonged to a previously given category. The central and/or peripheral objects were either neutral (such as plants, musical instruments) or phobia-relevant (such as insects). The reaction time analysis showed that untreated phobics, but not treated phobics or controls, identified phobia-relevant targets faster than neutral ones. Treated and untreated phobics were more distracted by phobia-relevant peripheral objects. In the case of negative decisions, phobics reacted more slowly when central or peripheral phobic objects were presented. In a second experiment, subjects had to decide whether words had been previously presented to them. In contrast to controls, phobic patients recognized phobia-relevant objects faster than control words. In addition, untreated phobics showed longer reaction times when they had to signal that a phobia-relevant word had not been previously presented.

Most relevant to the study of panic disorder is a series of experiments of Mathews, MacLeod, and coworkers on information processing in generalized anxiety disorder. Like panic patients, these patients suffer from severe anxiety not triggered by phobic situations. In reaction-time paradigms such as the Stroop color-naming task (Mathews and MacLeod 1985), dichotic listening (Mathews and MacLeod 1986), or a visual probe detection task combined with word reading (MacLeod et al. 1986), generalized anxiety patients showed an attentional bias for material representing social threat (words like "stupid," "hated") or physical threat (for example, "paralyzed" or "disease"). While patients shifted their attention to emotionally threatening material, controls tended to shift attention away from such material (MacLeod et al. 1986). The simultaneous presentation of threatening material interfered more with the patients' task performance than with that of controls (Mathews and MacLeod 1985, 1986). Interestingly, these attentional shifts could occur without the subjects' awareness: Patients could not recall or recognize the threat words better than controls (Mathews and MacLeod 1985, 1986) although they had responded to them differently.

In contrast to the consistent findings on attentional bias, evidence for memory bias in generalized anxiety is less clear. Mogg et al. (1987) studied active recall and recognition memory for positive and threatening adjectives that were either presented as self-relevant or relevant to another person. Previous findings in depression and students with social or test anxiety had suggested a self-referent recall bias favoring threatening words. However, anxiety patients tended to remember threatening material *less* well than controls. This finding is consistent with the trends found by Watts et al. (1986b) in spider phobics, and contrary to Mogg et al.'s predictions.

The findings on information processing in anxiety disorders can be summarized as follows: Patients with anxiety disorders detecd anxiety-relevant information in unattended material better or faster than neutral information (Burgess et al. 1981; Foa and McNally 1986; MacLeod et al. 1986; Mathews and MacLeod 1986; Streblow et al. 1985), while control groups did not show this response pattern. When anxiety patients were presented with task-irrelevant but anxiety-relevant information, larger interference with task performance was found than in controls, even when subjects were told to ignore this information (Watts et al. 1986a; Mathews and MacLeod 1985, 1986; Streblow et al. 1985). One interesting aspect concerns the type of stimulus material used: The studies in phobics or obsessive-compulsives used individualized material "tailored" to the specific content of the patients' fears, whereas the studies of the Mathews group used more general threat words that would probably be considered threatening by most subjects. While one could argue that the findings using individualized stimulus material were due to the fact that the material was irrelevant (not threatening) to the controls, but relevant (threatening) to the patients, this does not hold for the attentional bias found in generalized anxiety disorder.

Memory processess are probably less strongly affected than attentional processes in anxiety disorders. The studies cited above did not show differences in recognition memory for unattended material (Mathews and MacLeod 1985, 1986) even though differences in attention were found. If there is a memory bias, it operates in a different direction than the patients' attentional bias. It appears that anxious or phobic subjects may remember threatening material less well (Watts et al. 1986b; Mogg et al. 1987). Note that these authors used measures of the quality of recognition (number of correct answers or measures of discrimination), whereas Streblow et al. (1985) assessed the speed of recognition. In the latter study, phobic patients showed *faster* recognition of phobia-relevant words in the verification condition and *slower* recognition in the negative decision case. Unfortunately, hit/false alarm rates were not reported in the Streblow et al. study, and positive and negative decisions are combined in the data reported by Mogg et al. and Watts et al. Thus, the data from these different studies cannot be directly compared. Negative decisions seem to be a more complex task requiring more accurate and complex encoding of the material. It appears that the overall pattern of findings is consistent with the idea of poorer processing of threat material in anxiety disorders. The mechanisms of impaired processing such as poor focused attention, superficial processing, physiological defense reactions, or inhibition by cognitive avoidance strategies remain to be studied (cf. Mogg et al. 1987; Watts et al. 1986b). Overall, different biases seem to operate at different stages of information processing in anxiety disorders. Anxiety-relevant stimuli recruit attentional resources, but seem to be poorly processed.

The results reported here are directly relevant to the study of panic disorder. They might help in explaining the occurrence of panic attacks in the apparent absence of situational triggers. If panic disorder patients show similar attentional biases to threat cues as generalized anxiety patients, it is possible that information processing of threat cues without the patient's awareness is involved in triggering panic (cf. Mathews and MacLeod 1986). In terms of the psychophysiological model presented in Fig. 1, this would mean that we would have to assume an interaction between the perception of an internal or external cue and its association with danger: cues related to threat would more easily be detected.

We have started a research program designed to study attentional bias in panic patients and infrequent panickers (see also the chapter by Margraf and Ehlers in this book). In a first series of experiments (Ehlers et al., in press), we used a modified Stroop color-naming task similarly to the study of Mathews and MacLeod (1985). Subjects were asked to color-name cards (size A4) on which 96 words were written in red, blue, green, or yellow. Each card contained 12 different words. This series of words was repeated eight times in random order. Three of the six cards contained words related to threat of three categories: *Physical* threat words (such as "disease" or "fatal"; the word list used by Mathews and MacLeod 1985) were chosen because psychophysiological models emphasize the patient's fear of bodily symptoms or disease. Words related to *separation* ("separation," "lonely") were included because of Klein's theory that panic disorder is a form of separation anxiety (Klein 1980; for a review Margraf et al. 1986a). Finally, words related to social *embarrassment* were tested because of the patients' frequent reports that they are afraid of doing something embarrassing when having a panic attack in public. For each of the cards, a control card was constructed with neutral or positive words matched for word frequency and length (such as "leisure," "alert," "faithful," or "optimism"). The cards were presented in balanced order with the instruction to name the word colors as fast as possible without making mistakes, and without attending to the word content. The time it took subjects to color-name each of the cards was taken (in s). After the test, subjects answered a recognition questionnaire containing the 72 words shown on the cards plus 72 other (distractor) words.

Table 1 shows a comparison of 24 patients with panic disorder and 24 controls. The time it took subjects to color-name physical threat words and control words is presented. In an overall ANOVA comparing the two groups (group factor, patients vs controls), the experimental conditions (threat vs control word), and type of threat (physical vs separation vs embarrassment), we found significant group × condition ($P < 0.005$) and type × condition ($P < 0.05$) interactions. Further analyses showed that the group × condition interaction resulted from larger interference with threat words in the patient

Table 1. Stroop color-naming task. Mean time (s) and standard deviations

	Patients		Controls	
	M	SD	M	SD
Physical threat words	76.3	15.6	70.8	13.0
Control words	72.1	15.3	71.0	9.6

group. However, significantly larger interference was only found for *physical* threat, not for the two social threat conditions.

In another study comparing nonclinical panickers and controls, we also found larger interference in panickers when color-naming physical threat words than in controls. Responses to neutral control words and standard Stroop task (color words) were similar in both groups. In neither study, a difference in recognition memory between the groups was found. On the recognition questionnaire, both groups identified more threat words correctly than control words.

Thus, there is preliminary evidence for selective information processing of physical threat cues in panic disorder. Panic disorder patients as well as nonclinical panickers showed an attentional bias towards threat-related material. That physical threat words had a larger impact on the patient's performance than social threat words underlines the role of the association between bodily symptoms and danger in panic disorder postulated by psychophysiological models.

Summary and Conclusions

Evidence supporting a psychophysiological perspective of panic attacks is rapidly accumulating. Questionnaire and interview studies, experimental procedures, and treatment trials have yielded converging results. A challenge for future specifications of current models is to *predict* whether a person will have a panic attack in a given period of time. At present, the psychophysiological model seems most powerful in explaining panic attacks retrospectively.

We have outlined two areas of research that seem promising in specifying psychophysiological models. First, the role of interoception should be studied since the models give bodily sensations a central role in the positive feedback loop assumed to lead to panic. In this chapter, we have discussed the relation of self-reported and objectively assessed cardiac awareness in panickers and controls. We found that while panic patients report more than controls that they are generally very aware of sensations from their heart, they are not generally better cardiac perceivers in objective tests of cardiac awareness. Several open questions need to be answered. First, what do patients mean when they say that they are generally very aware of sensations from their heart? Do they mean that they feel their heart beat usually, often, or sometimes? When they speak of sensations from their heart, do they mean heart beats, changes in their heart rate, or arrhythmias? Or is it rather that their pulse sensations make them anxious? These different aspects of self-reported interoception should be distinguished (see the concept of anxiety probability and sensitivity, Reiss and McNally 1985).

Future studies are needed to clarify the role of accurate vs inaccurate interoception in panic disorder. It is possible that only in some patients accurate perceptions of internal cues trigger panic. Our studies have shown that only a subgroup of panic disorder patients seems to show accurate cardiac perception. Nevertheless, this variable could be an important factor in the maintenance of their panic attacks. This subgroup of patients is likely to perceive changes in their cardiac function like fast or strong heart beats that could trigger panic attacks depending on the different factors described above. The etiology of panic attacks in patients who believe that they perceive their heart beat accurately, but who are objectively poor cardiac perceivers might be quite different. One factor contributing to attacks might be that the majority tends to underestimate their heart rates. Therefore, they might overrespond when their heart beat becomes perceptible, for instance, when lying in bed.

Future studies should also investigate the state-dependence of cardiac perception. It is possible that while most panic patients cannot monitor their cardiac function accurately in the usual laboratory condition, they may be more likely than controls to become aware of their heart beat under certain conditions such as changes in posture, drug intake, or anxiety. Another possibility is that while panic patients may usually not be more aware of their heart rate they might be more sensitive to changes in other cardiac parameters like stroke volume.

At present, the reasons for why there are higher percentages of good cardiac perceivers among patients with panic disorder compared to infrequent panickers remain unknown. It is possible that good cardiac perception in patients reflects a consequence of the disorder. For example, panic patients might train their cardiac perception by taking their pulse frequently. At the same time, good cardiac perception may be one of the factors increasing the probability for an infrequent panicker to develop more frequent panic attacks. Only prospective longitudinal studies can decide which of the interpretations is valid. We are currently studying this question in our prospective study of infrequent panickers.

A second area of great interest is the role of possible attentional and/or memory biases in panic disorder. Results from studies in other anxiety disorders point to two possible mechanisms that could account for the fact that patients are often not able to report triggers of their panic attacks. First, patients could have an attentional bias to threat cues that operates withouth their awareness. Second, they could show poor recall of triggering events because of impaired processing of these cues. Preliminary support for an attentional bias to physical threat cues comes from our Stroop experiments described above. However, there are alternative explanations for these results, such as differences in response bias or impaired performance efficiency by increased arousal (anxiety induction) in the panic groups. Therefore, we have to wait for replications using other paradigms before we can draw final conclusions. We are currently using the visual probe detection paradigm described by MacLeod et al. (1986) that rules out these alternative explanations. Furthermore, the paradigms described above have only used verbal stimulus material. Since psychophysiological models emphasize the role of bodily sensations as anxiety triggers it is desirable to study attentional bias to bodily cues directly.

Acknowledgements: Preparation of this paper was supported in part by the German Research Foundation (grant Eh 97/1-1 to Anke Ehlers) and by the Medical Research Service of the Veterans Administration. We thank Sylvia Davies, Gerhard Jakschik, Frank Wrobel, and Peter Zezula for their assistance in data collection, and Franziska Schneider and Peter Zezula for technical support.

References

American Psychiatric Association (1987) Diagnostic and statistical manual of mental disorders. Third edition – revised. APA Press, Washington, DC

Arnow BA, Taylor CB, Agras WS, Telch MJ (1986) Enhancing agoraphobia treatment outcome by changing couple communication patterns. Behav Ther 16:452–467

Barlow D (1986) A psychological model of panic. In: Shaw BF, Cashman F, Segal ZY, Yallis TM (eds) Anxiety disorder: theory, diagnosis, and treatment. Plenum, New York

Barlow DH, Cohen AS, Waddell Mt, Vermilyea BB, Klosko JS, Blanchard EB, DiNardo PA (1984) Panic and generalized anxiety disorders: Nature and treatment. Behav Ther 15:431–449

Bass C, Kartsoumis L, Lelliott P (in press) Hyperventilation and its relationship with anxiety and panic. Integrative Psychiatry

Beck AT, Laude R, Bohnert M (1974) Ideational components of anxiety neurosis. Arch Gen Psychiatry 31:319-325

Beck AT, Emery GD, Greenberg R (1985) Anxiety disorders and phobias: a cognitive perspective. Basic, New York

Bonn JA, Harrison J, Rees W (1973) Lactate infusion in the treatment of "free-floating" anxiety. Therapeutic application. Br J Psychiatry 119:468-470

Bonn JA, Readhead CPA, Timmons BA (1984) Enhanced adaptive behavioral response in agoraphobic patients pretreated with breathing retraining. Lancet 1984:665-669

Boulenger JP, Uhde TW, Wolff EA, Post RM (1984) Increased sensitivity to caffeine in patients with panic disorder. Arch Gen Psychiatry 41:1067-1071

Breggin PR (1964) The psychophysiology of anxiety. J Nerv Ment Dis 139:558-568

Buller R, Maier W, Benkert O (1978) Das Herzangst-Syndrom - ein Subtyp der Panik-Syndroms. In: Nutzinger DO, Pfersmann D, Welan T, Zapotoczky HG (eds) Herzphobie. Enke, Stuttgart, pp 42-49

Burgess IS, Jones LM, Robertson SA, Radcliff WN, Emerson E (1981) The degree of control exerted by phobic and non-phobic verbal stimuli over the recognition behaviour of phobics and non-phobic subjects. Behav Res Ther 19:233-243

Burns LE, Thorpe GL, Cavallero A, Gosling J (1983) Agoraphobia eight years after behavioral treatment: A follow-up study with interview, questionnaire and behavioral data. World Congress of Behavior Therapy, Washington, DC

Chambless DL, Caputo GC, Bright P, Gallagher R (1984) Assessment of fear of fear in agoraphobics: the Body Sensations Questionnaire and the Agoraphobic Cognitions Questionnaire. J Consult Clin Psychol 52:1090-1097

Clark DM (1986) A cognitive approach to panic. Behav Res Ther 24:461-470

Clark DM (1988) A cognitive model of panic attacks. In: Rachman S, Maser J (eds) Panic: psychological perspectives. Erlbaum, Hillsdale

Clark DM, Salkovskis PM, Chalkley AJ (1985) Respiratory control as a treatment for panic attacks. J Behav Ther Exp Psychiatry 16:23-30

Charney DS, Heninger GR (1986) Abnormal regulation of noradrenergic function in panic disorders. Arch Gen Psychiatry 43:1042-1054

Cohen AS, Barlow DH, Blanchard EB (1985) Psychophysiology of relaxation-associated panic attacks. J Abn Psychol 94:96-101

Ehlers A, Margraf J, Roth WT (1986a) Experimental induction of panic attacks. In: Hand I, Wittchen HU (eds) Panic and phobias: empirical evidence of theoretical models and long-term efficacy of behavioral treatments. Springer, Berlin Heidelberg New York, pp 53-66

Ehlers A, Margraf J, Roth WT, Taylor CB, Maddock RJ, Sheikh J, Kopell ML, McClenahan KL, Gossard D, Blowers GH, Agras WS, Kopell BS (1986b) Lactate infusions and panic attacks: do patients and controls respond differently? Psychiatry Res 17:295-308

Ehlers A, Margraf J, Roth WT, Taylor CB (1987) Psychophysiology of panic attacks. 27th Annual meeting of the Society for Psychophysiological Research, Amsterdam

Ehlers A, Margraf J, Roth WT, Taylor CB, Birbaumer N (1988a) Anxiety induced by false heart rate feedback in patients with panic disorder. Behav Res Ther 26:1-11

Ehlers A, Margraf J, Roth WT (1988b) Interaction of expectancy and stressors in a laboratory model of panic. In: Hellhammer C, Florin I, Weiner H (eds) Neurobiological approaches to human disease. Huber, Toronto, pp 379-384

Ehlers A, Margraf J, Davies S, Roth WT (in press). Selective processing of threat cues in subjects with panic attacks. Cognition and Emotion.

Emmelkamp PMG, Kuipers ACM (1979) Agoraphobia: A follow-up study four years after treatment. Br J Psychiatry 143:352-355

Epstein S (1972) The nature of anxiety with emphasis on its relationship to expectancy. In: Spielberger CD (ed) Anxiety. Academic, New York

Evans IM (1972) A conditioning model of common neurotic pattern - fear of fear. Psychother Theor Res Pract 9:238-241

Fenichel O (1945) Psychoanalytic theory of the neuroses. Norton, New York

Fiegenbaum W (1986) Longterm efficacy of exposure therapy in cardiac phobia. In: Hand I, Wittchen HU (eds) Panic and phobias: Empirical evidence of theoretical models and long-term efficacy of behavioral treatments. Springer, Berlin Heidelberg New York, pp 81-89

Foa EB, Kozak MJ (1986) Emotional processing of fear: exposure to corrective information. Psych Bull 99:20-35

Foa EB, McNally RJ (1986) Sensitivity to feared stimuli in obsessive-compulsives: a dichotic listening analysis. Cogn Ther Res 10:477-485

Frankl VE (1975) Paradoxical intention and dereflection. Psychotherapy 12:226-237

Freud S (1895) Über die Berechtigung von der Neurasthenie einen bestimmten Symptomkomplex als "Angstneurose" abzutrennen. In: Freud S (1952) Gesammelte Werke, vol 1. (Standard Edition, vol 3, p 85, Hogarth, London)

Gitlin B, Martin J, Shear MK, Frances A, Ball G, Josephson S (1985) Behavior therapy for panic disorder. J Nerv Ment Dis 173:742-743

Goldstein AJ (1982) Agoraphobia: Treatment successes, treatment failures, and theoretical implications. In: Chambless DL, Goldstein AJ (eds) Agoraphobia: multiple prespectives on theory and treatment. Wiley, New York

Goldstein AJ, Chambless DL (1978) A reanalysis of agoraphobia. Behav Ther 9:47–59

Griez E, van den Hout MA (1983) Treatment of phobophobia by exposure to CO_2-induced anxiety symptoms. J Nerv Ment Dis 173:742–743

Griez E, van den Hout MA (1986) CO_2 inhalation in the treatment of panic attacks. Behav Res Ther 24:145–150

Guttmacher LB, Nelles C (1984) In vivo desensitization of lactate-induced panic: a case study. Behav Ther 15:369–372

Hand I, Lamontagne Y, Marks I (1974) Group exposure (flooding) in vivo for agoraphobics. Br J Psychiatry 124:588–602

Hand I, Angenendt J, Fischer M, Wilke C (1986) Exposure in vivo with panic management: Treatment rationale and longterm outcome. In: Hand I, Wittchen HU (eds) Panic and phobias: empirical evidence of theoretica models and longterm efficacy of behavioral treatments. Springer, Berlin Heidelberg New York, pp 104–128

Harbauer-Raum U (1987) Wahrnehmung von Herzschlag und Herzarrhythmien – Eine Labor-Feldstudie an Patienten mit Herzphobie. In: Nutzinger DO, Pfersmann D, Welan T, Zapotoczky Hg (eds) Die Herzphobie, Enke, Stuttgart, pp 84–91

Hibbert GA (1984) Ideational components of anxiety. Br J Psychiatry 144:618–624

Jacob RG, Rapport MD (1984) Panic disorder: medical and psychological parameters. In: Turner SM (ed) Behavioral theories and treatment of anxiety. Plenum, New York

Jacob RG, Møller MB, Turner SM, Wall C (1985) Otoneurological examination in panic disorder and agoraphobia with panic attacks: a pilot study. Am J Psychiatry 142:715–720

Katkin ES (1985) Blood, sweat and tears: individual differences in autonomic self-perception. Psychophysiology 22:125–137

King R, Margraf J, Ehlers A, Maddock R (1986) Panic disorder – overlap with somatization disorder. In: Hand I, Wittchen HU (eds) Panic and phobias: empirical evidence of theoretical models and longterm efficacy of behavioral treatments. Springer, Berlin Heidelberg New York, pp 72–77

Klein DF (1980) Anxiety reconceptualized. Compreh Psychiatry 21:411–427

Lader MH, Mathews AM (1968) A physiological model of phobic anxiety and desensitization. Behav Res Ther 6:411–421

Lader MH, Mathews AM (1970) Physiological changes during spontaneous panic attacks. J Psychosom Res 14:377–382

Lazarus RS, Averill JR (1972) Emotion and cognition: With special reference to anxiety. In: Spielberger CD (ed) Anxiety. Academic, New York

Lelliott PT, Marks IM, Monteiro WO, Tsakiris F, Noshirvani H (1987) Agoraphobia 5 years after imipramine and exposure. Outcome and predictors. J Nerv Ment Dis 175:599–605

Ley R (1985) Agoraphobia, the panic attack and the hyperventilation syndrome. Behav Res Ther 23:79–81

Ley R (1987) Panic disorder: a hyperventilation interpretation. In: Michelson L, Ascher M (eds) Cognitive-behavioral assessments and treatment of anxiety disorders. Guilford, New York

MacLeod C, Mathews A, Tata P (1986) Attentional bias in emotional disorders. J Abn Psychol 95:15–20

Marchione KE, Michelson L, Greenwald M, Dancu C (1987) Cognitive behavioral treatment of agoraphobia. Behav Res Ther 25:319–328

Margraf J, Ehlers A (in press) Biological models of panic disorder and agoraphobia: Theory and evidence. In: Roth M, Burrows GD, Noyes R (eds) Handbook of anxiety, Vol. III. Elsevier, Amsterdam

Margraf J, Ehlers A, Roth WT (1986a) Biological models of panic disorder and agoraphobia: a review. Behav Res Ther 24:553–567

Margraf J, Ehlers A, Roth WT (1986b) Sodium lactate infusions and panic attacks: a review and critique. Psychosom Med 48:23–51

Margraf J, Ehlers A, Roth WT (1987a) Panic attack associated with perceived heart rate acceleration: a case report. Behav Ther 18:84–89

Margraf J, Taylor CB, Ehlers A, Roth WT, Agras WS (1987b) Panic attacks in the natural environment. J Nerv Ment Dis 175:558–565

Margraf J, Ehlers A, Roth WT (in press) Expectancy effects and hyperventilation as laboratory stressors. In: Florin I, Weiner H, Hellhammer D (eds) Frontiers of stress research. Huber, Toronto

Marks I (1987) Fears, phobias and rituals. Oxford University Press, New York

Mathews AM, MacLeod C (1985) Selective processing of threat cues in anxiety states. Behav Res Ther 23:563–569

Mathews AM, MacLeod C (1986) Discrimination of threat cues without awareness in anxiety states. J Abn Psychol 95:131–138

Mathews AM, Teasdale J, Munby M, Johnston DW, Shaw P (1977) A home-based treatment program for agoraphobia. Behav Ther 8:915–925

McFarland RA (1975) Heart rate perception and heart rate control. Psychophysiology 12:402-405

McNally RJ, Foa EB (1987) Cognition and agoraphobia: bias in the interpretation of threat. Cogn Ther Res 11:567-582

McNally RJ, Lorenz M (1987) Anxiety sensitivity in agoraphobics. J Behav Ther Exp Psychiatry 18:3-11

McPherson FM, Brougham I, McLaren S (1980) Maintenance of improvement of agoraphobic patients treated with behavioural methods - four year follow-up. Behav Res Ther 18:150-152

Melzack R, Wall PD (1973) The challenge of pain. Basic, New York

Michelson L, Mavissakalian M, Marchione K (1985) Cognitive and behavioral treatments of agoraphobia: Clinical and behavioral, and psychophysiological outcomes. J Consult Clin Psychol 53:913-925

Mogg K, Mathews A, Weinman J (1987) Memory bias in clinical anxiety. J Abn Psychol 96:94-98

Munby M, Johnston DW (1980) Agoraphobia: the long-term follow-up of behavioral treatment. Br J Psychiatry 137:418-427

Öst LG (1988) Applied relaxation vs progressive relaxation in the treatment of panic disorder. Behav Res Ther

Ottavani R, Beck AT (1987) Cognitive aspects of panic disorder. J Anxiety Disorders 1:15-28

Porges SW, Raskin DC (1969) Respiratory and heart rate components of attention. J Exp Psychol 81:497-503

Rachman S, Levitt K, Lopatka C (1987) Panic: the links between cognitions and bodily symptoms - I. Behav Res Ther 25:411-423

Rapee RM (1985a) A case of panic disorder treated with breathing retraining. J Behav Ther Exp Psychiatry 16:63-65

Rapee RM (1985b) Distinction between panic disorder and generalised anxiety disorder: clinical presentation. Aust N Z J Psychiatry 19:227-232

Rapee RM (in press) The psychological treatment of panic attacks: theoretical conceptualization and review of evidence. Clin Psychol Review

Rapee RM, Mattick R, Murrell E (in press) Cognitive mediation in the affective component of spontaneous panic attacks. J Behav Ther Exp Psychiatry

Reiss S, McNally RJ (1985) Expectancy model of fear. In: Reiss S, Bootzin RR (eds) Theoretical issues in behavior therapy. Academic, New York, pp 107-121

Salkovskis PM, Jones DRO, Clark DM (1986) Respiratory control in the treatment of panic attacks: replication and extension with concurrent measurement of behaviour and pCO_2. Br J Psychiatry 148:526-532

Sanderson WC, Rapee RM, Barlow DH (submitted) The influence of an illusion of control on panic attacks via inhalation of 5,5% carbon dioxideenriched air.

Sartory G (1985) Vagal innervation techniques in the treatment of panic attacks. 15th Annual meeting of the European Association for Behaviour therapy, Munich

Schandry R (1981) Heart beat perception and emotional experience. Psychophysiology 18:483-488

Schandry R (1983) On the relation between the improvement of cardiac perception and the increase of emotional experience. Psychophysiology 20:468

Shands HC, Schor N (1982) The modern syndrome of phobophobia and its management. In: Dupont RL (ed) Phobia: a comprehensive summary of modern treatments. Brunner and Mazel, New York

Shear MK, Fyer A (1987) Effects of cognitive-behavioral treatments on sodium-lactate response of panic patients. Preliminary findings. Symposium treatments of panic and phobias, Ringberg

Stalmann H, Hartl L, Pauli P, Strian F (1987) Perception of pathological cardiac activity. Psychophysiology 24:614

Streblow H, Hoffmann J, Kasielke E (1985) Experimentalpsychologische Analyse von Gedächtnisprozessen bei Phobikern. Z Psychol 193:147-161

Taylor CB, Sheikh J, Agras WS, Roth WT, Margraf J, Ehlers A, Maddock RJ, Gossard D (1986) Ambulatory heart rate changes in patients with panic attacks. Am J Psychiatry 143:478-482

Taylor CB, King R, Ehlers A, Margraf J, Clark D, Roth WT, Agras WS (in press) Treadmill exercise test and ambulatory monitoring in patients with panic attacks. Am J Cardiol

Telch MJ, Agras WS, Taylor CB, Roth WT, Gallen CC (1985) Combined pharmacological and behavioral treatment for agoraphobia. Behav Res Ther 23:325-335

Tyrer P, Lee I, Alexander J (1980) Awareness of cardiac function in anxious, phobic and hypochondriacal patients. Psychol Med 10:171-174

van den Hout MA (1988) The explanation of experimental panic. In: Rachman S, Maser J (eds) Panic: psychological perspectives. Erlbaum, Hillsdale

van den Hout MA, Griez E (1982) Cognitive factors in carbon dioxide therapy. J Psychosom Res 26:209-214

van den Hout MA, Griez E (1983) Some remarks on the nosology of anxiety states and panic disorder. Acta Psychiat Belg 83:33-42 van der Molen GM, van den Hout MA, Vroemen J, Lousberg H, Griez E (1986) Cognitive determinants of lactate-induced anxiety. Behav Res The 24:677–680

Waddell MT, Barlow DH, O'Brien GT (1984) A preliminary investigation of cognitive and relaxation treatment of panic disorder: effects on intense anxiety vs "background" anxiety. Behav Res Ther 22:393–402

Watts FN, McKenna FP, Sharrock R, Trezise L (1986a) Colour naming of phobia-related words. Br J Psychol 77:97–108

Watts FN, Trezise L, Sharrock R (1986b) Processing of phobic stimuli. Br J Clin Psychol 25:253–259

Westphal C (1871) Die Agoraphobie, eine neuropathische Erscheinung. Arch Psychiat Nervenkrankh 3:138–161

Whitehead WE, Drescher VM, Heriman P, Blackwell B (1977) Relation of heart rate, heart rate control and heart rate perception. Biodfeed Self-Reg 2:371–392

13. Tests of a Cognitive Theory of Panic

D. M. Clark, P. M. Salkovskis, M. Gelder, C. Koehler, M. Martin, P. Anastasiades, A. Hackmann, H. Middleton, and A. Jeavons

Panic attacks are one of the most distressing of all forms of anxiety. The sudden onset of attacks and the intense bodily sensations which accompany them often lead patients to think they are about to die, go crazy, or suffer some other catastrophe. The fact that some attacks also appear to occur without warning is additionally alarming to patients and was initially interpreted by research workers as an indication that the central disorder in panic is a neurochemical disturbance. This point of view received further support from work on the pharmacological induction and treatment of panic. However, a number of investigators (Barlow, in press; Beck et al. 1985; Clark 1979, 1986; Griez and van den Hout 1984; Margraf et al. 1986; Rapee 1987, Seligman 1988) have recently proposed psychological theories which can also account for the main features of panic. In the present paper we provide a brief overview of one of the these theories – the cognitive theory described by Clark (1986) – and describe a series of experiments testing central predictions derived from this theory. Readers who would like a more detailed exposition of the theory are referred to Clark (1986, 1988) and Salkovskis (1988).

Overview of a Cognitive Theory of Panic

The cognitive theory states that individuals who experience panic attacks do so because they have a relatively enduring tendency to interpret certain bodily sensations in a catastrophic fashion. The sensations which are misinterpreted are mainly those which can be involved in normal anxiety responses (e.g., palpitations, breathlessness, dizziness, parasthesias), but also include some other sensations. The catastrophic misinterpretation involves perceiving these sensations as much more dangerous than they really are, and in particular, interpreting the sensations as indicative of an *immediately* impending physical or mental disaster. For example, perceiving a slight feeling of breathlessness as evidence of impending cessation of breathing and consequent death; perceiving palpitations as evidence of an impending heart attack; perceiving a pulsing sensation in the forehead as evidence of a brain haemorrhage; or perceiving a shaky feeling as evidence of impending loss of control and insanity.

The specific sequence of events which it is suggested to occur in a panic attack is shown in Fig. 1. A wide range of stimuli appear to provoke attacks. These stimuli can be external (such as a supermarket) but more often are internal (body sensation, thought or image). If these stimuli are perceived as a sign of danger, a state of apprehension results. This state is associated with a wide range of bodily sensations. If these anxiety-produced sensations are interpreted in a catastrophic fashion, a further increase in apprehension occurs. This produces a further

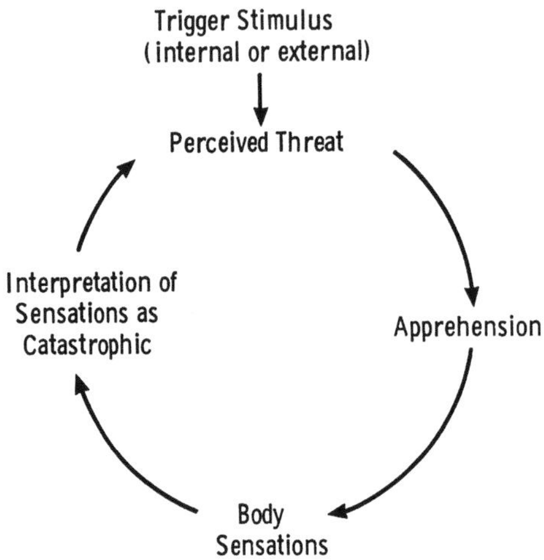

Fig. 1. The suggested sequence of events in a panic attack. (Reprinted with permission from Clark 1986, p 463)

increase in body sensations, leading to a vicious circle which culminates in an attack.

Once an individual has developed a tendency to catastrophically interpret bodily sensations, two further processes contribute to the maintenance of a panic disorder. First, because patients are frightened of certain sensations, they become hypervigilant and repeatedly scan their body for signs of danger. This internal focus of attention allows them to notice sensations which many other people would not be aware of. Once noticed, these sensations are taken as further evidence of the presence of some serious physical or mental disorder. Second, certain forms of avoidance also tend to maintain patients' negative interpretive style. This is true not only of patients who suffer from panic disorder with agoraphobia, but also of patients who suffer from panic disorder without agoraphobic avoidance. As Salkovskis (1988) has pointed out, these patients often engage in subtle forms of avoidance which tend to maintain their negative beliefs. For example, a patient who was preoccupied with the idea he may be suffering from cardiac disease avoided exercise (such as digging the garden) whenever he noticed a palpitation. He believed that this avoidance helped to prevent him from experiencing a heart attack. However, as he had no cardiac disease, it is more likely that the avoidance simply maintained his somatic preoccupation.

Different Types of Panic Attack

The model shown in Fig. 1 can account for both panic attacks which are preceded by a period of heightened anxiety and panic attacks which are not but instead appear "out of the blue." In both types of attack it is assumed that the crucial event is a misinterpretation of bodily sensations. In attacks preceded by heightened anxiety, these sensations are a consequence of the preceding anxiety, which in turn is due to anticipation of an attack *or* to some anxiety-evoking event which is unrelated to panic; such as an arguement with a spouse, or worrying about a work deadline. In the case of panic attacks which are not preceded by a period of heightened anxiety, the bodily sensations which are misinterpreted are initially caused either by a different emotional state (anger, excitement) or by some innocuous event such as drinking coffee (palpitations), getting up suddenly from a sitting position (dizziness, palpitations), or exercise (breathlessness, palpitations). In such attacks patients often fail to distinguish between the triggering bodily sensations and the subsequent panic attack and so perceive the attack as having no cause and coming "out of the blue." As Clark (1988) points out, this explanation can also be used to account for the occurrence of night-time attacks, in which the patient wakes up in a panic. Studies by Oswald (1966) have shown that we monitor the external world for personally significant sounds while asleep and tend to have our sleep disturbed or be woken by such sounds. It seems reasonable to suppose that we also monitor our *internal* environment for significant events. If this is the case, then an individual who is concerned about his heart might have a panic attack triggered by a palpitation which was detected and misinterpreted during sleep. He would then wake up in a state of panic[1].

Cognitive Theory and the Main Features of Panic

In previous reviews (Clark 1986, 1988), we have shown that the cognitive theory is consistent with most existing information on the nature of panic, including the sequence of events in an attack, the role of hyperventilation in panic, the success of sodium lactate and other pharmacological agents at inducing panic, and the results of existing research investigating possible biological dysregulation in panic disorder. Clark (1988) has also outlined the ways in which the cognitive theory differs from a simple fear of fear model and the hypothesized differences between the thinking of panic and non-panic hypochondriacal patients. An additional challenge for the cognitive theory is the apparent success of some pharmacological treatments for panic. Although still controversial (see, Telch 1988), it would appear that imipramine is effective in alleviating the attacks of some patients. This poses two questions for a cognitive theory. The first question is how to account for reductions in panic attacks which occur while patients are taking imipramine (or any other drug). This is relatively easy. Inspection of Fig. 1 reveals that there are several ways in which drugs could be effective in reducing the frequency of panic attacks. Blockade of, or exposure to, the bodily sensations which accompany anxiety, and a reduction in the frequency of bodily fluctuations which can trigger panic could all reduce panic while an individual is taking drugs. The second question is how can the theory account for any continued improvement in panic after drug withdrawal. When this occurs, the cognitive theory would hypothesize that the patients' thinking style has changed. It seems plausible that this might occur in some patients given drug treatment. For example, imagine a patient who initially believes that the cardiac sensations he experiences in an attack indicate he is suffering from a serious cardiac disease. If this patient sees a psychiatrist, is given a drug (such as imipramine) which he knows is not intended as cardiac medication and improves, he may revise his opinion and conclude that he does not have a cardiac disease. As therapists giving drug treatments do not specifically aim to promote cognitive change, we would expect that only a proportion of patients who improve while on drugs would change their pattern of thinking. The cognitive theory would predict that these patients would be particularly likely to remain well after discontinuation of the drug, while those patients who did not achieve cognitive change would relapse.

Experiments Testing Predictions Derived from the Cognitive Theory

The cognitive theory states that catastrophic misinterpretation of bodily sensations plays a causal role in the production of panic attacks. At least four major predictions follow from this statement.

---

[1] The authors are grateful to Donald Klein for pointing out that Freud's observation (in *The Interpretation of Dreams*) that individuals with a full bladder often dream that they are on the toilet is consistent with the notion that during sleep people scan their internal environment for personally significant sensations.

1. Panic patients will be more likely to interpret bodily sensations in a catastrophic fashion than individuals who do not experience panic attacks (such as non-panic anxious patients and normal controls).
2. During panic attacks, patients should experience thoughts concerned with the catastrophic interpretation of bodily sensations.
3. Within panic patients conditions which activate catastrophic misinterpretations should lead to an increase in anxiety and panic.
4. Panic attacks can be prevented by reducing patients' tendency to interpret bodily sensations in a catastrophic fashion.

Recently, we have started a programme of research which will test these predictions. The preliminary results of our research and some relevant research from other research groups are described below.

Prediction 1

Two experiments have tested this prediction. In the first experiment, we used a questionnaire to compare panic patients, other anxious patients, and normal controls in terms of the extent to which they were likely to interpret ambiguous events in a negative fashion. The questionnaire was a modified version of the questionnaire used by Butler and Mathews (1983) and by McNally and Foa (1987). Four types of ambiguous events were presented. These were:

1. descriptions of bodily sensations which the cognitive model predicts will be particularly likely to be misinterpreted by panic patients (e.g. "You notice your heart is beating quickly and pounding");
2. ambiguous social events (e.g. "You have visitors over and they leave sooner than you expected");
3. other ambiguous events (e.g. "A member of your family is late arriving home"), and
4. descriptions of bodily symptoms which should not be markedly misinterpreted by panic patients (e.g. "You have developed a small spot on the back of your hand").

The results are shown in Fig. 2. Consistent with prediction, panic patients were significantly more likely to interpret bodily sensations in a negative fashion than either other anxious patients ($P < 0.01$) or normal controls ($P < 0.01$). Furthermore,

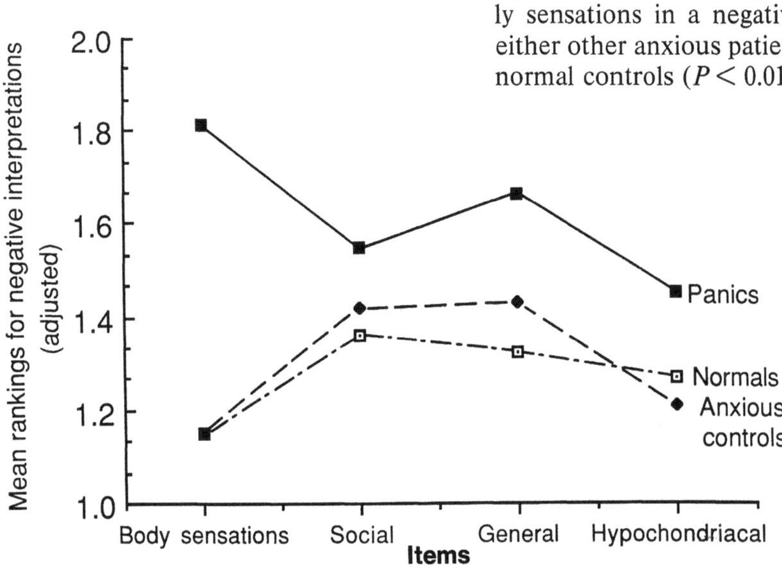

Fig. 2. Mean rankings for panic patients, anxious controls, and normals negative interpretations of four types of ambiguous events. Adjusted means were obtained from a two-way (groups × item) analysis of covariance with subjects' Spielberger State Anxiety scores used as covariates

Table 1. Pre-treatment and post-treatment means and standards deviations (in parentheses) for the negative interpretation of bodily sensations

Measure	Pre-treatment	Post-treatment	*t*
Negative interpretation of bodily sensations	2.23 (0.56)	1.35 (0.35)	4.74*

$n = 9$ patients; $*P < 0.01$

this appears to be a highly specific cognitive disturbance as, when equated for current levels of anxiety, panic patients did not differ from other anxious patients in their interpretation of the other ambiguous events (groups 2–4). Subsequently, we have retested a group of patients who have recovered from panic after psychological treatment. As predicted, these patients showed a marked reduction in their tendency to interpret bodily sensations in a catastrophic fashion (Table 1).

The results of this first experiment are clearly consistent with prediction 1. However, it could be argued that our questionnaire method of assessing catastrophic interpretations is rather artificial. Patients were specifically asked to provide interpretations of bodily sensations and were given an unlimited amount of time to do so. If misinterpretations occur in a panic attack they are much more likely to be automatic and to occur very quickly. In our second experiment we, therefore, used a task which was designed to detect fast and automatic interpretations of bodily sensations. This task is a modified version of the contextual priming task described by Fischler and Bloom (1979). Subjects were presented (on a VDU) with a sentence which was complete except for the last word. Having read this sentence frame, they were then presented with a single word and asked to read the word out loud as quickly as possible. Sentence frames and target words were constructed in such a way that the target word provided either a neutral or a negative interpretation of the bodily sensation specified in the target frame. Three frames are shown below, with their alternative target words italicized:

1. If I had palpitations I could be *dying.*
excited.
2. If I were breathless I could be *choking.*
unfit.
3. If my thinking were unusual I could be *insane.*
clever.

In a contextual priming task, subjects typically make faster word naming responses if the target word is one that they would expect from the sentence frame than if it is a word that they would not expect, given the sentence frame. If panic patients are particularly likely to make negative interpretations of bodily sensations we would, therefore, expect that, compared to controls, they would be relatively quicker at naming a word which completes a sentence if the sentence forms a negative interpretation of a bodily sensation than if it forms a neutral interpretation. Figure 3 shows that was in fact the case. Sixteen panic disorder patients were compared with 16 nonpatients of similar sex and age. In panic patients sentence completions with negative words were significantly faster than sentence completions with neutral words ($P < 0.05$). In normals completion times for the two word types were comparable. Two further analyses showed that panic patients' faster naming times for negative words preceded by a sentence frame were the result of making an interpretation

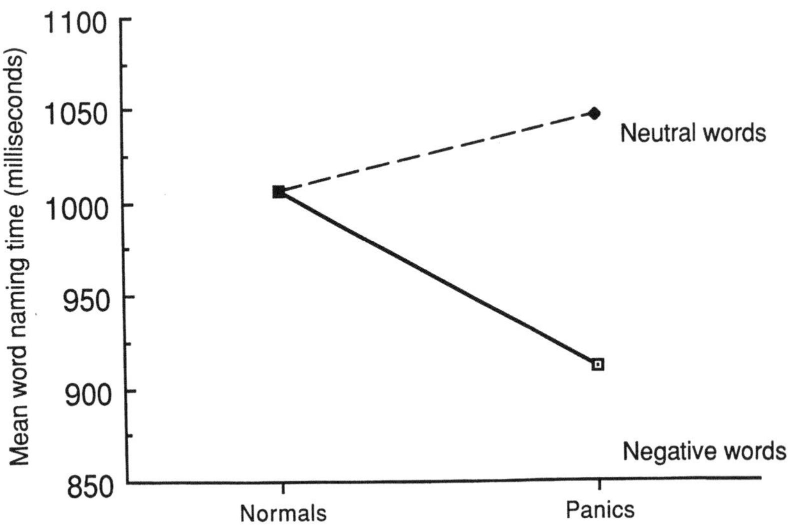

Fig. 3. Mean reaction times for negative and neutral words preceded by a sentence frame describing a bodily sensation. Means are based on a two-way (groups × item) analysis of covariance with subjects' Spielberger state anxiety scores used as covariates

rather than simply responding faster to negative words irrespective of their context. First, when word naming times were assessed in a condition in which words were preceded by a row of *x*'s instead of sentence frames, panic patients and normal controls were both significantly *faster* at naming neutral words than negative words. Second, the interaction shown in Fig. 3 remained significant when subjects' naming times in the *x*-frame condition was controlled for statistically using analysis of covariance.

Prediction 2

Rachman et al. (1987) have recently reported an experiment which provides some support for prediction 2. Panic disorder patients were asked to enter a series of feared situations and then complete checklists of cognitions and bodily sensations. As predicted, those cognitions which patients were able to report having experienced during attacks appeared to be meaningfully linked to the cluster of bodily sensations which were simultaneously being experienced. Furthermore, 12 out of 14 patients were able to identify catastrophic thoughts during some or all of their attacks.

The preceding experiments strongly suggest that panic patients are particularly likely to catastrophically misinterpret certain bodily sensations. However, it could be argued that this cognitive style does not play a causal role in the production of panic attacks but instead is epiphenomenal, perhaps arising as a consequence of an individual having experienced repeated attacks. In order to demonstrate that catastrophic misinterpretations play a causal role, it is necessary to experimentally manipulate patients' interpretations.

Prediction 3

Margraf et al. (1987) have recently reported a case study which provides support for the prediction that conditions which activate patients' catastrophic misinterpretations will lead to an increase in anxiety and panic. During the course of a laboratory experiment, a panic disorder patient was given false feedback indicating a sudden increase in heart rate. This provoked a full-blown panic attack. Similar feedback failed to lead to an increase in anxiety in normal controls (Ehlers et al. 1988).

In our own laboratory, we are using word-reading tasks in order to activate catastrophic misinterpretations. Patients and normal controls are each asked to read out loud series of paired associates. In the crucial conditions, the paired associates consist of various combinations of bodily sensations and catastrophes (e.g. breathlessness-suffocate; palpitations-dying; nausea-numbness; collapse-insane). Panic patients' negative belief systems should make these paired associates particularly anxiety-provoking and our preliminary results (see Table 2) suggest that this is indeed true. Panic disorder patients, recovered panic disorder patients (treated with cognitive therapy), and normal controls were asked to rate their anxiety before and after reading the cards and also to rate the extent to which they experienced an increase in any of the 12 DSM-III panic symptoms. Using the criterion of a sudden increase in anxiety reaching at least 50 on a 100-point scale and accompanied by four or more symptoms of an average intensity which is moderate or above, 10 out of 12 (83%) of panic patients, but no recovered patients or normal controls, had a panic attack while reading the cards ($P < 0.001$).

Prediction 4

If catastrophic misinterpretations of bodily sensations play a causal role in panic attacks, it should be possible to treat panic using a form of cognitive therapy which focusses on these specific cognitions. Such a treatment would have three main components:

a) identifying patients' negative interpretations of bodily sensations;
b) suggesting alternative non-catastrophic interpretations of the sensations; and
c) helping patients to test the validity of these alternative interpretations through discussion and behavioural experiments.

Several studies have adopted this treatment approach with apparent success.

Clark et al. (1985) concentrated on one particular alternative interpretation - the view that the bodily sensations which patients experience in a panic attack are the result of stress-induced hyperventilation, rather than the more catastrophic things which they usually fear (impending heart attack, insanity, loss of control). During the early phase of the treatment, patients were asked to voluntarily hyperventilate. If they recognised the

Table 2. Response to symptom and catastrophe cards

Measure	Subjects		
	Panic disorder patients	Recovered PD patients	Normals
Subjects experiencing a panic attack (%)	10/12 (83%)	0/8 (0%)	0/12 (0%)
Total symptom score[a]	13.2	4.8	2.2

[a] Symptom increases were rated as a 4-point scale on which "none" scored 0, "slight" scored 1, "moderate" scored 2 and "severe" scored 3

bodily symptoms induced by hyperventilation as similar to those experienced during naturally occurring attacks, this observation was used as the basis for a discussion in which the therapist tried to help the patients reattribute their panic sensations to stress-induced hyperventilation. This discussion was followed by training in controlled breathing techniques as a further validation of the hyperventilation explanation for sensations experienced during panic. We have reported two evaluations of this cognitive treatment. In the first evaluation (Clark et al. 1985), patients were selected who perceived a similarity between the effects of hyperventilation and naturally occurring panic attacks. Substantial reductions in panic attack frequency were observed during the first few weeks of treatment. These initial gains, which occurred in the absence of exposure to feared external situations, were improved upon with further treatment and were maintained at 2-year follow-up. Panic disorder patients (termed "non-situationals") did particularly well, all being panic free by the end of treatment.

In the second evaluation (Salkovskis et al. 1986), an unselected group of panic patients was studied. Again substantial reductions in panic frequency were observed. In addition, there was some evidence that outcome was positively correlated with the extent to which patients perceived a marked similarity between the effects of voluntary overbreathing and naturally occurring attacks. All patients improved. However, those who failed to perceive a marked similarity between the effects of hyperventilation and their naturally occurring attacks obtained relatively less benefit. For this reason, we have recently developed additional behavioural experiments for these patients.

Figure 4 shows the results of a pilot study in which seven panic disorder patients were given up to 12 sessions of cognitive therapy which included these new behavioural experiments. All patients showed substantial reductions in panic frequency with six out of seven becoming panic free at, or before, the 12th session. The remaining patient became panic free after additional sessions of cognitive therapy. None of these studies employed a waiting-list control group. However, it is unlikely that the observed improvements were due to spontaneous remission as, in the first two studies, a stable baseline was established before treatment and significant improvements from baseline took place in a treatment period shorter than the baseline.

Further support for the effectiveness of a cognitive approach to treatment comes from two recent case series and a controlled trial which have independently replicated the results obtained by Clark et al. (1985) and by Salkovskis et al. (1986). In Hungary, Kopp et al. (1986) found that a series of panic disorder and agoraphobia

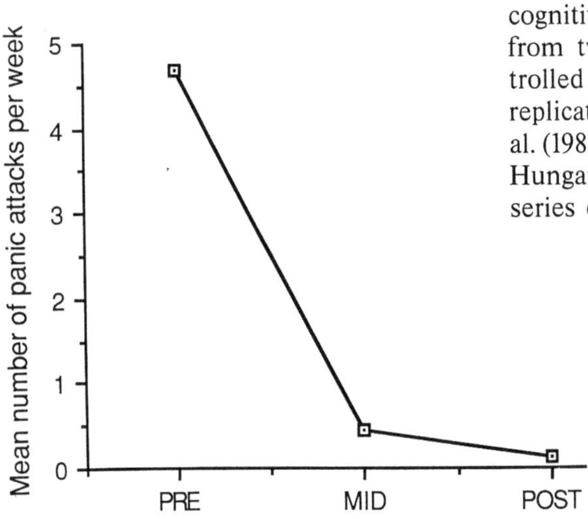

Fig. 4. Mean number of panic attacks, pre-treatment, mid-treatment and post-treatment

with panic patients showed substantial reductions in panic frequency during a 6-week application of the treatment of Clark et al. In the United States, Beck and colleagues incorporated this treatment within their cognitive therapy programme. In their first evaluation (Beck 1988), they found that a consecutive series of panic disorder patients showed substantial reductions in panic frequency during the course of treatment and these gains were maintained at 3-month follow-up. In their second evaluation (Sokol-Kessler and Beck 1987), cognitive therapy was found to be significantly more effective than brief supportive psychotherapy.

From these studies it would appear that a treatment package which aims to modify patients' misinterpretations of bodily sensations is effective in treating panic. This is consistent with prediction 4. However, the cognitive treatment is a complex package involving a mixture of cognitive and behavioural procedures. It could therefore be argued that the apparent effectiveness of cognitive therapy results from factors other than its emphasis on the modification of catastrophic misinterpretations of bodily sensations. Further studies are underway to investigate this question. In the meantime, a more direct test of prediction 4 might be single-session experiments which investigate the effectiveness of cognitive procedures in blocking panic induced by pharmacological agents. Rapee et al. (1986) have recently reported such an experiment. Patients who experienced recurrent spontaneous panic attacks were given single inhalations of 50% carbon dioxide/50% oxygen. One-half of the patients were allocated to a no explanation condition in which the minimal instructions about expected outcome were provided. The other half were given a more detailed explanation in which all possible sensations were described and attributed to the effects of the gas. This explanation was intended to block patients' naturally occurring tendency to catastrophically interpret CO_2-induced sensations. The results were consistent with prediction 4. Subjects given no explanation reported significantly more panic than patients given an explanation. However, the experiment was not entirely conclusive, as it is possible that the explanation group, knowing the likely effects of the gas, held their breath for a shorter time, thereby reducing the degree of gas exchange and the subsequent intensity of the experienced sensations. Such an artifactual explanation would not apply to a similar study which used sodium lactate rather than CO_2 inhalation as a provocation procedure. For this reason, we and other workers (van den Hout 1988) are investigating the effects of cognitive manipulations on lactate-induced panic.

Conclusion

A cognitive theory of panic has been presented. The theory is consistent with the major features of panic and with existing research findings. However, a theory must stand or fall on the accuracy of its predictions. Several experiments have been reported which test predictions derived from the cognitive theory. The results of these experiments are as predicted and further work is underway to test additional predictions. In the meantime, it is encouraging to note that the theory has generated what appears to be a highly successful, non-pharmacological treatment for panic.

Acknowledgement: The authors are grateful to the Medical Research Council of the United Kingdom for its support

References

Barlow DH (in press) Current models of panic disorder and a view from emotion theory. In Review of psychiatry, volume 7. American Psychiatric Press, Washington, DC

Beck AT (1988) Cognitive approaches to panic disorder: theory and therapy. In: Rachman S, Maser JD (eds) Panic: Psychological perspectives. Erlbaum, Hillsdale

Beck AT, Emery G, Greenberg RL (1985) Anxiety disorders and phobias: a cognitive perspective. Basic Books, New York

Butler G, Mathews AM (1983) Cognitive processes in anxiety. Adv Behav Res Ther 5:51-63

Clark DM (1979) Therapeutic aspects of increasing PCO_2 by behavioural means. Unpublished M Phil thesis, University of London

Clark DM (1986) A cognitive approach to panic. Behav Res Ther 24:461-470

Clark DM (1988) A cognitive model of panic attacks. In: Rachman S, Maser JD (eds) Panic: psychological perspectives. Erlbaum Hillsdale

Clark DM, Salkovskis PM, Chalkley AJ (1985) Respiratory control as a treatment for panic attacks. J Behav Ther Exp Psychiatry 16:23-30

Ehlers A, Margraf J, Roth WT, Taylor CB, Birbaumer N (1988) Anxiety produced by false heart rate feedback in patients with panic disorder. Beh Res Ther 26:1-11

Fishler I, Bloom PA (1979) Automatic and attentional processes in the effects of sentence contents on word recognition. J Verb Learn Verb Behav 18:1-20

Griez E, van den Hout MA (1984) Carbon dioxide and anxiety: an experimental approach to a clinical claim. Unpublished doctoral dissertation, Rijksuniversiteit, Maastricht, The Netherlands

Hout van den MA (1988) Metabolism, reflexes and cognitions in experimental panic. In: Rachman S, Maser JD (eds) Panic: psychological perspectives. Erlbaum, Hillsdale

Kopp M, Milhaly K, Vadasz P (1986) Agoraphobics es panikneurotikus betegek legzesi kontroll keyelese. Ideggyogyaszati Szemle 39:185- 196

Margraf J, Ehlers A, Roth WT (1986) Biological models of panic disorder and agoraphobia: a review. Behav Res Ther 24:553-567

Margraf J, Ehlers A, Roth WT (1987) Panic attack associated with perceived heart rate acceleration: a case report. Behav Ther 18:84-89

McNally RJ, Foa EB (1987) Cognition and agoraphobia: bias in the interpretation of threat. Cogn Ther Res

Oswald I (1966) Sleep. Penguin Books, Harmondsworth

Rachman S, Levitt K, Lopatka C (1987) Panic: the links between cognitions and bodily symptoms I. Behav Res Ther 25:411-423

Rapee RM (1987) The psychological treatment of panic attacks: theoretical conceptualisation and review of evidence. Clin Psychol Rev 7:427-438

Rapee RM; Mattick R, Murrell E (1986) Cognitive mediation in the affective component of spontaneous panic attacks. J Behav Ther Exp Psychiatry 17:245-253

Salkovskis PM (1988) Phenomenology, assessment and the cognitive model of panic. In: Rachman S, Maser JC (eds) Panic: psychological perspectives. Erlbaum Hillsdale

Salkovskis PM, Jones DRO, Clark DM (1986) Respiratory control in the treatment of panic attacks: replication and extension with concurrent measurement of behaviour and pCO_2. Br J Psychiatry 148:526-532

Seligman MEP (1988) Competing theories of panic. In: Rachman S, Maser SD (eds) Panic: psychological perspectives. Erlbaum, Hillsdale

Sokol-Kessler MS, Beck AT (1987) Cognitive therapy for panic disorder. Paper presented at the 140th Annual Meeting of the American Psychiatric Association, May 9-14, Chicago, Illinois

Telch MJ (1988) Combined pharmacological and psychological treatments for panic sufferers. In: Rachman S, Maser JD (eds) Panic: psychological perspectives. Erlbaum Hillsdale

14. What Cognitions Differentiate Panic Disorder from Other Anxiety Disorders?*

E. B. Foa

Phobias, characterized by intense anxiety to circumscribed stimuli and a strong tendency to their avoidance, have attracted much attention by learning theorists and behavior therapists. Interestingly, neither the early theoretical formulations nor the treatment procedures have distinguished among types of pathological fear. Thus, for example, the most popular theory of the acquisition and maintenance of *phobias,* Mowrer's (1939) two-stage theory, was adopted by Dollard and Miller (1950) to explain obsessive-compulsive symptoms. In the same vein, systematic desensitization (Wolpe 1958), the first behavioral procedure aiming at reduction of phobic fear, was employed not only with simple phobics but also with agoraphobics and with obsessive-compulsives, as it was expected to have similar effects on *all* manifestations of neurotic anxiety. Consonant with this assumption, many of the early behavior therapy outcome studies employed samples of mixed phobias (e.g., Gelder et al. 1967; Marks et al. 1968), again reflecting the belief that all neurotic fears are governed by the same mechanisms and, thus, will respond similarly to therapy.

The assumption of equivalence among fears has proved problematic in the face of empirical findings, pointing to an interaction between the type of fear and response to treatment. For example, systematic desensitization was found effective with simple phobics (e.g., Cooper et al. 1965; Marks and Gelder 1965), but not with obsessive-compulsives (Beech and Vaughn 1978) or with agoraphobics (Jansson and Ost 1982). Likewise, flooding proved more effective than systematic desensitization with agoraphobics, but equally effective with simple phobics (Marks et al. 1971). The differential effects of therapeutic procedures with different anxiety disorders suggest that these disorders represent different types of fear.

Parallel to the "lumping" approach, several researchers have attempted to categorize anxiety patients along phenomenological aspects (e.g., Marks 1969). More recently the American Psychiatric Association has devoted much effort to the development of such a classification. Indeed, the DSM-III (APA 1980) and its revision (APA 1987) include clear and reliable descriptions for identification of different anxiety disorders. Yet, this classification offers no theoretical framework for conceptualizing the similarities and differences among these disorders. In this chapter, I will briefly review a theory developed by Foa and Kozak (1985, 1986) that integrated available concepts of fear and anxiety, relevant experimental data, and clinical investigations. Anxiety disorders will be discussed in relation to this theory, and recent data about the differences between panic disorder and other anxiety disorders will be summarized.

---

* Preparation of this manuscript was supported in part by NIMH Grant No ROlMH40865-01 awarded to the author.

The Structure of Fear Memory

Colloquially, people seem to label heightened physiological activity as emotional when the context is perceived to be especially good or especially bad. Psychological theorists of emotion, for the most part, have adopted the notion that emotion is physiology plus interpretation of that physiology. Accordingly, fear, like any other emotion, includes physiological as well as meaning elements.

Adopting Lang's (1977, 1979) concept of fear, Foa and Kozak (1986) have suggested that fear is represented as a network in memory which includes three kinds of information:

a) information about the feared stimulus situation;
b) information about verbal, physiological, and overt behavioral responses; and
c) interpretive information about the meaning of the stimulus and response elements of the structure.

This information is conceived of as a program for escape or avoidance behavior.

Whereas Lang stressed the importance of the response elements in a fear structure, Foa and Kozak have focused on meaning elements. It stands to reason that if a fear structure is a program to escape danger, then it must involve information that stimuli and/or responses are *dangerous,* in addition to information about physiological activity which is preparatory for escape. Thus, a fear structure is distinguished from other information structures not only by response elements, but also by the meaning information it contains. For example, the program for running ahead of a competitor who carries a baton during a race is similar to the program of running away from an assailant on that same race track: both involve similar stimulus and response information. *That* which distinguishes the fear structure is the meaning of the stimuli and the responses: only the fear structure involves escape from threat.

The Structure of Pathological Fear

Most people experience fear in some circumstances, thus implying the activation of a fear structure. "Normal" fear occurs when one perceives actual threat that disappears when the danger is removed.

Fear becomes pathological when its intensity disrupts daily functioning and when it persists despite information that it is unrealistic. In other words, pathological structures involve excessive response elements (e.g., avoidance, physiological activity, etc.) and are resistant to modification. If a fear is unrealistic, it must imply that the underlying fear structure contains stimulus-stimulus (S-S) associations which do not accurately represent relationships in the world. For example, for the obsessive-compulsive washer who fears contamination by rabies, the backyard is strongly associated with rabies and therefore avoided. In reality, rabies is rarely encountered in one's backyard. Associations between harmless *stimuli* and escape or avoidance *responses* are also disordered: escape from a supermarket or a tunnel does not enhance the organism's survival. In some individuals, disordered response-response (R-R) associations are also observed. An example is the agoraphobic who fears tachycardia.

Some of the erroneous meaning of the pathological fear structure is embedded in these disordered associations. Additional erroneous meaning is coded semantically as interpretive elements in the structure. Several types of erroneous evaluations can be evidenced in the fear structures of anxiety-disordered individuals. First, a common belief among these individuals is that anxiety will persist forever unless escape of the feared situation is realized.

Second, the fear stimuli and/or fear responses are estimated to have an unrealistically high potential for causing either psychological (e.g., losing control) or physical (e.g., dying, being ill) harm. Third, the anticipated consequences have relatively high negative valence, i.e., are extremely aversive for the individual.

The Relationship Between Fear Structures and Anxiety Disorders

The various anxiety disorders can be viewed as representing different fear structures. For example, the presence of a relationship between certain situations, such as department stores and fear responses in panicky agoraphobics indicates a disordered link among stimulus and response elements of their underlying fear structure. In this respect they are similar to the simple phobic who dreads heights. What distinguishes the structure of agoraphobia from that of simple phobia and other anxiety disorders is the presence of erroneous evaluations of fear responses. Agoraphobics commonly perceive anxiety itself to be dangerous - since they typically expect anxiety responses to cause physical or psychological harm. Stimulus elements (e.g., supermarkets) are not evaluated as intrinsically threatening. Rather, the danger is perceived to lie in the anxiety which they evoke. In contrast, in simple phobias the potential harm is expected to stem from the stimulus situation itself (e.g., snakes, wasps, dogs). An agoraphobic fear structure is schematically illustrated in Fig. 1. It illustrates that response, but not stimuli, are associated with semantic elements of danger.

It is important to note that not all elements of an emotional structure are accessible by introspection. Certainly, individuals are aware of some aspects of their fear, and their beliefs and evalua-

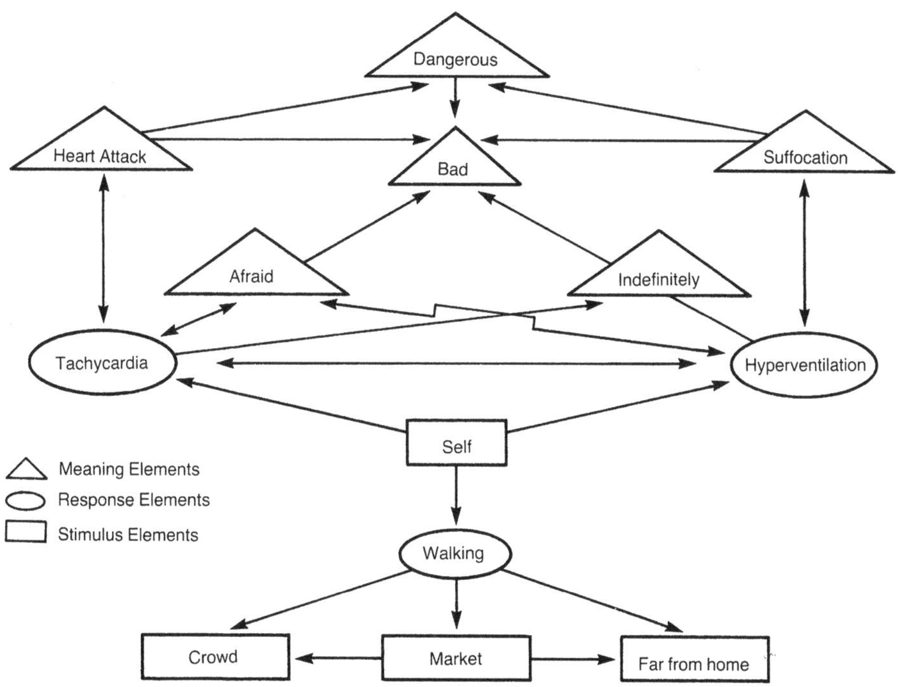

Fig. 1. Connecting vectors suggest directions for the various conceptual relations among the elements; e.g., tachycardia causes heart attack, heart attack brings tachycardia, self is walking in the market (Foa and Kozak 1986)

tions must reflect elements of their fear structures. However, this knowledge about their fear structure is imperfect. Theories of emotions must take into account what people tell us about their emotions. At the same time, these self-reports must be considered with caution. Thus, a satisfactory theory would encompass the content of self-reports without theoretical dependency on this content. Because of people's imperfect knowledge about their fear structures, nonintrospective assessment of emotional structures is also necessary.

"The Fear of Fear" Hypotheses: Further Evidence

The fear structure of agoraphobics has gained considerable attention with the emergence of the "fear of fear" hypothesis (Goldstein and Chambles 1978; Weekes 1977). This hypothesis holds that agoraphobics but not simple phobics fear interoceptive cues because they associate such cues with pending disasters, such as death. Three studies will be described next, exemplifying the use of various methodologies in examining the characteristics of the agoraphobics' fear structures in comparison with those of patients with other anxiety disorders and normals.

"Fear of Fear" in Anxiety Disorders: Questionnaire Data

An attempt to examine the extent to which different anxiety-disordered individuals associate interoceptive responses with danger was carried out by Dattilio and Foa (1987), comparing anxiety disorders and normals on a series of self-report instruments which tap the semantic structure of fear.

Specifically, Dattilio and Foa compared five groups of 20 subjects each: specific phobics, generalized anxiety disorder, panic disorder with and without agoraphobia, and nonanxious controls. All subjects received questionnaires assessing fear of fear via items which pertain to interoceptive cues and the harm anticipated from them. In addition, some questionnaires also included items about general fear situations that would be fearful to nonanxiety-disordered individuals as well. The results are summarized in Table 1.

Two questionnaires were adapted by Foa and McNally (1985) from Butler and Mathews (1983): the Subjective Probabili-

Table 1. Mean scores of anxiety threat and general threat for agoraphobia (Agora), panic disorders (PD), generalized anxiety disorders (GAD), simple phobia (SP), and normals (N)

Instrument	Agora	PD	GAD	SP	N
Subjective Probability Questionnaire					
Anxiety threat	41.90	36.70	26.20	29.25	13.30
General threat	17.80	25.50	22.95	26.20	18.50
Subjective Cost Questionnaire					
Anxiety threat	54.50	51.15	42.75	35.85	26.85
General threat	34.90	41.70	40.20	37.60	33.20
Anxiety Sensitivity Index	34.22	38.21	25.90	19.41	11.65
Body Sensations Questionnaire	2.97	2.89	2.24	2.41	1.74
Interpretation Questionnaire					
Anxiety threat	7.60	7.80	4.70	3.95	1.60
General threat	8.20	7.60	6.25	3.95	1.95

ty Questionnaire and the Subjective Cost Questionnaire. They measure the degree of bias in estimating the occurrence of certain bodily sensations and external negative events, as well as the relative aversivenes associated with them. Both panic-disordered groups scored higher than all other groups when asked to estimate the probability that bodily sensations would occur; however, they did not differ from the others in anticipating general fear events. The same pattern emerged for ratings of valence or cost: the panic-disordered groups rated interoceptive cues as more aversive than did the other groups. And again, they did not differ from others on rating the aversiveness of external fear-evoking situations.

Two other instruments, the Anxiety Sensitivity Index (ASI; Reiss et al. 1986) and the Body Sensations Questionnaire (BSA; Chambless et al. 1984) were used. Both measures are concerned with anxiety-related physical sensations and their anticipated consequences. As expected, the panic-disordered groups scored higher than the other three groups on both instruments.

A fifth instrument, the Interpretive Questionnaire (adapted by Foa and McNally 1986; from Butler and Mathews 1983) was also administered to the five groups. It includes imagined vignettes each of which could be interpreted as either dangerous or nondangerous. Some scenarios focus on interoceptive cues, others on external events. A somewhat different picture emerged from these data. In brief item questionnaires (as expected), panic-disordered groups differed from other groups on "fear of fear," but not on external fear items. When presented with more elaborate scenarios, however, the panic-disordered groups scored higher than the other groups on *both* internal and external situations. Perhaps imagined vignettes are more successful in evoking fear than brief questions, regardless of fear content. And once the physiology of fear is evoked in panic-disordered patients, response-threat associations are accessed, thus priming an association of threat with external as well as with internal events.

"Fear of Fear" in Agoraphobia and Simple Phobics: Experimental Data

Strong support for the hypothesis that agoraphobics, but not simple phobics, show especially strong associations between interoceptive responses and threat, comes from a psychophysiology study of imagery with eight agoraphobics and eight simple phobics (Mansueto et al. 1987).

Subjects were presented with four types of scenes:

a) external fear stimuli, such as supermarkets or snakes, which constituted each subject's most feared object or situation;
b) interoceptive fear responses, such as heart rate or breathing changes, which constituted the responses most associated with fear for each individual;
c) stimulus plus response scenes, combining the external and interoceptive propositions for each person; and
d) neutral (nonfear) stimuli.

Self-report and heart rate (HR) were used to assess fear. Each scene was presented twice in a random order. Data for each scene were then averaged over the two presentations.

It was hypothesized that agoraphobics will be fearful while imagining external, interoceptive (internal), and combined scenes, but not when imagining neutral material. Simple phobics, on the other hand, whose fear structure is not distinguished by response-threat associations were hypothesized to evidence fear only while imagining external and combined scenes.

Table 2. Mean self ratings of fear for agoraphobics and simple phobics

Type of scenarios	Type of Anxiety disorders Agoraphobics	Simple phobics
Neutral	0.9	0.7
External	4.1	4.8
Internal	4.1	2.0
Internal and external	4.2	4.5

Table 3. Mean heart rate for agoraphobics and simple phobics

Type of scenarios	Type of anxiety disorders Agoraphobics	Simple phobics
Neutral	76.9	77.2
External	79.5	82.5
Internal	80.2	78.0
Internal and external	79.2	82.5

Self-report as well as heart rate data strongly supported the hypotheses; they are depicted in Tables 2 and 3, respectively:

As shown in Table 2, agoraphobics rated the external, internal, and combined scenes as more fearful than the neutral scene. Simple phobics also reported being fearful when imagining their feared stimuli-situation either alone or in combination with fear responses. However, in contrast to agoraphobics, they did not report the image of fear responses alone to be more fearful than neutral material. The same pattern emerged from the heart rate data (Table 3): agoraphobics, but not simple phobics, evidenced significantly higher heart rates when imagining their fear responses than when imagining neutral material. Both groups show increased heart rate when imagining external fear.

The psychophysiological results of the study described above converge with the questionnaire data of Dattilio and Foa (1987): the agoraphobics' fear structures, unlike those of simple phobics, are characterized by a particular interpretive meaning that interoceptive responses are dangerous. This convergence of introspective and physiological data suggests that people's beliefs about the nature of their fears reflect elements of their structures.

"Fear of Fear" in Agoraphobics: Before and After Effective Treatment

Further support for the hypothesis that agoraphobics' fear structures are distinguished by response-threat associations emerged in a study conducted by McNally and Foa (in press). In this study nine untreated agoraphobics were compared with nine normal controls and nine agoraphobics who had been treated successfully via anxiety-management techniques. All three groups received questionnaires with items pertaining to fear of interoceptive cues and the harm anticipated from them, as well as items about general fear situations that might also disturb nonanxiety disordered individuals. The questionnaires were the same as those used by Dattilio and Foa (1987) described above. The results are summarized in Table 4.

Table 4. Mean scores of anxiety threat and general threat for treated and untreated agoraphobics and normal controls

Instrument	Untreated Agoraphobics	Treated Agoraphobics	Normals
Subjective Probability Questionnaire			
Anxiety threat	6.48	3.24	2.63
General threat	4.82	2.63	4.46
Subjective Cost Questionnaire			
Anxiety threat	6.48	3.24	3.83
General threat	4.82	2.63	4.46
Anxiety Sensitivity Index	46.67	16.44	
Body Sensations Questionnaire	2.91	1.68	
Interpretation Questionnaire			
Anxiety threat	10.33	5.00	3.22
General threat	10.22	5.78	5.22

Despite differences between the studies in the scoring procedures of the subjective probability and cost questionnaires, the results of the two studies were consistent. Untreated agoraphobics scored higher than normals when asked to estimate the probability and cost of interoceptive cues, but did not differ from them in responding to external fear situations. When asked to consider scenarios describing either interoceptive responses or external stimuli, again consistent with Dattilio and Foa's study, this group interpreted *both* types of events as more threatening than did normals. Interestingly, the treated agoraphobics did not differ from normals on any of the measures. These results provide evidence for the relationship between the hypothesized agoraphobic fear structure and agoraphobic symptoms. Moreover, they suggest that change in the fear structure may explain therapy outcome. Accordingly, pathological fear structures are the target of treatment.

Further Considerations

The notion that agoraphobia is distinguished by an association between bodily sensation and threat was implicit in descriptions of this syndrome already in the last century, when the term agoraphobia was introduced by Westphal (1871) who described it as the "... impossibility of walking through certain streets or squares, or possibility of so doing only with *resultant dread of anxiety*" (italics ours). In the past 20 years, researchers have shifted their construal of agoraphobia from fear of external situations to fear of fear responses (e.g., Goldstein and Chambless 1978). What, then, is the theoretical and practical advantage in assimilating the "fear of fear" hypothesis about agoraphobia into a general theory of emotional processing of fear?

The usefulness of the emotional processing theory over S-R theories, cognitive theories, and Lang's bioinformation theory have been advocated elsewhere (Foa and Kozak 1986). Some specific gains for the conceptualization of anxiety disorders, including agoraphobia, lie in its explication of the mechanisms involved in maintenance and reduction of fear. For example, this theory accounts for the relationship among short- and long-term habituation, fear ideation, and treatment outcome. From this account, in turn, one can derive specific hypotheses about differential effects of a given procedure on different fear structures. In addition to hypotheses regarding fear reduction, i.e., treatment, the conceptualization of anxiety disorders as fear structures has a heuristic value for generating hypotheses about psychopathology. For example, one could predict that certain propositions will be more strongly associated in one disorder than in another based on the hypothesis that specific fear structures underlie the different disorders.

Whereas many anxiety researchers have made important discoveries which constitute pieces of the anxiety puzzle, emotional processing theory and its notion of fear structures is an attempt to integrate these discoveries into a unified conceptual framework.

References

American Psychiatric Association (1980) Diagnostic and statistical manual of mental disorders, 3rd edn, Washington DC

American Psychiatric Association (1987) Diagnostic and statistical manual of mental disorders - revised. Washington, DC

Beech HR, Vaughn M (1978) Behavioral treatment of obsessional states. Wiley, New York

Butler G, Mathews A (1983) Cognitive processes in anxiety. Adv Behav Res Ther 5:51-62

Chambless DL, Caputo GC, Bright P, Gallagher R (1984) Assessment of fear of fear in agoraphobics: the body sensations questionnaire and the agoraphobic cognitions questionnaire and the agoraphobic cognition questionnaire. J Consult Clin Psychol Rev 4:431-457

Cooper JE, Gelder MG, Marks IM (1965) Results of behaviour therapy in 77 psychiatric patients. Br Med J [Clin Res] 1:1222-1225

Dattilio FM, Foa EB (1987) Fear of fear: a comparison of generalized anxiety disorder, panic disorder with and without agoraphobia, and simple phobia. Unpublished manuscript

Dollard J, Miller NE (1950) Personality and psychotherapy: an analysis in terms of learning, thinking, and culture. McGraw-Hill, New York

Foa EB, Kozak MJ (1985) Treatment of anxiety disorders: implications for psychopathology. In: Tuma AH, Maser JD (eds) Anxiety and the anxiety disorders. Erlbaum, Hillsdale

Foa EB, Kozak MJ (1986) Emotional processing of fear: exposure to corrective information. Psychol Bull 99:20-35

Foa EB, McNally RJ (1986) Sensitivity to feared stimuli in obsessive-compulsives: a dichotic listening analysis. Cogn Ther Res 10:477-485

Gelder MG, Marks IM, Wolff HH (1967) Desensitization and psychotherapy in the treatment of phobic states: a controlled enquiry. Br J Psychiatry 113:53-73

Goldstein AJ, Chambless DL (1978) A reanalysis of agoraphobia. Behav Res Ther 9:47-59

Jansson L, Ost L (1982) Behavioral treatment for agoraphobia: an evaluative review. Clin Psychol Rev 2:311-336

Lang PJ (1977) Imagery in therapy: an information processing analysis of fear. Behav Res Ther 8:862-886

Lang PJ (1979) A bio-informational theory of emotional imagery. Psychophysiology 16:495-512

Mansueto CS, Grayson JB, Foa EB (1987) Assessment of the "fear of fear" component in agoraphobic versus specific phobia patients. Unpublished manuscript

Marks I (1969) Fears and phobias. Academic, New York

Marks IM, Gelder MG (1965) A controlled retrospective study of behaviour therapy in phobic patients. Br J Psychiatry 111:571-573

Marks IM, Gelder MG, Edwards JG (1968) Hypnosis and desensitization for phobias: a controlled prospective trial. Br J Psychiatry 114:1263-1274

Marks IM, Boulougouris J, Marset P (1971) Flooding versus desensitization in the treatment of phobic disorders. Br J Psychiatry 119:353-375

McNally RJ, Foa EB (1985) Information processing during anxious mood. National Institute of Mental Health grant no MH 40191-01

McNally RS, Foa EB (to be published) Cognition and agoraphobia: bias the interpretation of threat. Cogn Ther Res

Mowrer OA (1939) Stimulus-response analysis of anxiety and its role as a reinforcing agent. Psychol Rev 46:553-565

Reiss S, Peterson RA, Gursky DM, McNally RJ (1986) Anxiety sensitivity, anxiety frequency, and the prediction of fearfulness. Behav Res Ther 24:1-8

Weekes C (1977) Simple effective treatment of agoraphobia. Hawthorne, New York

Wolpe J (1958) Psychotherapy by reciprocal inhibition. University Press, Stanford

15. Factors Relevant to Lactate Response in Panic Disorder

R. Buller, W. Maier, and O. Benkert

Introduction

Infusion of 0.5 molar sodium lactate has been reported to provoke panic attacks in patients with panic disorder, agoraphobia with panic attacks (Liebowitz et al. 1984, 1985a), and subjects with a previous history of panic attacks (Cowley et al. 1987b). On the other hand, normal controls and patients with social phobia (Liebowitz et al. 1985b), obsessive compulsive disorder (Gorman et al. 1985), or major depression without a history of panic attacks respond significantly less often with panic during the infusion procedure.

The nature of the mechanism for pharmacological induction of panic is unclear. Hypotheses explaining the panicogenic effects of lactate range from assumptions that the procedure represents merely nonspecific arousal to theories of an underlying biological disturbance or specific vulnerability which is tapped by lactate.

With the revision of DSM-III (Diagnostic and Statistical Manual, 3rd edition, revised; DSM-IIIR, APA 1987) the definition of panic disorder has become wider. Patients with a frequency of only a single panic attack can now receive the diagnosis of panic disorder if the attack has been followed by a period of at least 1 month of persistent fear of having another attack. In addition, subjects with concurrent depression are now given both diagnoses instead of being excluded from the category of panic disorder as was the rule in DSM-III (APA 1980).

For this more heterogeneous class of panic disorder little is known about lactate vulnerability. We, therefore, conducted a study with lactate infusions in patients meeting criteria for DSM-IIIR panic disorder. Since we were interested in the effects that can be attributed to sodium lactate itself, we took care to minimize nonspecific factors.

Methods

Thirteen female inpatients who met DSM-IIIR criteria for panic disorder were included in the study. Among these were seven patients with a concurrent major depressive episode (MDE). Five inpatients with a current MDE who had never experienced panic attacks served as controls. Patients in both groups were between 18 and 47 years old. They were free of medication (tricyclic antidepressants, MAO-inhibitors, alprazolam, or neuroleptics) for 2 weeks.

Physical illness was excluded by a full medical evaluation carried out by a senior internist who was informed about the study. Patients received routine laboratory tests as well as an ECG and chest X-ray. Patients gave consent to participate in a research project where they were to have a cortisol profile, a CRH-challenge, and an infusion of sodium lactate. All tests were performed in a fixed order with the cortisol profile and the CRH challenge on 1 day followed by the lactate provocation 2 days later. During the endocrine investigations, subjects had to remain in the research room for 11 h in a supine position. The room is very similar to a normal hospital room - cords and i.v. lines go to the adjacent control room where blood samples are handled and the recordings are made. Likewise, infusion bottles are in this room so that patients remain blind to which substance is infused at a certain time. The staff in the control room were able to watch the patient via video screen with the camera being visible to the patient.

Lactate infusions were given at noon after patients had had a light breakfast in the morning but abstained from caffeine.

Two i.v. lines were inserted; one for the infusion, the other for drawing blood samples. After initial infusion with 5% glucose in water for a varying amount of time, the infusion rate was increased for several minutes. Half-molar sodium lactate was then given at a dose of 10 ml per kg body weight within 20 min.

Patients were asked to report any changes or symptoms during the test procedure to a research physician who was present in the same room. Both were blind to the beginning of the lactate infusion. When the infusion was completed, patients were monitored for another 30 min and then transfered to their ward. A panic attack during the infusion was diagnosed by the research physician when the patient reported intense fear, discomfort or panic with at least four of the symptoms listed in DSM-IIIR.

A response that consisted of at least four panic symptoms unaccompanied by intense anxiety was termed "symptom attack."

Results

Four of the 13 patients with DSM-IIIR panic disorder responded with a panic attack (31%), of these, three suffered from concurrent MDE (see Table 1). In another seven patients there was a "symptom attack" without panic leaving merely two patients unaffected by significant physical or psychological symptoms during the infusion. In the control group with depressed patients, none responded with a panic or symptom attack. Symptoms known to be caused by lactate, such as increase in heart rate, tingling sensations, tremor, or urinary urgency were equally frequente in both groups. The total number of symptoms reported was significantly higher in patients with panic disorder. However, there were no differences between groups with respect to baseline, peak heart rate and blood pressure (systolic and diastolic).

Table 1. Lactate response in patients with DSM-IIIR panic disorder and depressed controls

	Panic disorder ($n = 13$)	Depressed controls ($n = 5$)
Panic attack	4 (31%)	0 (0%)
Symptom attack	7 (54%)	0 (0%)
Number of symptoms	5.0 ± 2.0	1.2 ± 1.0[1]
Heart rate		
Baseline	80 ± 12	78 ± 7 n.s.
Peak during lactate	108 ± 12	100 ± 9 n.s.
Blood pressure:		
Systolic		
Baseline	110 ± 16	104 ± 17 n.s.
Peak	122 ± 21	120 ± 11 n.s.
Diastolic		
Baseline	74 ± 14	73 ± 11 n.s.
Peak	77 ± 14	70 ± 13 n.s.

[1] $P < 0.01$

Discussion

Although in our study the panicogenic effect of the lactate infusion appears to be specific for patients with panic disorder when compared with depressed controls, the rate of 31% responding with a panic attack is much lower than in previous publications (Liebowitz et al. 1984). There is only one study (Gorman et al. 1985) that reports a similarly low lactate response in 36% of patients with panic disorder. However, Gorman et al. consider their finding as a chance occurrence in a small sample. Although the same explanation could apply to our results as well, the low rate of lactate-induced panic that is in the range of placebo response in patients or lactate response in healthy subjects could be caused by the careful control of situational and nonspecific factors.

Baseline heart rate was rather low and similar between groups, indicating that there was no increased arousal in our patients with panic disorder. Higher baseline anxiety has been reported to be responsible for higher rates of anxiety attacks during lactate (Ehlers et al. 1986). Expectancy biases leading patients to "overreport" panic attacks were reduced by a careful explanation of the procedure to the patients. This may not have been done in comparable detail in previous studies.

As a third alternative for explaining our finding, one might argue that our definition of panic attack may be too strict. However, we did not create new criteria, but merely recorded those symptoms that patients volunteered to tell us, wich we then classified according to DSM-IIIR criteria for panic attacks. We find that this procedure is appropriate, since the possibility of overreporting (tendency to say yes when being repeatedly asked for the presence of a symptom by questionnaire) is reduced. In addition, severe anxiety that led to premature termination of the lactate infusion was only found in three of the four panickers, but in none of the patients with symptom attacks.

The fact that an increased number of symptoms and symptom attacks was seen only in the group with panic disorder may indicate that there is a more intense arousal in the sense of a threshold specificity for an interaction between lactate and illness-related mechanisms. This interpretation is in line with a finding reported by Koenigsberg et al. (1987) that lactate can induce arousal when infused during sleep. In the waking state, such factors as being accustomed to the clinical setting, feeling safe or even bored, having a physician nearby or in the same room may then be important for the outcome of the provocation test. Since the lactate infusion is a procedure with an interplay between pharmacological, situational, nonspecific, and illness-related aspects, as was pointed out by Margraf et al. (1986), it is necessary to control for these variables in order to assess the biological effects of sodium lactate in patients with panic disorder.

References

American Psychiatric Association (1980) Diagnostic and statistical manual of mental disorders, 3rd edn. (DSM-III). American Psychiatric Association, Washington, DC

American Psychiatric Association (1987) Diagnostic and statistical manual of mental disorders, 3rd edn. revised (DSM-III-R) American Psychiatric Association, Washington, DC

Cowley DS, Dager SR, Dunner DL (1987b) Lactate infusions in major depression without panic attacks. J Psychiatr Res 21:3:243–248

Ehlers A, Margraf J, Roth WT et al (1986) Lactate infusions and panic attacks: do patients and controls respond differently? Psychiatry Res 17:295–308

Gorman JM, Liebowitz MR, Fyer AJ et al (1985) Lactate infusions in obsessive-compulsive disorder. Am J Psychiatry 142:7 864–866

Koenigsberg HW, Pollak C, Sullivan T (1987) The sleep lactate infusion: arousal and the panic mechanism. Biol Psychiatry 22:786–789

Liebowitz MR, Fyer AJ, Gorman JM et al (1984) Lactate provocation of panic attacks. Arch Gen Psychiatry 41:764–770

Liebowitz MR, Gorman JM, Fyer AJ et al (1985a) Lactate provocation of panic attacks. Arch Gen Psychiatry 42:709–719

Liebowitz MR, Fyer AJ, Gorman JM et al (1985b) Specificity of lactate infusions in social phobia vs panic disorders. Am J Psychiatry: 142:8:947–950

Margraf J, Ehlers A, Roth WT (1986) Sodium lactate infusions and panic attacks: a review and critique. Psychosom Med: 48:1/2:23–51

16. Do Anxiety Patients Differ in Autonomic Base Levels and Stress Response from Normal Controls?

M. Albus, A. Zellner, M. Ackenheil, S. Braune, and R. R. Engel

Introduction

During the past decade much attention has been focused on anxiety disorders. Progress has been made with regard to classification, therapy, and psychophysiology and biochemistry of underlying mechanisms. Challenge procedures are the most widely used approach to the biology of anxiety states, especially panic attacks, and have focused on several neurotransmitter systems. Besides the benzodiazepine-GABA-receptor complex (Dorow et al. 1983) and the adenosine receptor (Charney et al. 1985), the adrenergic system turned out to be a very promising one. Drug challenges with yohimbine (Charney et al. 1984, 1987), with isoproterenol (Nesse et al. 1984; Rainey et al. 1984), with lactate (Liebowitz et al. 1984; Fyer et al. 1985), and breathing CO_2 (Gorman et al. 1984) led to the assumption that pharmacologically or physiologically induced changes have a direct panic-inducing effect in anxiety patients, but not in healthy controls. However, these hypotheses are by no means proven. Counterhypotheses have emerged out of the findings of other research groups (Clark and Hensley 1982; van den Hout and Griez 1982; Hippert 1984; Ley 1985; Griez et al. 1986; Margraf et al. 1986; Ehlers et al. 1986). They suggest that panic attacks appear as a result of close interaction of biological factors, experimental setting, expectancy factors, and conditioning mechanisms.

Coming back to biological factors, there is empirical evidence that the adrenergic neurotransmitter systems are implicated in anxiety, but precise functions have not yet been delineated. The data for plasma catecholamines are equivocal. Some authors have reported elevated epinephrine base levels (Mathew et al. 1981; Nesse et al. 1984; Villacres et al. 1987) while others have found no differences between patients and controls (Kralik et al. 1982; Mathew et al. 1982; Gasic et al. 1985). Similar diverging results have been reported for norepinephrine and its major metabolite, MHPG: higher base levels (Mathew et al. 1981; Ballenger et al. 1984), as well as no differences between patients and controls (Mathew et al. 1982; Kralik et al. 1982; Gasic et al. 1985; Villacres et al. 1987; Pohl et al. 1987).

Also measurement of peripheral indices of autonomically mediated physiological activity has shown controversial results. Blood pressure, heart rate, and skin conductance have been reported to be higher at initial baseline in patients compared to controls (Freedman et al. 1984; Ehlers et al. 1986; Roth et al. 1986; Cowley et al. 1987). This is put in question by the findings of other groups, which have failed to find differences (Mathew et al. 1982; Gasic et al. 1985; Freedman et al. 1985; Cowley et al. 1987; Villacres et al. 1987; Woods et al. 1987; Yeragani et al. 1987). Both, the conflicting results of drug challenges and of baseline autonomic activation in these patients underscore the importance of the experimental setting. Thus, it points out the importance of a separate consideration of specific psychological responses and specific situational stresses. Direct measures of response to cognitive or active physical stressors have been used infrequently. This is especially surprising as stress is known to influence the adrenergic transmitter system (Dimsdale and Moss 1980; Ward et al. 1983; Albus et al. 1985, 1986). Until now, only Gasic et al. (1985) have investigated stress response of patients with cardiac phobia in comparison to controls, concluding that the patients respond to psychological stress with an inadequately sustained activation of the sympathetic nervous system. In a yohimbine challenge study with additional stress exposure (mental arithmetic and a continuous performance task), we found that yohimbine effects on electrodermal activity, cardiovascular system, and NE secretion overall did not differ between patients and controls. In contrast, patients rated a significant increase in anxiety and panicky feelings. However, they did not get panic attacks (Albus et al., in prep.). To further evaluate the role of stress exposure, we carried out two stress investigations comparing anxiety patients and controls.

Methods

Subjects

Stress I

Nine patients took part in the investigation, four met DSM-III criteria for agoraphobia and five met the criteria for generalized anxiety disorder. Six were women and three were men, with a mean age of 37 ± 8.5 years and with a duration of illness of 6.3 ± 2.8 years. All patients were off drugs for a minimum of 3 weeks before the stress test was administered. As controls, eight healthy subjects (five women, three men) with a mean age of 32.6 ± 12 years were obtained from referrals and determined to be free of mental disorder, none of them reported taking any psychoactive medication. None of the healthy subjects and patients reported a history of serious medical illness and they all had normal results of electrocardiogram, laboratory tests, and physical examination.

Stress II

Twenty-seven patients were investigated, 15 met DSM-III criteria for agoraphobia with panic attacks and 12 met the criteria for panic disorder; 15 were women and 12 were men with a mean age of 38.2 ± 8.9 years and a duration of illness of 4.3 ± 3.1 years. Again, all patients were off drugs for a minimum of 3 weeks before the stress test was administered. Controls were 10 healthy subjects (6 women, 4 men) with a mean age of 38.1 ± 5.3 years, free of mental disorder.

Procedure

Stress I

Subjects (Ss) stayed in a soundproof, electrically shielded test room. Fifteen minutes after insertion of an indwelling catheter the Ss had to undergo five tasks that were presented using a tape recorder:

1. Recall of an anxiety-provoking situation (Recall): Ss were told to remember a frigthening situation they had experienced in the past.
2. Mental arithmetic (MA): subtracting continuously 7 from 500 until they reached zero, starting again from 500 if they made a mistake.
3. Noise (MN): 5- to 15-s periods of pure tones alternated with environmental sounds (i.e., car crashes, soccer crowds), so as to retard habituation. The mean intensity was 95 dB, maximum peaks 105 dB.
4. Anticipation of an aversive stimulus (Anticipation): Ss were told that they would get a painful electrical stimulus. They did not know at what

time this was to be expected, they only knew that this would not occur within the next 2 min. The shock itself was not applied.

5. Ergometry (E): an ergometer was pedalled in a supine position with a load of 75 Watts.

Each task lasted for 3 min followed by a rest period of 8 min, with additional rest periods at the beginning (8 min) and end (15 min) of the test. After each stressor, subjects evaluated themselves on a 100-mm visual analogue scale (VAS). Additionally, after having entered the test room, at the beginning of the stress test, and after the trial, Ss completed a 48-item anxiety questionnaire, which was developed from the STAI-G (Spielberger 1975) and DES+A (Izard 1972) questionnaires.

Stress II

In this trial, four tasks were given each lasting for 3 min, followed by a rest period of 4 min with additional rest periods at the beginning and end of the tests. Since only MA was identical to stress I, only baseline and MA data will be reported here. Additional to the subjective ratings given in study I, Ss scored their anxiety and panicky feelings on a 100-mm visual analogue scale after stressors and during the rest periods.

Measures and Analysis

The following physiological parameters were recorded simultaneously and quantified on-line in 10-s periods: electrodermal activity (skin conductance reaction (SCR) and skin conductantce level (SCL), recorded from thenar and proximal hypothenar of the left hand; heart rate (HR), recorded over the cardiac axis (median part of the right clavicula and lower left costal arch); blood pressure, recorded automatically every minute using Riva-Rocci. Riva-Rocci's method. Blood samples for the analyses of NE and E were drawn 2 min after the beginning of each task and at the end of each rest period. Catecholamines were estimated by high pressure liquid chromatography and electrochemical detection.

For statistical evaluation, physiological data were averaged individually within stress and rest periods. To analyse differences between the groups for the different conditions, repeated measured analyses of variance were carried out for all parameters investigated as well as post-hoc Hotelling-t^2 tests for independent samples. Calculations were done with the program BMDP2V.

Results

Stress I

Biochemical and Physiological Data

Though NE secretion was higher in patients, due to the wide variation the ANOVA did not show overall group

Table 1. Norepinephrine (pg/ml) during rest (rest 1, initial rest period; rest 2, final rest period) and during five different stressors

Situations	Patients ($n = 6$) Mean	SD	Controls ($n = 8$) Mean	SD
Rest 1	318.28	106.19	270.63	60.96
Recall	334.86	99.92	237.25	60.38
Mental arithmetic	365.00	111.52	273.50	85.33
Noise	332.83	109.07	266.88	75.87
Anticipation	276.68	58.55	234.25	59.17
Ergometry	354.83	161.17	264.88	86.01
Rest 2	343.17	121.19	258.63	53.84

Table 2. Epinephrine (pg/ml) during rest (rest 1, initial rest period; rest 2, final rest period) and during five different stressors

Situations	Patients Mean	SD	Controls Mean	SD
Rest 1	106.46	97.89	28.88	21.40
Recall	68.10	105.03	25.88	23.31
Mental arithmetic	95.33	68.89	56.25	39.40
Noise	35.17	32.50	21.38	13.73
Anticipation	33.18	7.37	28.13	23.28
Ergometry	37.00	20.99	18.75	12.93
Rest 2	33.17	23.94	27.88	21.63

differences (Table 1). Post hoc *t*-tests showed significantly higher NE levels in the patient group during MA ($P < 0.05$). Also NE secretion increased significantly during MA and ergometry in both groups ($P < 0.05$, Table 1).

Patients had significantly higher E baseline secretion compared to controls ($P < 0.05$). MA led to an increase in E secretion, in the both groups, however, again due to the wide variation did not reach statistical significance (P 12; Table 2).

There was a significant group effect in the ANOVA ($P < 0.02$) as well as a significant situation effect ($P < 0.001$) due to the HR increase in MA and ergometry (Table 3).

The significant situation effect in the ANOVA for systolic BP ($P < 0.001$) was due to increases during MA and ergometry, whereas the significant situation ef-

Table 3. Heart rate (bpm) during initial rest period and during five different stressors

Situations	Patients Mean	SD	Controls Mean	SD
Rest	83.03	18.74	64.60	8.48
Recall	86.67	19.10	65.60	10.45
Mental arithmetic	102.53	21.18	81.08	16.60
Noise	81.03	17.29	64.40	8.96
Anticipation	82.86	20.00	67.01	11.21
Ergometry	106.59	8.67	89.88	15.42

Table 4. Systolic blood pressure (mmHg) during initial rest period and during five different stressors

Situations	Patients Mean	SD	Controls Mean	SD
Rest	113.88	13.51	113.38	10.48
Recall	116.50	15.10	113.50	12.20
Mental arithmetic	134.13	14.93	124.25	15.28
Noise	116.38	14.90	115.63	12.64
Anticipation	116.63	16.18	112.25	12.68
Ergometry	134.13	16.78	125.50	17.33

fect in diastolic BP ($P < 0.001$) was only due to an increase during MA. Again no significant differences between the groups were found (Tables 4 and 5).
The ANOVA showed a significant situation effect for both variables of the electrodermal activity ($P < 0.001$) due to an increase during MA (Tables 6 and 7).

Anxiety Ratings (DES + A)

For state anxiety the ANOVA showed a significant group effect ($P < 0.001$), as well as a significant interaction situation × group ($P < 0.003$) in patients having higher state anxiety levels, more pronounced at the beginning of the trial compared to controls. (Patients: initial rest, 91.89 ± 13.82; final rest, 76.89 ± 20.33. Controls: initial rest, 57.38 ± 4.84; final rest, 55.88 ± 6.01.) For trait anxiety a significant difference between patients and controls (patients, 77.22 ± 14,24; controls 48.50 ± 9.24) was found. Evaluation of stressors did not differ between patients and controls.

Table 5. Diastolic blood pressure (mmHg) during initial rest period and during five different stressors

Situations	Patients		Controls	
	Mean	SD	Mean	SD
Rest	77.50	9.15	76.13	6.85
Recall	79.50	11.94	78.25	6.25
Mental arithmetic	89.50	10.70	85.38	9.75
Noise	79.63	11.48	80.00	5.32
Anticipation	80.63	13.29	70.63	6.00
Ergometry	82.25	11.16	83.00	8.86

Table 6. Skin conductance reaction ($\mu s/cm^2$) during initial rest period and during five different stressors

Situations	Patients		Controls	
	Mean	SD	Mean	SD
Rest	0.44	0.43	0.38	0.20
Recall	0.53	0.38	0.45	0.26
Mental arithmetic	0.76	0.48	0.89	0.39
Noise	0.89	0.56	1.04	0.27
Anticipation	0.89	0.54	1.08	0.38
Ergometry	0.96	0.51	0.90	0.37

Table 7. Skin conductance level ($\mu s/cm^2$) during initial rest period and during five different stressors

Situations	Patients		Controls	
	Mean	SD	Mean	SD
Rest	28.92	15.56	31.49	8.52
Recall	30.22	15.57	31.55	10.66
Mental arithmetic	37.16	19.39	44.65	7.81
Noise	37.04	18.23	44.84	11.57
Anticipation	39.32	21.33	48.75	8.93
Ergometry	44.76	26.39	48.96	12.14

Stress II

In NE both patient groups showed significantly higher levels compared with controls ($P < 0.02$; Table 8). In E secretion, there were no significant differences between the three groups. Also in HR neither rest levels nor increases due to MA showed any difference between the groups investigated. MA led to a significant HR increase in all groups ($P < 0.001$). In ratings of panickiness both patient groups scored significantly higher than controls in all conditions. Agoraphobics scored significantly higher during initial rest compared to panic disorder patients and controls. Again, in anxiety ratings, both patients groups were higher compared to controls. Agoraphobics showed a significant decrease after MA as well as during the final rest period compared to baseline measures. In contrast, panic disordered patients showed a significant increase due to MA.

Besides the data listed in Table 8, anxiety patients again showed overall significantly higher levels in state and trait anxiety as compared to controls (measured by DES+A).

Discussion

Comparison of Base Levels

Consistently anxious patients had higher norepinephrine (NE) base levels in both studies, reaching statistical significance when increasing the number of patients investigated (stress II). This is in line with Mathew et al. (1981) and Ballenger et al. (1984), but seems to contradict the results of others (Kralik et al. 1982; Gasic et al. 1985; Pohl et al. 1987; Villacres et al. 1987). In study I we replicated the findings of Mathew et al. (1981), Nesse et al. (1984), and Villacres et al. (1987) of higher epiphrine (E) baseline secretion in anxious Ss. However, in study II baseline E secretion did not differ between patients groups and controls, a result already reported by Kralik et al. (1982) and Gasic et al. (1985). These diverging results for catecholamine secretion cannot be explained by differ-

Table 8. Means and standard deviations for norepinephrine (NE), epinephrine (E), heart rate (HR), panicky (panic) and anxiety feelings during initial rest (rest 1), final rest (rest 2), and mental arithmetic (MA)

		Agoraphobia with panic ($n = 15$)	Panic disorder ($N = 12$)	Controls ($n = 10$)
Rest 1	NE	316.36 ± 102.49	325.73 ± 62.08	235.70 ± 53.05
	E	46.29 ± 22.59	67.64 ± 34.26	59.70 ± 28.87
	HR	80.40 ± 10.39	76.91 ± 14.01	74.00 ± 7.00
	Panic	38.20 ± 28.42	18.41 ± 21.06	9.30 ± 11.30
	Anxiety	46.47 ± 23.10	25.92 ± 18.83	9.80 ± 11.30
MA	NE	345.60 ± 86.11	346.09 ± 60.33	256.70 ± 62.46
	E	58.71 ± 34.62	78.64 ± 30.20	68.70 ± 23.80
	HR	91.80 ± 12.68	93.30 ± 16.60	87.77 ± 8.80
	Panic	40.27 ± 27.30	28.92 ± 31.69	14.20 ± 18.78
	Anxiety	36.27 ± 26.99	37.00 ± 26.34	12.00 ± 14.58
Rest 2	NE	356.21 ± 109.14	316.18 ± 69.75	274.60 ± 57.06
	E	42.86 ± 19.83	58.64 ± 19.74	61.50 ± 36.00
	HR	78.13 ± 9.23	74.42 ± 7.91	76.22 ± 7.27
	Panic	17.20 ± 19.84	15.92 ± 26.20	5.22 ± 5.45
	Anxiety	23.40 ± 22.28	16.83 ± 24.83	4.77 ± 4.35

ences in the age and sex ratio, since they were comparable in all studies. More likely differences in arterial and venous NE and E content (Villacres et al. 1987), as well as differences in the diagnostic subgroups investigated contribute to those equivocal results. We found elevated NE levels in patients with panic disorder and agoraphobia with panic attacks. In contrast Kralik et al. (1982) as well as Gasic et al. (1985) investigated patients with generalized anxiety disorder and simple phobia. Thus, patients with panic attacks are most likely distinguished from normal controls and other diagnostic subgroups by higher activation of the periphera noradrenergic system. Moreover, the number of patients we investigated in study II was the highest compared to all other studies. Other factors responsible for the discrepancies are differences in refinement of methods in estimating catecholamines and postural effects.

In spite of these limitations our data suggest that anxious patients have a higher activation of the adrenal-medullary component as well as from postganglionic sympathetic nerves of the SNS. For now it is premature to draw any conclusions as to whether these results reflect state or trait phenomena associated with this disorder.

For heart rate (HR) our findings are controversial: In study I patients had significantly higher rest levels than controls, whereas in study II there were no differences between the groups. Since most authors report higher HR base levels (Freedman et al. 1984; Ehlers et al. 1986; Roth et al. 1986; Cowley et al. 1987) in the same diagnostic subgroups we investigated in study II, differences in experimental setting are most likely responsible for the diverging results. While in study I patients were only instructed that they will have to undergo several stress situations, instructions similar to those used in other studies with challenge procedures or habituation tasks, Ss in study II were instructed to cope with tasks requiring active behavior. Gasic et al. (1985), the only group that to date has carried out a stress procedure with anxious patients, also reported no differences in HR and BP. Thus, expectancy factors and differences in experimental setting with structured and time-limited tasks, in contrast to loosely structured challenge procedures have differential effects on base levels in HR and BP. Moreover, differences in drug off-time also have to be considered as a possible source for different findings. The same considerations can be applied to the result that both parameters of electrodermal activity, SCR and SCL, are not significantly different between patients and controls. Since our data are based on patients without panic attacks, whereas the elevation of those parameters reported by Roth et al. (1986) were derived from patients with panic attacks, differences in diagnostic subgroups could have influenced these conflicting findings.

Stress Response

Any conclusions drawn from the stress experiment must be tempered because of the relatively small sample size in study I. Nonsignificant increases in the response variables may have reached significance with a larger sample. Nevertheless, our findings demonstrate that MA leads to significant increases in NE and E. Thus, we have replicated the findings of Dimsdale et al. (1980); Ward et al. (1983); Albus et al. (1985). The most pronounced increase in NE secretion due to ergometry is in line with Gasic et al. (1985). It has to be pointed out that anxious patients have a similar secretion pattern in NE, however based on higher initial levels compared to controls. The possibility was considered first that patients are in a chronic state of maximal arousal and further increases cannot be reached. However, epinephrine

(E) levels, heart rate (HR), and indices of electrodermal activity (EDA) argue against this hypothesis. Moreover, in spite of higher base levels, NE secretion due to ergometry in higher in patients compared to controls. This more pronounced increase and a successive delayed decrease count for the higher NE levels in patients during the final rest period. Thus, this secretion pattern is likely due to an inappropriate sustained activation of sympathetic mechanisms.

Another limitation should be kept in mind for the stress response data. Ward et al. (1983) have shown that results of the repeated measurement ANOVA are inferior to those of a time-series analysis, since ANOVA requires random and independent observations and both catecholamine levels have an underlying trend and slow return to baseline after each intervention. This is also valid for the physiological parameters. In EDA, both groups showed a significant increase due to MA. While patients had a slight increase during ergometry, controls showed a decrease. These differences again reflect higher sympathetic activation to physical stress in the patient group. This is supported by the more pronounced increase in HR and systolic BP in ergometry in the patient group. In contrast, increases in HR, systolic and diastolic BP due to MA are comparable in both groups. These findings suggest that psychological stressors like MA, recall, and anticipation of an aversive situation did not induce different response patterns between patients and controls. The differences in patients and controls in base levels due to expectancy factors disappear, when patients have to undergo structured psychological stressors, where they focus on external stimuli and distract themselves from potentially threatening internal stimuli.

This is supported by the subjective ratings of state and trait anxiety. Here, highly significant differences between patients and controls occurred, a finding reported in all of the above-cited studies. Most strikingly, both, anxiety and panicky feelings were by far higher at the beginning of the test. In the agoraphobics base levels of anxiety and panicky feelings were so high that no further increase was registered due to additional stress such as MA. For anxiety patients the initial rest period is the condition with the highest stress and anxiety-provoking potency. In agoraphobics this ceiling effect suppresses further increases in anxiety due to additional stress, therefore these ratings drop to much lower values after MA and at the end of the trial.

On the present evidence, while differences emerge between anxious patients and controls one cannot link these to the disorder per se. Autonomic functioning and subjective evaluation is not a static property of the individual. It has a developmental course and is influenced by learning and psychological state. Further studies of cognitive and psychological contributions to baseline and response measures are necessary to clarify the role of those determinants.

References

Albus M, Ackenheil M, Engel RR, Müller-Spahn F, Stahl S (1985) Influence of beta-blockers and/or minor tranquilizers on autonomic stress reactions. Pharmacopsychiatry 18:15–16

Albus M, Stahl S, Müller-Spahn F, Engel RR (1986) Psychophysiological differentiation of two types on anxiety and its pharmacological modification by minor tranquilizer and beta-receptor-blocker. Biol Psychol 23:39–51

Ballenger JC, Peterson GA, Laraia M, Hueck A, Lake CR, Jimerson D, Cow DJ, Trockman C, Shipe JR, Wilkinson C (1984) A study of plasma catecholamines in agoraphobia and the relationship of serum tricyclic levels to treatment response. In: Ballenger JC (ed) Biology of agoraphobia. Psychiatric Press, Washington, DC, p 42

Charney DS, Heninger GR, Breier A (1984) Noradrenergic function in panic anxiety: effects of yohimbine in healthy subjects and patients with agoraphobia and panic disorder. Arch Gen Psychiatry 41:752–763

Charney DS, Heninger GR, Breier A (1984) Noradrenergic function in panic anxiety. Arch Gen Psychiatry 41:751-763

Charney DS, Heninger GR, Jatlow PI (1985) Increased anxiogenic effects of caffeine in panic disorders. Arch Gen Psychiatry 42:233-243

Charney DS, Woods SW, Goodman WK, Heninger GR (1987) Neurobiological mechanisms of panic anxiety: biochemical and behavioral correlates of Yohimbine-induced panic attacks. Am J Psychiatry 144:8:1030-1036

Clark DM, Hensley DR (1982) The effect of hyperventilation: individual variability and its relation to personality. J Behav Ther Exp Psychiatry 13:41-47

Cowley DS, Hyde TS, Dager SR, Dunner DL (1987) Lactate infusions: the role of baseline anxiety. Psychiatry Res 14:169-179

Dimsdale JE, Moss J (1980) Short-term catecholamines response to psychological stress. Psychosom Med 52:5:493-497

Dorow R, Horowski, Paschelke G et al. (1983) Severe anxiety induced by FG 7142, a β-carboline ligand for benzodiazepine receptors. Lancet II:98-100

Ehlers A, Margraf J, Torth WT, Taylor CB, Maddock RJ, Sheikh J, Kopell ML, McClenahan KL, Gossard D, Blowers GH, Agras WS, Kopell BS (1986) Lactate infusions and panic attacks: do patients and controls response differently? Psychiatry Res 17:295-308

Freedman RR, Ianni P, Ettedgui E, Pohl R, Rainey JM (1984) Psychophysiological factors in panic disorder. Psychopathology 17:1:66-73

Freedman RR, Ianni P, Ettedgui E, Puthezhath N (1985) Ambulatory monitoring of panic disorder. Arch Gen Psychiatry 42:244-248

Fyer AJ, Liebowitz MR, Gorman JM et al (1985) Lactate vulnerability of remitted panic patients. Psychiatry Res 14:138-143

Gasic S, Grünberger J, Korn A, Oberhummer I, Zapotoczky HG (1985) Biochemical physical and psychological findings in patients suffering from cardiac neurosis. Neuropsychobiology 13:12-16

Gorman JM, Askanazi J, Liebowitz MR et al (1984) Response to hyperventilation in a group of patients with panic disorder. Am J Psychiatry 141:857-861

Griez EJL; Lousberg H, van den Hout MA, van der Molen GM (1986) Psychiatry Res 20:87-95

Hibbert GA (1984) Ideational components of anxiety: their origin and content. Br J Psychiatry 144:618-624

Izard CE (1972) Patterns of emotions. Academic, New York

Kralik PM, Ho BT, Mathew JR, Taylor DL, Weinman ML (1982) Effects of adrenaline administration on platelet MAO of anxious and normal subjects. Neuropsychobiology 8:205-209

Ley R (1985) Agoraphobia, the panic attack and the hyperventilation syndrome. Behav Res Ther 23:79-82

Liebowitz MR, Fyer AJ, Gorman JM, Dillon D, Appleby IL, Anderson S, Levitt M, Palij M, Davies SO, Klein DF (1984) Lactate provocation of panic attacks: I. Clinical and behavioural findings. Arch Gen Psychiatry 41:764-770

Margraf J, Ehlers A, Roth WT (1986) Sodium lactate infusions and panic attacks: a review and critique. Psychosom Med 48:23

Mathew RJ, Ho BT, Kralik PM, Taylor DL, Claghorn JL (1981) Catecholamines and monoamine oxidase activity in anxiety. Acta Psychatr Scand 63:245-252

Mathew RJ, Ho BT, Francis DJ, Taylor DL, Weinman ML (1982) Catecholamines and anxiety. Acta Psychiatr Scand 65:142-147

Nesse RM, Cameron OG, Curtis GC, McCann DS, Huber-Schmith (1984) Adrenergic function in patients with panic anxiety. Arch Gen Psychiatry 41:771-776

Pohl R, Ettedgui E, Bridges M, Lycaki H, Jimerson D, Kopin I, Rainey JM (1987) Plasma MHPG levels in lactate and isoproterenol anxiety states. Biol Psychiatry 22:1127-1136

Rainey JM, Pohl RB, Williams M, Knitter E, Freedman RR, Ettedgui E (1984) A comparison of lactate and isoproterenol anxiety states. Psychopathology 17 (1):74-82

Roth WT, Telch MJ, Taylor CB, Sachitano JA, Gallen CC, Kopell ML, McClenahan KL, Agras WS, Pfefferbaum A (1986) Autonomic characteristics of agoraphobia with panic attacks. Biol Psychiatry 21:1133-1154

Spielberger CD (1975) Anxiety: state-trait-process. In: Spielberger CD, Sarason IG (eds) Stress and anxiety, vol 1, Wiley, New York

Van den Hout MA, Griez E (1982) Cognitive factors in carbon dioxide therapy. J Psychosom Res 26:209-214

Villacres EC, Hollified M, Katon WJ, Wilkinson CW, Veith RC (1987) Sympathetic nervous system activity in panic disorder. Psychiatry Res 14:313-321

Ward MM, Mefford IN, Parker SD, Chesney MA, Taylor CB, Keegan DL, Barchas JD (1983) Epinephrine and norepinephrine responses in continuously collected plasma to a series of stressors. Psychosom Med 45:6:471-486

Woods SW, Charney DS, McPherson CA (1987) Situational panic attacks. Arch Gen Psychiatry 44:365-375

Yeragani VK, Pohl R, Rainey JM, Balon R, Ortiz A, Lycaki H, Gershon S (1987) Pre-infusion heart rates and laboratory-induced panic anxiety. Acta Psychiatr Scand 75:51-54

17. Comorbidity of Panic Disorder and Major Depression: Results from a Family Study

W. Maier, R. Buller, and J. Hallmayer

Introduction

Familial clustering of anxiety disorders was found in several studies: for anxiety neurosis (Noyes et al. 1978), panic disorder and agoraphobia (Harris et al. 1983; Crowe et al. 1983; Crowe 1985; Noyes et al. 1986; Hopper et al. 1987), and generalized anxiety disorder (Noyes et al. 1987). Twin studies have demonstrated that genetic factors are relevant for the familial clustering of panic disorder/agoraphobia (Crowe 1985). Psychosocial factors may also be relevant, for the concordance rate for monozygotic twins is only 60% (Torgersen 1983).

Though familial clustering of panic disorder is common, "sporadic" cases also are reported (Van Valkenburg et al. 1984) and the extent of clustering is heterogeneous. Carefully designed family studies are tools for dissolving this heterogeneity. Factors modifying the familial rate of particular disorders can be isolated by family studies. An example for the utility of family studies in solving the problem of etiologic heterogeneity is the Yale Family Study in depressive disorders (Leckman et al. 1983a; Price et al. 1987), where it was observed that panic attacks occurring in patients with a lifetime history of major depression substantially increased the familial risk of major depression. This result stimulates a hypothesis concerning the factors modifying the familial rate and being responsible for the genetic heterogeneity of panic disorders: patients with both panic disorder and major depression have a higher familial risk for panic disorder than patients with panic disorder only. Investigating this hypothesis requires refraining from using the hierarchical procedure in differentiating between anxiety and depressive disorders (symptoms of anxiety due to - i.e., occurring during - an affective episode - are neglected for diagnosis); DSM-IIIR offers a non-hierarchical manner of classification (APA 1987). Family studies of panic disorder addressing this issue of comorbidity of depressive and anxiety disorders have not been published yet.

We report lifetime diagnoses of firstdegree relatives of patients with panic disorder (DSM-IIIR) with and without additional lifetime diagnosis of major depression (DSM-IIIR). The control group in this report are families of patients with major depression without a lifetime diagnosis of anxiety syndromes.

The data to be presented are preliminary results from an ongoing family study including patients with anxiety and affective disorders and control subjects. Because of the small number of completely interviewed families, we are not able to distinguish the probands by sex and by generations (parents, siblings, children). Only diagnoses obtained by personally interviewing the probands, blindly for the diagnosis of other family members are reported.

Patients, Probands and Procedure

In- and outpatients (aged 20–70 years) admitted to the Psychiatric University Hospital in Mainz with a present major depression (DSM-IIIR) or a present panic disorder (DSM-IIIR) received a structured lifetime interview using the SADS-LA. Patients with a lifetime history of delusions, hallucinations, schizophreniform disorders, schizoaffective disorders, psychotic affective disorders, an episode of mania (bipolar major depression), obsessive-compulsive disorder, or dependence on alcohol or drugs (DSM-IIIR) were excluded. All other patients with at least one living first-degree relative were asked for consent in participating in this study; all first-degree relatives older than 14 years were asked for consent in participation.

Family members agreeing to participate were interviewed using a structured clinical interview (SADS-LA) performed by trained research assistants (the training had at least 20 sessions, kappa for reliability in the major diagnoses - major depression, panic disorder - was about 0.80). The interviews of different members of a family were carried out independently by different interviewers who were blind for the diagnoses of other family members (including the patient).

Family members not agreeing to participate were diagnosed using the family history method. Families without first - degree relatives available to be interviewed personally with the SADS-LA were excluded from this report.

The final DSM-IIIR diagnoses of each proband were assigned by experienced psychiatrists based on the data obtained from the SADS-LA, charts - as far as they were available - and other informations (e.g., the general practitioner treating the family). Conflicting diagnostic information was handled according to the rules of the "best estimate diagnosis" (Leckman et al. 1982).

Fifteen patients with panic disorder without a history of major depression, 27 patients with panic disorder and major depression, and 29 patients with major depression without a history of anxiety disorders with families fulfilling these conditions were recruited. In order to keep the groups comparable, the three groups to be compared were matched for sex and age (± 3 years); for each of the 15 patients with pure panic disorder, one patient in each of both other groups was selected. We came up with 15 patients and their families in each of the three groups.

Relatives and patients were diagnosed according to DSM-IIIR. In patients only definite diagnoses were counted; in relatives the diagnoses were based on the definite as well as probable cases; panic disorder was diagnosed if the attacks were accompanied by at least two symptom criteria. Relatives whose attacks occurred less frequently than once per week for 3 weeks were also assigned to panic disorder; major depression was diagnosed if at least three of the eight symptom criteria for major depression were present in previous episodes or if at least four of eight symptom criteria for major depression were present for a current episode.

Results

Fifteen patients and their families in the subsample of patients with major depression and panic disorder and equally 15 patients and their families in the subgroup of patients with major depression alone were matched by age and sex to the 15 patients with pure panic disorder (Table 1). All three groups to be compared have in addition similar numbers of first-degree relatives; the mean age and the sex distribution of the first-degree relatives is not significantly different ($P < 0.05$) between the three groups (U-test, Chi-square test).

Table 1. Age and sex in the patients and their first-degree relatives

	Panic disorder alone ($n = 15$)	Major depression + panic disorder ($n = 15$)	Major depression alone ($n = 15$)
Probands:			
Mean age (years)	39.6	40.6	40.9
Sex (m:f)	5:10	5:10	5:10
Relatives:			
First-degree relatives (n)	62	58	56
Personally interviewed (n)	45	45	46
Mean age (years)	43.7	46.2	44.9
Sex (m:f)	20:25	22:23	20:26

Consequently, we are justified in comparing the familial loadings in the three groups without adjusting for differences in age distributions and sex ratios between the groups; the frequencies of disorders in the family can be used instead of morbid risks (Andreasen et al. 1987).
The familial patterns of panic disorder (probable or definite) and of major depression (probable and definite) behave along the following lines (Table 2):

1. Major depression (definite or probable) as well as panic disorder (definite or probable) are more frequent in families of patients with both major depression (definite) and panic disorder (definite) than in families with a lifetime diagnosis of either major depression (definite) or panic disorder (definite).
2. Major depression is more frequent in families of patients with major depression (21%) than in panic patients without a history of major depression (11%).
3. Panic disorder is more frequent in families of patients with panic disorder (15%) than in families of depressed patients without a history of anxiety disorders (11%).

The identical patterns can be observed if major depression is substituted by all kinds of affective disorders (DSM-IIIR including labile personality and minor depression according to RDC) in relatives and if panic disorder is substituted by all kinds of anxiety disorders (DSM-IIIR including adjustment disorders with anxiety) in relatives (Table 3).

Taking all kinds of psychiatric disorders together as they are listed in DSM-IIIR (axis I) and assessed by the SADS-LA (including labile personality and minor depression), families of patients with panic disorder as well as major depression show the highest prevalence of psychiatric

Table 2. Panic disorder (DSM-IIIR) and major depression (DSM-IIIR) in the first-degree relatives of patients with panic disorder and major depression

Diagnoses in patients' relatives	Panic disorder alone ($n = 15$)	Major depression + panic disorder ($n = 15$)	Major depression alone ($n = 15$)
Panic disorder	15	18	11
Major depression	11	21	19
Both disorders	7	13	10

Table 3. Anxiety and affective disorders (DSM-IIIR) in the first-degree relatives of patients with panic disorder and major depression

Diagnoses in probands' relatives	Panic disorder alone ($n = 15$)	Major depression + panic disorder ($n = 15$)	Major depression alone ($n = 15$)
Anxiety disorder	19	25	14
Affective disorders	16	28	24
Both	11	20	12

Table 4. Psychiatric disorders (DSM-IIIR) in the first-degree relatives of patients with panic disorder and major depression

Diagnoses in patients' relatives	Panic disorder alone ($n = 15$)	Major depression + panic disorder ($n = 15$)	Major depression alone ($n = 15$)
Psychiatric disorders	31	45	38

disorders (45%; Table 4), families of patients with panic disorder and without a history of major depression show the lowest prevalence of psychiatric disorders (31%; Table 4).

These trends are not clearly significant because of the limited sample size; the twofold sample size will be necessary to reach significance for the characteristic family patterns described above.

Discussion

The distinction between panic disorder (DSM-IIIR) and major depression (DSM-IIIR) is supported by the family data reported in this study: the prevalence of panic disorder in families of patients with panic disorder is higher than in families of patients without a history of panic attacks; equally the prevalence of major depression in families of depressed patients is higher than in families of patients without a history of major depression.

Unfortunately the rates for major depression and panic disorder in families of nonpsychiatric control probands are not available at present. Compared to lifetime prevalence of panic disorder in epidemiological samples, the prevalence of panic disorder in families of patients with major depressions is higher than is reported for the general population (Wittchen, Chapter 1, Robins et al. 1984). Our finding is in contrast to other family studies (Noyes et al. 1986; Van Valkenburg et al. 1984). The lower prevalences for panic disorder in these family studies may be explained by methodological differences with our family study. We used non - hierarchical diagnostic schedules; the less sensitive family history method instead of a family study method was used in the study of Van Valkenburg et al. (1984).

An increased prevalence of major depression in families of patients with panic disorder but without a history of major depression compared to rates in the general population (Wittchen, Chapter 1; Robins et al. 1984) was also observe. The interpretation of this finding is difficult. One explanation is that panic disorder per se is associated with an increased familial risk of major depression; another possible explanation is that the increased familial risk is due to lowdegree depressed mood in the probends with panic disorder but not severe enough to be classified as affective disorders. Noyes et al. (1986) also found an increased familial risk for (secondary) major depression in panic and agoraphobic patients. Van Valkenburg et al. (1984) are not in agreement with these results. Again methodological differences may explain this discrepancy.

The increased rates for major depression in families of panic disorder patients and for panic disorder in families of depressed patients support the hypothesis of an overlap in the etiologies of panic and affective disorders. This hypothesis is also supported by a series of biological studies (e.g., Uhde and Stein, Chapter 2). On the other hand, the differences of the familial loadings between the pure panic and the pure depression group show that there is only a partial overlap in the etiologies of panic and depressive disorders.

The comorbidity of panic and depressive disorders was associated with an increased risk for panic disorder and major depression, for anxiety and depressive disorders, and for the total group of psychiatric disorders. This trend did not reach significance because of the limited sample size. These findings are in line with the Yale Family Study (Leckman et al. 1983), demonstrating a superadditive effect of the comorbidity on major depression; however, the comparison group of the mixed states was only a group of purely depressed patients; a group of patients without depressive disorders was not a included in the Yale Family Study. On the other hand, Van Valkenburg et al. (1984) could not find an increased risk of pure depression in mixed states relative to pure depressive disorder; equally they could not find an increased risk of panic disorder in mixed states relative to pure panic disorder. The discrepancies between these and our findings may be due to the family history method used by Van Valkenburg et al.; this method is less sensitive than the family study method and is more prone to biases in reporting the symptomatology.

The limitation of this study is the small sample size in each group ($n = 15$). Though this shortcoming is partly compensated by the matched-pairs technique, the trends observed did not reach significance. A twofold larger sample size in each group will be necessary so that each of the trends reported can show significance.

References

American Psychiatric Association (APA) (1987) DSM-III. 3rd edn. (DSM-IIIR). American Psychiatric Association, Washington DC

Andreasen NC, Rice J, Endicott J, Coryell W, Grove WM, Reich T (1987) Familial rates of affective disorders. Arch Gen Psychiatry 44:461–472

Crowe RR, Noyes R, Pauls DL, Slymen D (1983) A family study of panic disorder. Arch Gen Psychiatry 40:1065–1069

Crowe RR (1985) The genetics of panic disorder and agoraphobia. Psychiatr Develop 2:171–186

Harris EL, Noyes R, Crowe RR, Chandry DR (1983) Family study of agoraphobia. Arch Gen Psychiatry 40:1061–1064

Hopper JL, Judd FK, Burrows GD (1987) Family study of panic disorder. Genet Epidemiol

Leckman JF, Sholomskas D, Thompson WD, Balanger A, Weissman MM (1982) Best estimate of lifetime psychiatric diagnosis: a methodological study. Arch Gen Psychiatry 39:879–883

Leckman JF, Weissman MM, Merkangas KR, Pauls DL, Prusoff BA (1983) Panic disorder and major depression: increased resk of depression, alcoholism, panic and phobic disorders in families of depressed probands with panic disorder. Arch Gen Psychiatry 40:1055–1060

Noyes R, Clancy J, Crowe R, Hoenk PR, Slymen DJ (1978) The familial prevalence of anxiety neuroses. Arch Gen Psychiatry 35:1057–1060

Noyes R, Crowe RR, Harris EL, Hamra BJ, McChesney CM, Chaudhry DR (1986) Relationship between panic disorder and agoraphobia. A family study. Arch Gen Psychiatry 43:227–232

Noyes R, Clarkson C, Crowe RR, Jates WR, McChesney CM (1987) A family study of generalized anxiety disorder. Am J Psychiatry 144:1019–1024

Price RA, Kidd KK, Weissman MM (1987) Early onset (under age 30 years) and panic disorder as markers for etiologic homogeneity in major depression. Arch Gen Psychiatry 44:434–440

Robins LN, Helzer ZE, Weissman MM, Orvaschel H, Gruenberg E, Burke JD, Regier DA (1984) Lifetime prevalence of specific psychiatric disorders. Arch Gen Psychiatry 41:949–958

Torgersen S (1983) Genetic factors in anxiety disorders. Arch Gen Psychiatry 40:1085–1089

Van Valkenburg C, Akiskal HS, Puzantian V (1984) Anxious depression: clinical, family history and naturalistic outcome - comparisons with panic and major depression disorder. J Affective Disord 6:67–82

18. Anxiety and Sensitization: A Neuropsychological Approach

F. Strian and L. Hartl

In view of the growing controversy about panic attacks in the context of the new operationalization in DSM-IIIR over biologically and behaviorally oriented approaches to anxiety, we present a neuropsychological approach to the etiology and classification of anxiety attacks. Pathological anxiety always results from the interplay of psychological and physiological factors. Consequently, failure to consider this interaction can be detrimental to both diagnosis and treatment.

We would like to describe the role of the limbic structures that may be called a "biological alarm system," and their reciprocal interaction with - in the broadest sense - extralimbic system which represent environmental, organismic, cognitive, and behavioral influences on anxiety attacks.

As early as 1952, Mulder and Daly reported that anxiety was found to be a frequent symptom in 100 patients with temporal lobe disorders, including 24 tumors. They pointed out that "temporal" anxiety occurs as ictal as well as interictal anxiety. Harper and Roth (1962) were not able to delineate significant differences between anxiety in temporal lobe epilepsy and anxiety occurring in the context of the neurotic "phobic anxiety depersonalization syndrome." Differences between the two manifestations of anxiety rather concerned the presence of absence of precipitating factors and the underlying personality. Remarkably, the explicit symptomatology of panic attacks diagnosed according to DSM-III has recently been reported to occur with temporal lobe disorders (Dietch 1984, Wall et al. 1985, Ghadirian et al. 1986). Since slowly growing tumors of the base of the skull such as gliomas and meningiomas frequently present with psychopathological symptoms alone - a "pseudoneurotic" prodromal stage - anxiety attacks may be the only symptom over a prolonged period of time. The organic pathogenesis is confirmed only when anxiety attacks later become the aura of complex partial seizures in addition to being still present as isolated anxiety attacks.

Recent reports concerning changes of regional cerebral blood flow and metabolism in patients with typical panic attacks determined by positron emission tomography (PET) are of particular interest in this context. Reimann et al. (1986) describe an increase in blood flow, blood volume, and oxygen consumption in the right parahippocampal region in patients with lactate-induced panic attacks. Reivich et al. (1983) demonstrated an increase of glucose utilization in the right frontodorsal area. Although these findings need further confirmation, they may represent a promising additional approach as far as topical aspects of anxiety are concerned.

The morphological as well as the electroencephalograpic demonstration of functional disturbances related to cerebral anxiety attacks meets with special difficulties. For example, an underlying gliosis of the mediobasal temporal lobe may be visualized only by nuclear magnetic resonance imaging (NMR) and not by cranial computerized tomography (CCT).

The electroencephalographic demonstration of paroxysmal anxiety appears to be equally difficult, since hypersynchronous activity of mediobasal temporal lobe structures is by no means necessarily visible in surface EEG recordings. Occasionally, this activity has been successfully demonstrated with special recording techniques from the base of the skull such as sphenoidal (Kristensen and Sindrup 1978) or, although invasive, infraorbital leads (Wieser et al. 1985).

Recently, the improvement of depth electrode recordings, the so-called stereo-EEG, has provided further topical insights. With stereotactic stimulation of mediobasal temporal regions, anxiety is the emotion evoked by far the most frequent (Fig. 1). As compared to other ictal phenomena, symptoms of anxiety are about three times as frequent as the next most frequent symptom (visual hallucinations) and occur approximately ten times as often as the next most common emotion (depression, Gloor et al. 1982). Depth electrode recordings during spontaneous anxiety showed that hypersynchronous activity was frequently recorded in the mediobasal temporal lobe exclusively, while surface-EEG tracings remain unnoticed. Weingarten et al. (1977) demonstrated by depth electrode recordings that paroxysmal activity was associated with anxiety only and that anxiety was followed by a complex partial seizure as soon as the ictal activity spread to neighboring limbic structures. Obviously, anxiety can be elicited not only from the amygdaloid nucleus but also from other temporal and limbic structures, particularly the hippocampal region. If localized in the temporopolar region, seizures are associated - in addition to anxiety - with pronounced autonomic reactions. Using depth electrode recordings, Stodieck and Wieser (1986) documented sudden excessive heart rate changes resembling those of panic attacks (Cohen et al. 1985).

On the basis of extensive depth electrode recordings in temporal lobe epilepsy, Wieser (1983) was able to detect characteristic pathways of spread of hypersynchroneous activity. Symptoms of anxiety appear to be associated predominantly with a temporobasal and a temporopolar pathway. The prevailing path of spread allows certain conclusions as far as addi-

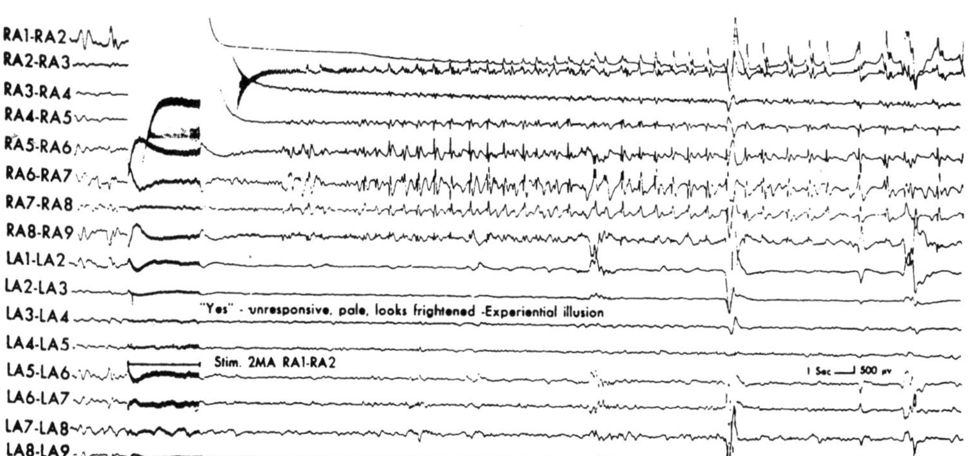

Fig. 1. Stereotactic stimulation of the right amygdala (RA1-RA2) elicits a complex experiential response and an aftercharge involving limbic and neocortical structures of the right temporal lobe. During stimulation with a higher intensity (3mA) the same patient reported being extremely frightended. (Gloor et al. 1982).

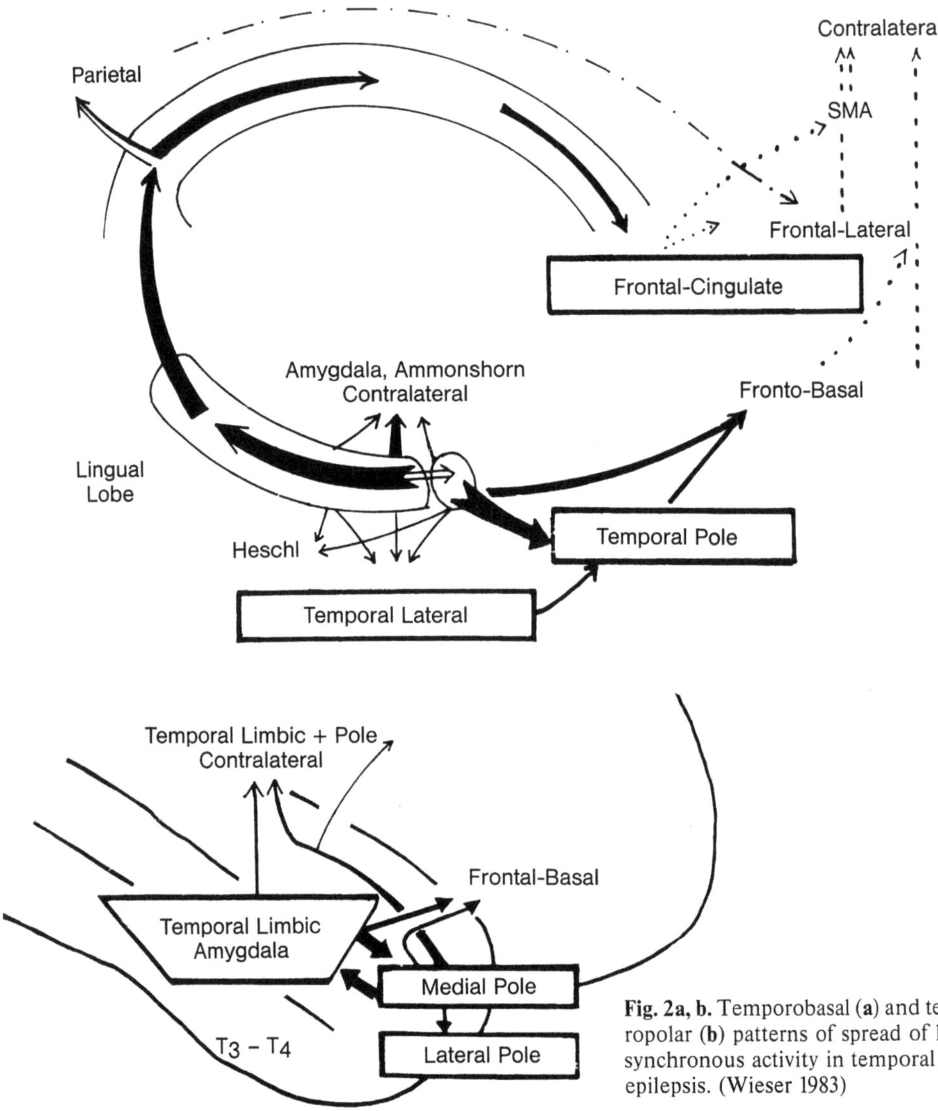

Fig. 2a, b. Temporobasal (**a**) and temporopolar (**b**) patterns of spread of hypersynchronous activity in temporal lobe epilepsis. (Wieser 1983)

tional symptoms associated with an anxiety attack are concerned, such as feelings of derealization or depersonalization, hallucinations, and clouding of consciousness, on the one hand, and autonomic reactions, on the other (Fig. 2a, b).

The clinical and electrobiological observations described here lend support to the assumption that certain limbic structures are a central component of a biological alarm system which is normally turned on by an external threat, but that may also be activated by a functional disturbance of these structures themselves. In the latter case, the ensuing symptoms are those of spontaneous, paroxysmal anxiety to which a subset of panic attacks may possibly also be attributed. All other manifestations of anxiety arise from perceptive-cognitive "pathways of threat,"

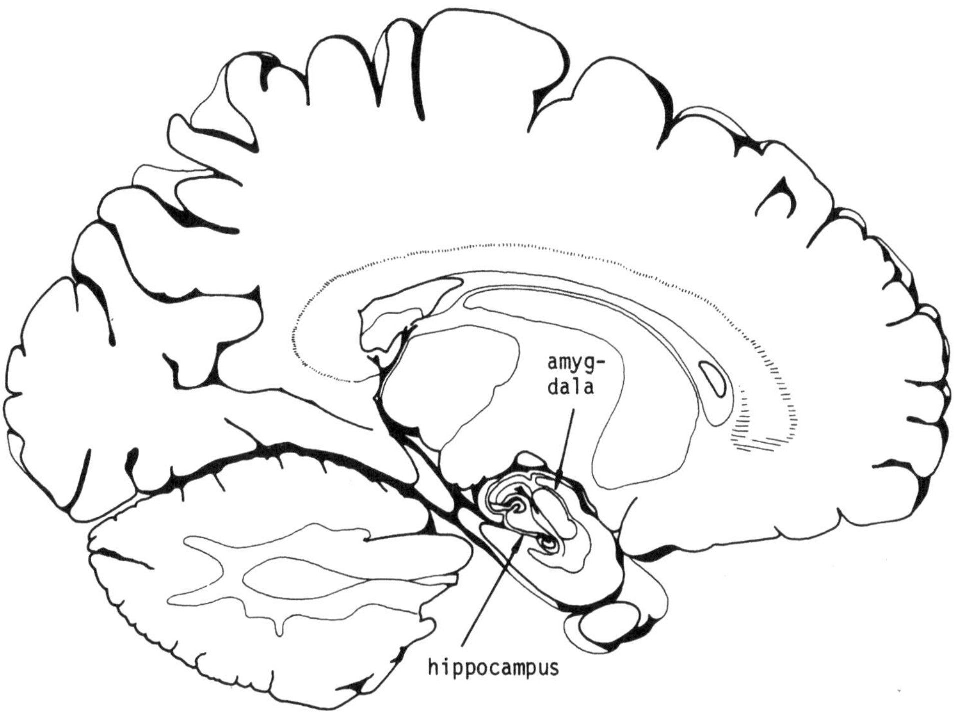

Fig. 3. The paramedian section of the cerebrum shows the hidden topography of the hippocampal and amygdaloid structures

specifically via sensory or visceral perception, or on the basis of behavioral or cognitive factors. Several of the neuroanatomical and functional features of certain limbic structures, particularly of the hippocampus and the amygdaloid nucleus, may be interpreted in the context of these hypotheses (Fig. 3).

Neuroanatomically, there are extensive reciprocal connections of limbic structures via the inner and outer cingulum and via the septal-hypothalamic-mesencephalic axis which includes noradrenergic projections from the locus ceruleus and serotonergic projections from the raphe nuclei. Furthermore, the hippocampus and the amygdaloid nucleus receive multimodal sensory afferences from the primary sensory areas of the cerebral cortex. Since these afferences are always indirect projections, the sensory input is highly convergent. Therefore, hippocampus and amygdala represent entry ports for preprocessed information from all sensory modalities. Simultaneously, the hippocampus and the amygdaloid nucleus project to subcortical and neocortical, particularly prefrontal regions. Consequently, the hippocampus and the amygdaloid nucleus represent an interface between external and internal perception and the cortical and subcortical mechanisms concerned with the regulation of behavior.

Thus, from a neuroanatomical point of view, the mediobasal temporal structures appear to be predisposed for the discrimination between irrelevant and relevant, unconditioned and conditioned, indifferent and emotional, as well as neutral and threatening information from the external environment and from the organism itself.

Functionally, hippocampus and amygdala show some peculiar features that appear to be relevant to emotional reactions and to the processing of threatening information. These are the phenomena of synaptic facilitation, long-term potentiation, low seizure threshold, kindling, and the fact that ictal symptoms are readily elicited. Synaptic facilitation denotes and enhancement of transsynaptic excitation of relatively short duration; long-term potentiation (LTP) is an increase of synaptic excitability for hours to weeks (McNaughton et al. 1978). Since these phenomena are probably caused by the cooperative action of different neurons, it appears likely that an associative coupling of simultaneous stimuli is induced and that, in addition, a reinforcement of neighboring synapses occurs (Andersen and Hvalby 1986). The enhancement of synaptic excitability may, therefore, be the basis for the conditioning mechanisms characteristic for emotional behavior. (In addition, LTP has been proposed to represent an important mechanism in the formation of permanent memory traces.) Finally, synaptic facilitation effective for a prolonged period of time, and lowering of the threshold in the hippocampus, may be a direct substrate of emotional reactions, since these reactions also outlast the initiating stimulus and require facilitation and a certain latency period (Creutzfeld 1983). Similar functional features are also characteristic for the amygdaloid nucleus.

Since anxiety is a complex experience and behavior and is determined by a multitude of external, internal, biographical, ethological, behavioral, and cognitive factors, the central nervous system mechanisms involved may be expected to be equally complex. On the other hand, anxiety, particularly pathological anxiety, always appears to involve mediobasal temporal lobe structures and the associated symptoms - this is consistent with the clinical experience that anxiety never occurs without its physical features which are essential to the irresistible and overwhelming character of anxiety.

The cerebral approach to anxiety described here may therefore serve as a basis for a neuropsychologically oriented classification of clinical anxiety states. Pathological anxiety may be defined as anxiety occurring without any perception of threat - i.e., in the absence of a present or preceding threatening situation - or as anxiety out of proportion to the present threat. In addition, anxietysolving behavior (Caspar 1983).

Spontaneous paroxysmal anxiety probably most closely corresponds to a functional disturbance of the limbic structures themselves, including the noradrenergic and serotonergic projections of the locus ceruleus and the raphe nuclei, respectively. All other manifestations of anxiety arise from an interaction of "extralimbic" and may also arise from behavioral and decision-making conflicts occurring as a consequence of competing coping strategies that inhibit problem-"limbic" structures (Fig. 4).

In the latter case, three pathogenetic pathways are conceivable:

a) Anxiety arises from threatening sensory, i.e., environmental, information or sensory information that is erroneously considered to be threatening.
b) Anxiety arises from threatening visceral, i.e., internal information, or visceral information that is erroneously considered to be threatening.
c) Anxiety arises from behavioral and decision-making conflicts blocking adequate coping strategies.

Conceivably, the development of anxiety states is always characterized by reciprocal interactions of pathogenetic pathways. On the one hand, a disturbance of limbic function may lead to an abnormal, phobic processing of environmental situations (see also the discussion of acquired and innate factors in the development of

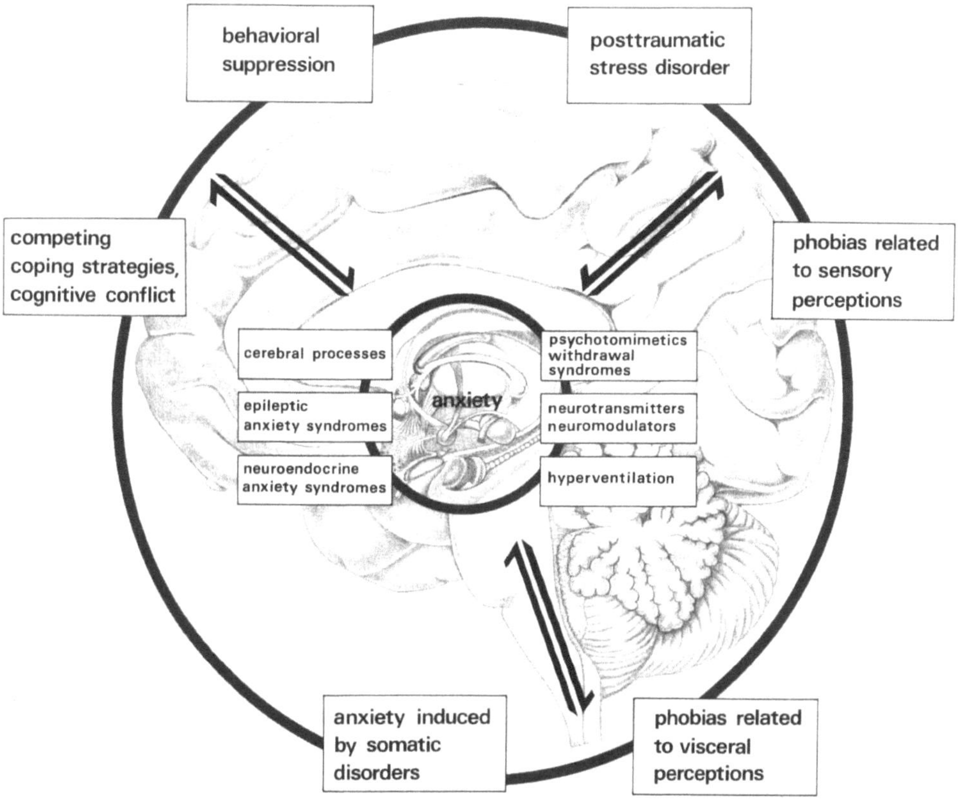

Fig. 4. This pathogenetic model of anxiety shows the reciprocal interaction of limbic and extralimbic conditions

phobias by Seligman 1971). In this model, the phobic avoidance behavior arises from a sensitization and generalization of situations and conditions associated with the panic attacks. The development of agoraphobic symptoms following initial panic attacks may be an example. On the other hand, spontaneous panic attacks, following excessively threatening experiences, such as situations of war and persecution or airplane hijackings, point to an opposite direction of the pathogenetic pathway. In this case, environmental events appear to induce a persistent limbic "sensitization" predisposing to the development of panic attacks. Equivalent reciprocal relationships are also conceivable concerning visceral perceptions (e.g., cardiac phobia vs organic cardiac disease) or conflict of behavior and decision making (behavioral suppression is the most important animal model of anxiety).

The presentation of clinical, neuropsychological, and psychological findings supporting this interpretation of anxiety emphasizing central nervous system mechanisms are beyond the scope of this article. However, a neuropsychological approach to anxiety and clinical syndromes of anxiety will hopefully eliminate traditional, presently irreconcilable dichotomies between psychological, biological, genetic, etc. aspects and may provide more reliable criteria for therapeutic decisions. The clinical relevance of these models for the development of pathological anxiety has yet to be determined. The interactions of the neuropsychological model described here not only provide a basis for an understanding of the development of anxiety states as sensitization processes, but may also serve as a plausible explanation for the success of behaviorally oriented therapeutic interventions in the sense of reconditioning processes.

References

Andersen P, Hvalby O (1986) Long-term potentiation: problems and possible mechanisms. In: Isaacson RL, Pribram KH (eds) The hippocampus, vol 3. Plenum, New York, pp 169-186

Caspar F (1983) Verhaltenstherapie der Angst. In: Strian F (ed) Angst - Grundlagen und Klinik. Springer, Berlin Heidelberg New York, pp 383-428

Cohen AS, Barlow DH, Blanchard EG (1985) Psychophysiology of relaxation-associated panic attacks. J Abnorm Psychol 94:96-101

Creutzfeldt OD (1983) Cortex cerebri. Leistung, strukturelle und funktionelle Organisation der Hirnrinde. Springer, Berlin Heidelberg New York

Dietch JT (1984) Cerebral tumor presenting with panic attacks. Psychosomatics 25:861-863

Ghadirian AM, Gauthier S, Bertrand S (1986) Anxiety attacks in a patient with a right temporal lobe meningioma. J Clin Psychiatry 47:270-271

Gloor P, Olivier A, Quesney Lf, Andermann F, Horowitz S (1982) The role of the limbic system in experimental phenomena of temporal lobe epilepsy. Ann Neurol 12:129-144

Harper M, Roth M (1962) Temporal lobe epilepsy and the phobic anxiety-depersonalization syndrome. Part I: a comparative study. Compr Psychiatry 3:129-151

Kristensen O, Sindrup EH (1978) Psychomotor epilepsy and psychosis. Electroencephalographic findings (sphenoidal electrode recordings). Acta Neurol Scand 57:370-379

McNaughton BL, Douglas RM, Goddard GV (1978) Synaptic enhancement in fascia dentata: cooperativity among coactive afferents. Brain Res 157:277-293

Mulder DW, Daly D (1952) Psychiatric symptom associated with lesions of temporal lobe. JAMA 150:173-176

Reiman EM, Raichle ME, Robins E, Butler FK, Herscovitch P, Fox P, Perlmutter J (1986) The application of positron emission tomography to the study of panic disorder. Am J Psychiatry 143:469-477

Reivich M, Gur R, Alavi A (1983) Positron emission tomographic studies of sensory stimuli, cognitive processes and anxiety. Hum Neurobiol 2:25-33

Seligman MEP (1971) Phobias and preparedness. Behav Res Ther 2:307-321

Stodieck RG, Wieser HG (1986) Autonomic phenomena in temporal lobe epilepsy. J Auton Nerv Syst [Suppl]:611-621

Wall M, Tuchman M, Mielke D (1985) Panic attacks and temporal lobe seizures associated with a right temporal lobe arteriovenous malformation: case report. J Clin Psychiatry 46:143-145

Weingarten SM, Cherlow DG, Halgren E (1977) Relationship of hallucinations of the depth structures of the temporal lobe. In: Sweet WH, Obrador S, Martin-Rodriguez JG (eds) Neurosurgical treatment in psychiatry, pain and epilepsy. University Park Press, London, pp 553-568

Wieser HG (1983) Electroclinical features of the psychomotor seizure. Fischer, Stuttgart

Wieser HG, Elger CE, Stodiek SRG (1985) The "foramen ovale electrode„ a new recording method for the preoperative evaluation of patients suffering from mesio-basal temporal lobe epilepsy. Electroencephalogr Clin Neurophysiol 61:314-322

Part IV

Specific Variables Affecting Treatment Outcome of Anxiety Disorders: Clinical, Psychosocial, and Interactional Factors

19. Failures in Exposure Treatment of Agoraphobia: Evaluation and Prediction

M. Fischer, I. Hand, J. Angenendt, H. Büttner-Westphal, and Ch. Manecke

Introduction

Failures in behavior therapy of agoraphobics have been largely neglected during the 1970s and early 1980s when research interest was mainly focussed on proving the effectiveness of behavioral treatments (Marks 1969; Chambless and Goldstein 1982; Thorpe and Burns 1983; Strian 1983; Foa et al. 1984; Tearnan and Telch 1984; Marks 1987a). Several long-term follow-up studies have confirmed exposure in vivo to be the treatment of choice for some 70% of agoraphobic patients who participated in such a treatment (Marks 1971; Emmelkamp and Kuipers 1979; McPherson et al. 1980; Munby and Johnston 1980; Cohen et al. 1984; Fiegenbaum 1986; Hand et al. 1986). Most of these studies found a significant and stable reduction of agoraphobic and other symptomatology for up to 9 years after treatment. When assessed at all, an improved private and social adjustment was evident. This high effectiveness turns out to be even more important as:

1. Agoraphobia shows a chronic course without treatment (Agras et al. 1972; Wittchen and von Zerssen 1987).
2. Agoraphobic patients are highly restricted in their daily-life activities and have to depend on significant others as accompanying persons (Marks 1987).
3. Agoraphobic patients without behavioral treatment run a considerable risk for secondary alcohol or tranquilizer dependence (Smail et al. 1984; Fyer et al. 1987).

Foa and Emmelkamp (1983) were the first to shift the main emphasis from successes to failures in behavior therapy. They consider the problem of failures "as an invaluable source of information for elucidating the mechanisms underlying our interventions, for perfecting existing procedures, and for inventing new ones" (Foa et al. 1983).

In agoraphobia the currently popular concept is of endogenous panic whereby depression may explain some failures from exposure treatment, but it certainly cannot be regarded as *the main* explanatory model for these patients (see review papers in Hand and Wittchen 1986; Marks 1987a, b).

Although gains from behavioral treatments for agoraphobics are manifold, few follow-up-studies have been conducted with separate analyses for the 20%–35% of failures (Emmelkamp and Kuipers 1979; Emmelkamp and van der Hout 1983; Hand et al. 1986).

To identify pretreatment characteristics of patients related to *short-term* outcome, some studies have analyzed personality variables (Watson and Marks 1971; Stern and Marks 1973; Mathews et al. 1974), depression (Marks 1969), or social anxiety (Emmelkamp 1980) - but correlations with outcome were low. In analyzing sociodemographic, symptom-, and personality-variables, Emmelkamp and Kuipers (1979) did not find any (pretreatment) differences between failures and successes 4 years after treatment. In another study (Emmelkamp and van der Hout

1983), a variety of pretreatment variables of 11 success- and 5 failure patients were analyzed. Low marital satisfaction appeared the only predictor for poor outcome. Because of the small number of patients (n = 16: 11 successes, 5 failures) the authors themselves are cautious with regard to the relevance of this result.

The main aim of this study is to identify variables from pre- and posttreatment ratings that may allow prediction of long-term outcome. The question "What type of treatment should be given to what patient in order to minimize therapeutic failure?" (Emmelkamp and Foa 1983) should ideally be answered before treatment starts in order to avoid unnecessary or even harmful interventions. Yet, in a short-term treatment it makes sense to additionally look for treatment process and immediate outcome variables for prediction of long-term development. Furthermore, even variables from the follow-up period may serve to support the predictive power of the identified predictor variables from pre- to posttreatment ratings.

Long-term failures, predictable immediately after exposure, may stand a good chance for improvement when alternative, more adequate treatments could be offered immediately thereafter.

Design of the Follow-Up Studies and Identification of Failures at Follow-Up

From 1976 to 1983 some 260 agoraphobic patients were referred to or had applied for treatment in our unit. After an intensive behavioral analysis, 24% of these patients had either refused or dropped out of an exposure study (Fischer et al. 1987); 198 patients completed all five exposure sessions of the standard program.

The analyses presented in this chapter are based on two follow-up studies of these 198 agoraphobics (Fig. 1). As different sets of self-rating scales for neurotic multi-symptomatology were introduced between 1976–1979 and 1980–1983, patients had to be split into two groups (Fig. 1):

1. Eighty patients treated between 1980 and 1983 (1–4 years follow-up; study 1); 75 of them (88%) participated in this follow-up (Hand et al. 1986; Fischer et al. 1988)
2. One hundred thirteen patients treated between 1976 and 1979 (6–9 years follow-up; study 2); 90 (80% of the sample) participated in this follow-up (Büttner-Westphal 1986; Manecke 1986)

Patients

Patients were diagnosed as agoraphobics in the clinical intake interviews. The diagnosis was evaluated several months later (waiting list of 2–12 months) by the therapists who were supervised weekly. This ensured homogeneity of diagnostic criteria throughout the unit and over the

Table 1. Demographic data

	Study 1 (n = 75)	**Study 2** (n = 90)
Gender		
Female	63 (84%)	75 (83%)
Male	12 (16%)	15 (17%)
Age (years)	$\bar{x}$ = 32.40 (range, 18–54)	$\bar{x}$ = 34.40 (range, 19–61)
Matrial status		
With spouse	59 (79%)	77 (86%)
Without spouse	16 (21%)	12 (14%)
Occupational status		
Work outside family	42 (56%)	54 (60%)
Housewife	19 (25%)	26 (29%)
Unemployed	10 (13%)	2 (2%)
Sick leave/ pension	2 (3%)	7 (8%)
Missing data	2 (3%)	1 (1%)
History of illness behavior		
Symptom duration (years)	$\bar{x}$ = 6.8 (range, 1–19)	$\bar{x}$ = 7.2 (range, 1–31)
Treatment prior to exposure	71 (95%)	-
Psychotropic medication	60 (80%)	-

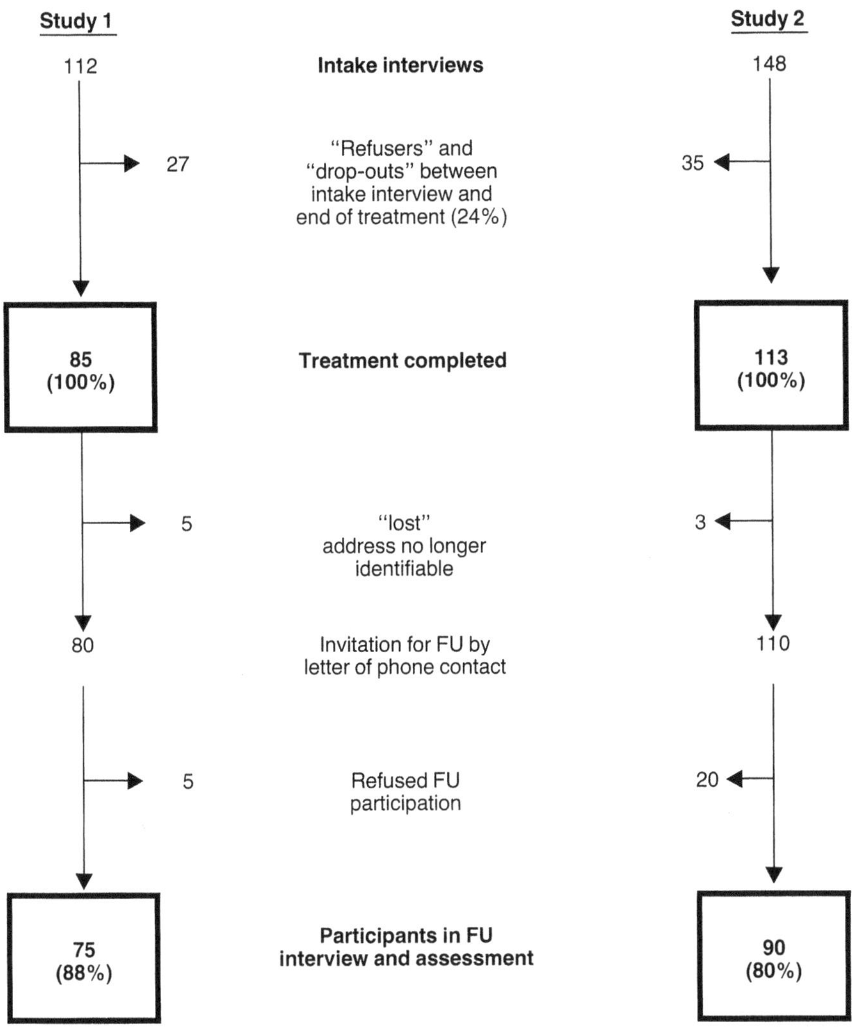

Fig. 1. Agoraphobic patients in the Hamburg Behavior Therapy Outpatient Unit 1976–1983

years. Some 50% of the patients showed agoraphobia with panic attacks (DSM-III, APA 1980) or panic disorder with agoraphobia (DSM-IIIR, 1987).

Demographic data of study 1 and study 2 patients are shown in Table 1. Patients are comparable to those of previous studies with regard to sociodemographic and symptom-related characteristics (Thorpe and Burns 1983; Marks 1987). Most of them were female, about 33 years old, and living with a spouse. They had had agoraphobic symptoms for some 7 years; 90% had sought professional help prior to behavior therapy. More than 80% had been treated with psychotropic medication (mainly tranquilizers).

Treatments

Behavioral treatments consisted of 6–8 h behavioral and motivational analysis, plus:

1. Either: four therapist-aided and one self-conducted exposure in vivo sessions (with 4–7 h per session) individually (13 patients in study 1, 39 patients in study 2)
2. Or: Four therapist-aided and one self-conducted exposure in vivo sessions conducted in cohesive groups (Hand et al. 1974; 43 patients in study 1, 51 patients in study 2)
3. Or: the manual-aided home-based treatment program for agoraphobia (Mathews et al. 1977, 1981) consisting of self-directed daily exposure sessions with assistance of a spouse or partner and of program-counseling by a therapist once a week (19 patients of study 1)

The first two modes of exposure were conducted over a period of 2 weeks, the latter one over a period of 4 weeks. A detailed description of the treatment concept for therapist-guided exposure, including panic and depression (emotional distress) management as well as fostering of high group cohesion for mutual support and motivation, is given by Hand et al. (1974, 1986).

Assessments

Both studies consisted of a prospective (patients' self-rating scales on neurotic multisymptomatology) and a retrospective (assessors' semistructured follow-up interview) part. The prospective part was different in both studies as a new set of self-rating scales was introduced in 1980 to assess multiple neurotic symptomatology in a systematic way (Hand and Zaworka 1982).

Study 1 instruments:

1. Agoraphobia: Fear Survey Schedule, FSS-P, subscale agoraphobia (Hallam and Hafner 1978)
2. Hindrance of daily-life activities by phobia: 99 mm visual analog scale
3. Behavioral resistance, i.e., the extent to which daily-life activities are carried on when phobic anxiety/panic occurs (reversed formulation of avoidance behavior): 99 mm visual analog scale
4. Social phobia: Fear Survey Schedule, FSS-S (Hallam and Hafner 1978)
5. Depression: Depression Scale, D-S (von Zerssen and Koeller 1976)
6. Obsessions and compulsions: Hamburger Zwangsinventar (Hamburg O-C Inventory; Zaworka et al. 1983; Klepsch 1987)
7. Personality variables: Freiburger Persönlichkeitsinventar, FPI-A (Fahrenberg et al. 1973, 1984)

Study 2 instruments:

1. Agoraphobia: Watson and Marks (1971) 0–8 scale
2. Hindrance of daily-life activities by phobia: Watson and Marks (1971) 0–8 scale
3. Avoidance behavior in phobic situations: Watson and Marks (1971) 0–8 scale
4. Personality variables: Freiburger Persönlichkeitsinventar, FPI-A (Fahrenberg et al. 1973, 1984)

In both groups, the prospective assessment instruments were given to the patients at pretreatment, posttreatment, 6 months after treatment, and the long-term follow-up.

The retrospective semistructured interview was identical in both studies and included additional qualitative information about treatments after behavior therapy and hindrance in daily-life activities.

Operationalization of Failure

Emmelkamp and Foa (1983) classified failures into: refusals, drop-outs, nonresponders, and relapses. In this chapter, those patients who did not *complete* behavior therapy are excluded. We only analyzed *nonresponders* and *relapses.* A study with the other two groups is currently underway (first results in Fischer et al. 1987).

In identifying failures at the last follow-up, we decided to use a clinically derived cut-off point on the FSS agoraphobia scale, but the inidvidual pretreatment ratings vary from little to extremely above this point. Emmelkamp and van der Hout (1983) suggested a definition of success using a minimum of 3 points reduction on the Watson-Marks scale ranging from 0–8, but a reduction from 8 to 5 may not reflect a change comparable to a reduction from 4 to 1. For methodological as well as clinical reasons we decided to use the cutoff point of the agoraphobia self-rating scales (detailed explanation of our choice in Hand and Zaworka 1982; Hand et al. 1986).

Study 1

Existence of high agoraphobic anxiety was defined by a rating on the FSS subscale agoraphobia (Hallam and Hafner 1978) of ≧ 18. This cutoff point was derived as the mean rating of an unselected clinical population of 126 untreated agoraphobics. Only patients with pretreatment ratings of ≧ 18 were taken into our research projects. Following this definition, *failures* rated ≧ 18 points at the last follow-up:

1. *Nonresponders* were those patients who had rated ≧ 18 at pre- and posttreatment and remained on this high anxiety level at the last follow-up.
2. *Relapses* were those patients whose ratings were ≧ 18 at pre- and < 18 right after treatment, but were back to ≧ 18 at the long-term follow-up.

Study 2

Existence of high agoraphobic anxiety was defined by a rating ≧ 4 on the Watson-Marks scale (0–8; Watson and Marks 1971). *Failures* rated ≧ 4 on this scale, at the long-term follow-up, with *nonresponders* and *relapses* being defined as in study 1.

Results

Presentation of data will focus on the following questions:

1. What is the percentage of failures in both follow-up studies and to what extent are they relapses or nonresponders?
2. Are there pretreatment predictors of long-term outcome, e.g., do failures and successes show differences in sociodemographic variables, illness development variables, and neurotic symptomatology at pretreatment?
3. Do failures and successes reveal differences in response to treatment which can serve as additional predictors for patients' development over the whole follow-up period or which can enhance the predictive power of pretreatment variables, e.g., are failures at follow-up mainly nonresponders to treatment or relapses during follow-up?
4. Do other indicators of failure – apart from patients' ratings on the FSS agoraphobia scale – like hindrance in daily-life activities, additional treatment and use of psychotropic medication during or at follow-up, and a global self-rating of improvement support our operationalization of failure and success, on which the study is based?

Failures: Nonresponders and Relapses

Excluding 11 patients with mild (<18) agoraphobia at pretreatment (Hand et al. 1986) from this analysis, there were 23 failures in study 1 (32% of total group of 75 patients and 37% of the 64 severe agoraphobics) and 17 in study 2 (24% of the 82 patients who had filled out the self-rating scales). These results largely resemble those from previous studies (Marks 1971; Emmelkamp and Kuipers 1979; McPherson et al. 1980; Munby and Johnston 1980; Emmelkamp and van der Hout 1983; Cohen et al. 1984; Fiegenbaum 1986).

Nonresponders seem to be preponderant among failures in exposure treatment for anxiety disorders (Foa et al. 1983) especially when covert avoidance is involved during exposure treatment (Emmelkamp and van der Hout 1983). When relapse occurs in phobics, this may be due to depressive episodes or a new confrontation with events resembling those at first onset of the phobia (Marks 1987; Lelliott et al. 1986). In our two studies, results are almost contradictory to each other regarding the respective percentage of relapses and nonresponders (Fig. 2).

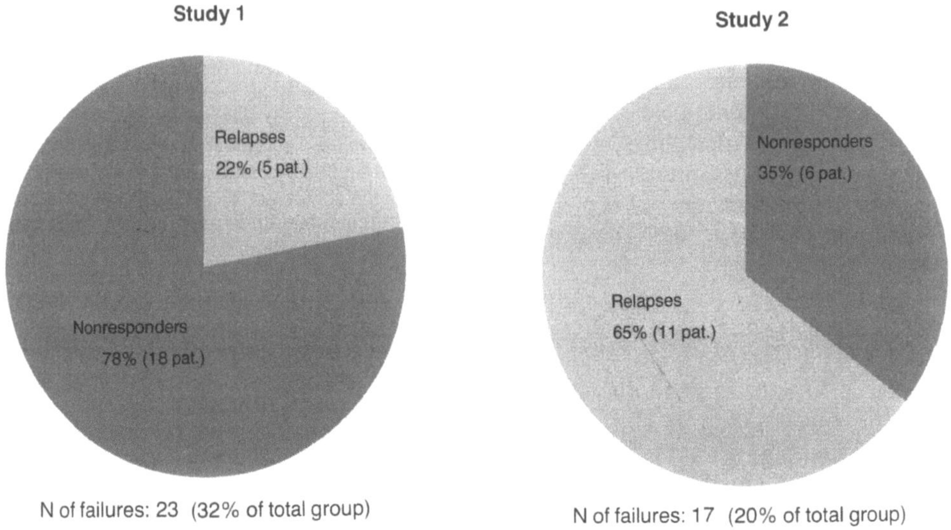

Fig. 2. Percentage of nonresponders and relapses

In *study 1,* we found a rate of 78% ($n = 18$) nonresponders among failure patients. Relapses ($n = 5$; 22%) turned out to be reactions to severe life-events in four cases (rape, death of relative or spouse) and to enduring unemployment in two cases.

In *study 2,* only 6 of the failure patients were nonresponders (35%) and 6 were relapses (35%). Data for five patients were missing for posttreatment. Retrospective interview data suggest those patients to be also relapses. Thus we found 65% relapses among study 2 failures. At the moment we have no explanation for these differences between the studies. To gain further information, we have started single-case reanalysis of nonresponders and relapses.

Predictors for Long-Term Failure

Pretreatment Variables

In both studies, demographic, symptom, and personality variables were checked for prognostic validity. "History-of-illness" variables were analyzed for study 1 additionally. Results are summarized in Table 2.

In all variables, including indicators for help-seeking behavior, ratings of failures are numerically higher than those of successes. But, except for the item "number of contacts with psychiatrists during the 2 years before behavior therapy," these differences between failures and successes were statistically not significant. Nevertheless, it may indicate that the later failures from behavior therapy had already previously shown more illness behavior than the later successes.

Among the symptom variables, only severity of agoraphobic anxiety was a predictor for poor outcome: failures rated significantly higher anxiety than successes (in study 1 on the FSS agoraphobia, in study 2 on the Watson-Marks (WM) scale, both correlating 0.84).

These findings seem to contradict the results of Emmelkamp and Kuipers (1979), who did not find higher anxiety as a predictor for poor long-term outcome – using different criteria for poor outcome in a smaller sample of patients.

Table 2. Prognostic variables

	Study 1			Study 2		
	Success	Failure	Test	Success	Failure	Test
Gender						
Female	42	21		52	15	
Male	10	2	Chi	13	2	Chi
Age (years) $\bar{x}$	31.3	34.6	*t*	34.5	36.4	*t*
Spouse						
Yes	41	18		54	16	
No	11	5	Chi	10	1	Chi
Occupation						
Yes	33	13		-	-	
No	19	10	Chi	-	-	
Symptom duration (years) $\bar{x}$	6.3	7.6	*t*	7.1	8.3	*t*
Inpatient treatment "yes"	5	7	Chi	-	-	
2 years before BT	$\bar{x}$	$\bar{x}$		$\bar{x}$	$\bar{x}$	
N contacts to						
Psychiatrists	7.5	18.7	*t**	-	-	
Psychotherapists	9.8	11.1	*t*	-	-	
N days with						
Psychotropic medication	227.4	343.2	*t*	-	-	
Unable to work	78.9	166.4	*t*	-	-	
Symptom scales						
Agoraphobia (FSS/WM)	22.93	26.52	*t**	5.79	6.59	*t**
Behavioral resistance/avoidance behavior	39.59	39.70	*t*	5.93	6.46	*t*
Interference	70.24	69.87	*t*	6.00	6.44	*t*
Social phobia	9.12	10.13	*t*	-	-	
Total phobia	60.17	67.96	*t*	-	-	
Depression	22.51	19.95	*t*	-	-	
Obsessions and compulsions	3.25	3.35	*t*	-	-	
Personality variables						
Depression	6.17	6.45	*t*	6.36	6.77	*t*
Social inhibition	6.48	6.59	*t*	6.47	6.38	*t*

*, $P < 0.05$ **, $P < 0.01$ ***, $P < 0.001$ - not assessed

Treatment Variables

Since at least FSS agoraphobia ratings showed predictive power to indicate long-term failures, the questions arises whether failure was due to treatment nonresponse or follow-up relapse.

Study 1 failures showed significant immediate treatment responses in agoraphobia, hindrance by phobia, and obsessions and compulsions. Yet, in spite of the significant reduction of their initial extreme phobia ratings, their respective posttreatment ratings were almost as high as

Table 3. Treatment response to exposure

	Study 1				Study 2			
	Success		Failure		Success		Failure	
	T1	T2	T1	T2	T1	T2	T1	T2
	$\bar{x}$	$\bar{x}$	$\bar{x}$	$\bar{x}$	$\bar{x}$	$\bar{x}$	$\bar{x}$	$\bar{x}$
Symptom scales								
Agoraphobia (FSS/WM)	22.93	13.05***	26.52	21.68**	5.79	2.71***	6.59	3.80***
Behavioral resistance/avoidance	39.59	71.59***	39.70	52.91	5.93	2.50***	6.46	3.54***
Interference	70.24	39.05***	69.87	56.18**	6.00	2.67***	6.44	3.53***
Social phobia	9.12	7.03**	10.13	9.45	-	-	-	-
Total phobia	60.17	43.19***	67.96	61.14	-	-	-	-
Depression	22.51	14.44***	19.95	18.10	-	-	-	-
Obsessions/compulsions	3.25	2.45***	3.35	2.59*	-	-	-	-
Personality variables								
Depression	6.19	6.00	6.67	6.67	6.36	6.38	6.77	6.46
Social inhibition	6.47	5.91*	6.66	6.09	6.47	6.09	6.38	6.69

T1, pretreatment T2, posttreatment *, $P < 0.05$ **, $P < 0.01$ ***, $P < 0.001$

pretreatment ratings of long-term successes. Failures showed no response in their depression ratings - although this was initially numerically lower than that of successes! They also showed no response in behavioral resistance and social phobia. In contrast, successes showed significant immediate reductions on all these scales (Table 3).

In *study 2,* the results are similar with regard to reductions in agoraphobic anxiety and hindrance in successes as well as in failures. At posttreatment, phobia ratings of failures were higher than those of successes, but reduction of phobia and hindrance was highly significant for both. Study 2 results differ with regard to phobic avoidance (resistance), with failures showing a significant treatment response. Unfortunately, patients in this study were not given the other symptom self-rating scales (for depression, social anxiety and obsessive-compulsive symptoms; see above).

In both studies, on personality scales for depression and social inhibition no significant or clinically relevant changes were found during treatment, mean ratings remaining within the range of the "normal" population.

Follow-Up Variables

During the follow-up period, in both studies successes showed further significant gains, while failures did not improve in any of the variables. Failures even developed some (statistically not significant) deterioration after the 6-months follow-up. Significant changes in the personality scales (reduction of depression in successes of both studies, and a reduction of social inhibition in study 2 patients) occurred within the "normal population" range (Table 4).

Table 4. Follow-up response to exposure

	Study 1				Study 2			
	Success		Failure		Success		Failure	
	T3	T4	T3	T4	T3	T4	T3	T4
	$\bar{x}$	$\bar{x}$	$\bar{x}$	$\bar{x}$	$\bar{x}$	$\bar{x}$	$\bar{x}$	$\bar{x}$
Symptom scales								
Agoraphobia (FSS/WM)	11.85	9.05**	20.63	23.54	2.61	1.61***	3.78	5.01
Behavioral resistance/avoidance	78.29	78.59	52.47	51.08	2.49	1.66*	4.16	4.87
Interference	27.76	24.08**	47.84	63.00	2.53	1.53**	3.92	4.88
Social phobia	7.12	5.26**	8.50	9.50	-	-	-	-
Total phobia	39.79	32.56**	60.68	62.63	-	-	-	-
Depression	12.47	8.71**	19.11	18.54	-	-	-	-
Obsessions/ compulsions	2.24	1.94**	2.47	2.48	-	-	-	-
Personality variables	T2	T4	T2	T4	T2	T4	T2	T4
Depression	6.03	4.94**	6.55	6.40	6.38	5.00**	6.46	6.00
Social inhibition	5.97	5.59	5.95	5.70	6.09	5.18***	6.69	5.77*

T2, posttreatment; T3, 6 months after treatment; T4, long-term follow-up; *, $P < 0.05$; **, $P < 0.01$; ***, $P < 0.001$

Additional Indicators of Failure at Follow-Up

The clinical relevance of our cut-off point on the phobia scales is supported by additional indicators of failure and success.

Hindrance in Daily-Life Activities

In the follow-up interviews, patients rated hindrance in daily-life activities, occupation, psychological well-being, leisure activities, social contacts, spouse and family relationships (on a 0 to 8 point Watson-Marks scale). This was done retrospectively for the time before behavioral treatment, and for their current situation at follow-up. Details of these ratings are given in Table 5 and in Fig. 3 (follow-up ratings). As retrospective pretreatment ratings are rather weak data, no methods for testing significance were employed.

Not surprisingly, daily-life hindrance before treatment was more severe in areas requiring activities outside home (in failures as well as in successes). At follow-up, failures show medium to severe impairment, while successes rate no to minimal hindrance. The comparability of study 1 and study 2 failures is shown clearly in these hindrance assessments.

Treatments During Follow-Up

Retrospective assessment of therapist contacts over the follow-up period proved very difficult. Results are probably not reliable, and they need to be evaluated with great caution. Failures are overrepresented in those patients with additional consultations with psychiatrists and psychotherapists during the follow-up period. Nineteen of the 23 study 1 failures (83%) and all 17 study 2 failures had been seeking professional help, in more than one-half of the cases at least of two different kinds. For successes the same was true for some 50%.

Reported intensity of therapist contacts (frequency per year) varied extremely.

Table 5. Hindrance in daily-life activities: pretreatment (retrospectively) and follow-up

	Study 1				Study 2			
	T1		T4		T1		T4	
	Success $\bar{x}$	Failure $\bar{x}$	Success $\bar{x}$	Failure $\bar{x}$	Success $\bar{x}$	Failure $\bar{x}$	Success $\bar{x}$	Failure $\bar{x}$
Occupation	5.82	6.13	1.83	4.13**	5.05	5.19	1.19	3.88***
Psychological well-being	6.75	7.26	2.00	4.87***	6.62	6.41	1.95	4.88***
Leisure activities	5.72	6.87	1.33	4.82***	6.23	6.06	1.56	4.88**
Social contacts	4.39	4.56	0.58	3.04***	4.47	4.18	0.98	3.29***
Spouse relationship	3.87	3.14	1.12	2.71*	2.66	2.88	0.83	3.19**
Family relationship	3.40	3.77	0.72	2.27**	3.23	3.94	0.84	3.41***

T1, pretreatment (retrospectively); T4, long-term follow-up; *, $P<0.05$; **, $P<0.01$; ***, $P<0.001$

Most successes reported very few additional contacts, whereas among failures quite a number had additional outpatient or inpatient treatments. Like exposure, these additional treatments did not change agoraphobic and other symptomatology in failures.

Does this mean, that failures from exposure have a general resistance to change – regardless of treatment mode?

Psychotropic Medication

The number of patients with psychotropic medication at follow-up is given in Table 6.

More than one-half of the failures (52% and 65%) – in contrast to about 20% of the successes – were taking psychotropic medication at follow-up. As more than 80% of our total sample had been taking psychotropic medication at pretreatment, this indicates that some 20%–30% of failures had stopped their medication after exposure treatment. According to patients' attribution, this resulted from the "panic and emotional distress management training" in our exposure in vivo program (Hand et al. 1986).

All of the 12 *study 1* failures with medication received tranquilizers, two took additional antidepressants, and another two additional low-dose neuroleptics. In *study 2,* out of 11 failures with medication, eight received tranquilizers, one additional low-dose neuroleptics, and three antidepressants only. The small number of only five patients on antidepressant medication is surprising compared to 20 failures with anxiolytic medication.

Table 6. Patients with psychotropic medication at long-term follow-up

Study 1		Study 2	
Success	Failure	Success	Failure
7 (17% of 23)	12 (52% of 23)	16 (23% of 73)	11 (65% of 17)
Σ 19 (25% of 75)		Σ 27 (30% of 90)	

Global Self-Rating of Improvement

On the self-rating scale "Do you feel better, unchanged, or worse compared to the time before behavior therapy?", a surprisingly high number of failures (48% in study 1 and 53% in study 2) rated subjective improvement. This rating, togeth-

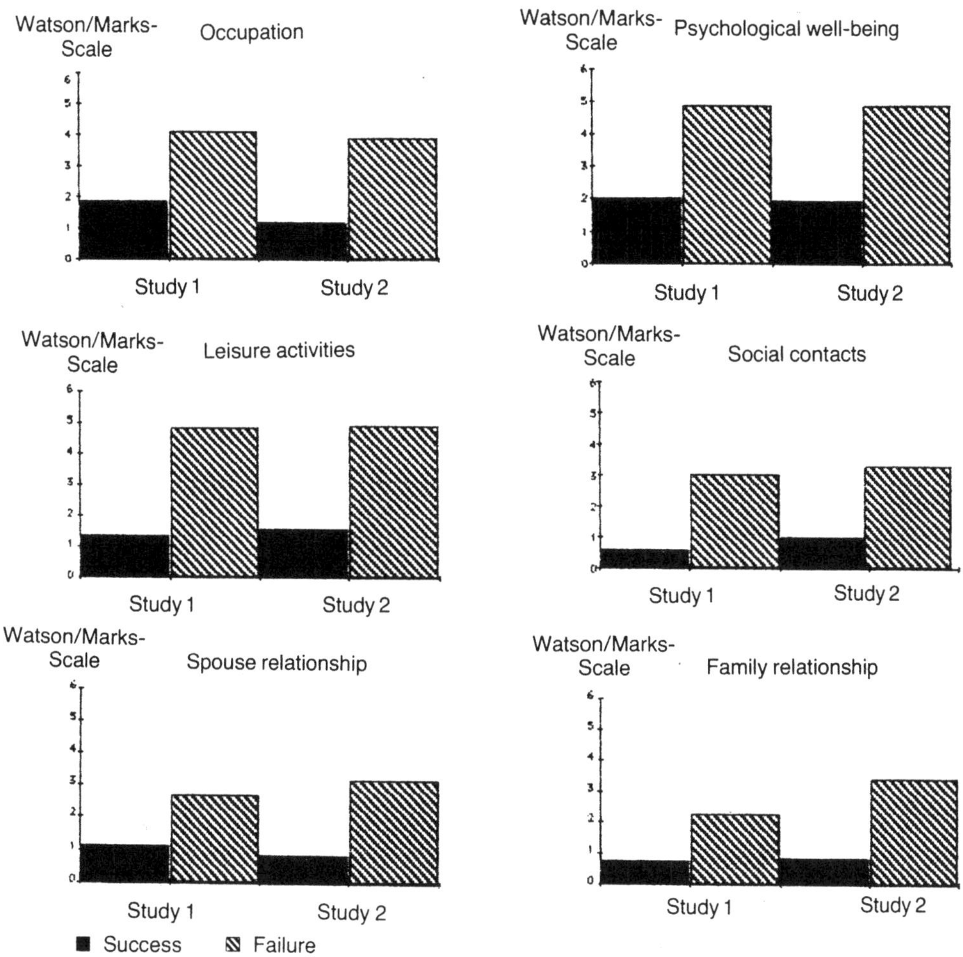

Fig. 3. Hindrance in daily life activities at follow-up (0 = no hindrance at all: 6–8 = severe hindrance)

er with the reduction in medication, indicates that exposure (and or follow-up treatments?) had some beneficial effects even in failure patients.

For failures and successes together, this scale gives a total rate of improvement of 79% (study 1) and 88% (study 2; Table 7).

Summary and Discussion

In two long-term (1–9 years) follow-up studies with a total of 165 agoraphobics, the general outcome regarding failures – about 28% in both studies together – confirms the results in previous studies from other groups. Symptom ratings in agoraphobics again were useful and easy-to-obtain indicators of a variety of other illness behaviors.

Our operationalization of failure and success by means of a clinically derived cutoff point on the FSS agoraphobia scale proved surprisingly valid with regard to separation of failures and successes on other symptom scales, in illness behaviors, and in daily-life activities. Reanalyses of all pretreatment to last follow-up ratings of success and failure patients separately clearly produces much more

Table 7. Global self-rating about improvement

	Study 1		Study 2	
	Success	Failure	Success	Failure
Better	48 (92%)	11 (48%)	70 (97%)	9 (53%)
Unchanged	4 (8%)	9 (39%)	2 (3%)	6 (35%)
Worse	-	3 (13%)	-	2 (12%)
Σ	52 (100%)	23 (100%)	72 (100%)	17 (100%)

useful information than the usual total sample analyses. As our analyses show (cf. also Hand et al. 1986), the "average" agoraphobic hardly exists after exposure treatment - rather, patients are either failures or successes. Successes reach normal or almost normal ratings on the decisive symptom scales (phobic anxiety and depression), while failures remain very disturbed. The mean outcome of both - as usually published in treatment studies - is clinically misleading. Reanalyses of failures and successes also reveal, that successes show further significant reduction of multisymptomatology during follow-up, while failures do not do so or even deteriorate. This follow-up result with successes strongly confirms the tentative first results in patients from high cohesion groups in the Hand et al. study (1974).

At what point in time (after exposure) patients become failures cannot be answered from our studies. Whereas in study 1 about 78% of the long-term failures were treatment nonresponders compared to 22% relapses, in study 2 almost the reverse outcome was found. We are trying to find the reasons for this difference.

Regarding *prediction of failure* from exposure treatments, the following results are to be emphasized:

1. Very high *initial phobic anxiety* predicts poor long-term outcome.
2. *Nonresponse in depression* (during exposure) predicts poor long-term outcome. The initial depression rating by itself does not do so!
3. *Multisymptomatic response* (during exposure) predicts further, significant symptom reduction during follow-up - and vice versa.

The first result was found in both studies, with different self-rating scales for agoraphobia. The other two results only came from study 1 (failures: n = 23), being the only one with repeated multisymptomatic assessments.

The higher predictive value of posttreatment levels of anxiety and depressions as compared to pretreatment levels - i.e. the decisive role of (short-term) treatment response for prediction of longterm behavior therapy outcome - has already been noted in our earlier studies (Hand et al., 1986) and has now been replicated by Chambless and by Steketee (in this volume).

The impact of depression on treatment outcome in our studies appears to depend on its functionality: Initial depression (even when high) in successes follows the agoraphobia ratings (eventually down to normal levels), whereas in failures, depression (even when comparatively low) does not respond during exposure, in spite of phobia reduction.

In the intake interviews and assessments we may have misdiagnosed some of these failures as agoraphobics - their depression actually not having been secondary to agoraphobia but to other symptoms or problems. This assumption is supported by:

a) the result in study 1, that failures did not respond (during exposure) in

depression, social anxiety, and behavioral resistance, while there were responses in all other symptom ratings;
b) in study 1 and 2, at last follow-up failures showed significantly higher social anxiety than successes.

In spite of a careful diagnostic procedure, in spite of specific interventions for social anxiety in agoraphobics being part of our exposure program (cf. "social spin-off from exposure" in Hand et al. 1974), and in spite of the availability of a specific exposure in vivo program for social phobics in our unit, we may have misdiagnosed some multisymptomatic social phobics as agoraphobics, or we may not have paid enough attention to the social anxiety in the exposure treatment of some of our agoraphobic failures.
Of course, nonresponse in depression in some patients may also have been due to an "endogenous" panic disorder or to a "neurotic conflict" situation, both of which may not have been assessed correctly.
The poor outcome for the extremely agoraphobic patients (independent of their depressions ratings) may also be taken as evidence for an endogenous panic disorder.

To summarize: About 30% of agoraphobics who participated in exposure treatment are long-term failures. Repeated multisymptomatic assessments over time reveal that extreme initial phobic anxiety, on the one hand, and treatment nonresponse in depression and social anxiety/inhibition on the other hand, may be crucial predictors for failure in agoraphobia. To investigate this hypothesis and to detect possible causes for this symptomatic phenomenon, clinical reassessments are currently underway in a single-case design. Particular emphasis is put on the endogenous panic concept on the one hand, and functional, motivational, and systemic analyses on the other.

References

Agras WS, Chapin HN, Oliveau D (1972) The natural history of phobia. Arch Gen Psychiatry 26:315-317

American Psychiatric Association (ed) (1980) Diagnostic and statistical manual of mental disorders, 3rd edn (DSM III). Washington, DC

American Psychiatric Association (ed) (1987) Diagnostic and statistical manual of mental disorders, 3rd edn, revised (DSM-IIIR). Washington, DC

Büttner-Westphal H (1986) Agoraphobie: Verläufe und Tendenzen 6-9 Jahre nach der Kurzzeit-Verhaltenstherapie. Psychology thesis, University of Hamburg

Chambless DL, Goldstein AJ (eds) (1982) Agoraphobia: multiple perspectives on theory and treatment. Wiley, New York

Cohen SD, Monteiro W, Marks IM (1984) Two-year follow-up of agoraphobics after exposure and imipramine. Br J Psychiatry 144:276-287

Emmelkamp PMG (1980) Agoraphobics' interpersonal problems: their role in the effects of exposure in vivo therapy. Arch Gen Psychiatry 37:1303-1306

Emmelkamp PMG, Foa EB (1983) Failures are a challenge. In: Foa EB, Emmelkamp PMG (eds) Failures in behavior therapy. Wiley, New York

Emmelkamp PMG, Kuipers AC (1979) Agoraphobia: A follow-up study four years after treatment. Br J Psychiatry 134:352-355

Emmelkamp PMG, Van der Hout A (1983) Failure in treating agoraphobia. In: Foa EB, Emmelkamp PMG (eds) Failures in behavior therapy. Wiley, New York

Fahrenberg J, Hampel R, Selg H (1973) Das Freiburger Persönlichkeitsinventar FPI. Handanweisung. Hogrefe, Göttingen
und der teilweise geänderten Fassung FPI-A. Hogrefe, Göttingen

Fiegenbaum W (1986) Agoraphobie. Theoretische Konzepte und Behandlungsmethoden. Westdeutscher Verlag, Opladen

Fischer M, Hand I, Angenendt J (1987) Long-term developments of agoraphobics who refused or dropped out of exposure treatment. 17th Annual meeting of the European Association for Behaviour Therapy, Amsterdam

Fischer M, Hand I, Angenendt J (1988) Langzeiteffekte von Kurzzeit-Verhaltenstherapien bei Agoraphobie. Z Klin Psychol (in press)

Foa EB, Emmelkamp PMG (eds) (1983) Failures in behavior therapy. Wiley, New York

Foa EB, Steketee G, Grayson JB, Doppelt HG (1983) Treatment of obsessive-compulsives: When do we fail? In: Foa EB, Emmelkamp PMG (eds) Failures in behavior therapy. Wiley, New York

Foa EB, Steketee G, Young MC (1984) Agoraphobia: phenomenological aspects, asociated characteristics, and theoretical considerations. Clin Psychol Review 4:431–457
Fyer A, Liebowitz M, Gorman J, Compeas R, Levin A, Davis S, Götz D, Klein D (1987) Discontinuation of alprazolam treatment in panic patients. Am J Psychiatry 144:303–308
Hallam RS, Hafner RJ (1978) Fears of phobic patients: factor analyses of self-report data. Behav Res Ther 16:1–6
Hand I (1986) Verhaltenstherapie und kognitive Therapie in der Psychiatrie. In: Kisker KP, Lauter H, Meyer J-E, Müller C, Strömgen E (eds) Psychiatrie der Gegenwart, vol I. Springer, Berlin Heidelberg New York
Hand I, Wittchen HU (eds) (1986) Panic and phobias. Empirical evidence of theoretical models and longterm effects of behavioral treatments. Springer, Berlin Heidelberg New York
Hand I, Zaworka (1982) An operationalized multisymptomatic model of neuroses (OMMON): toward a reintegration of diagnosis and treatment in behavior therapy. Arch Psychiatrie Nervenkrankheiten 232:359–379
Hand I, Lamontagne Y, Marks IM (1974) Group exposure (flooding) in vivo for agoraphobics. Br J Psychiatry 124:588–602
Hand I, Angenendt J, Fischer M, Wilke C (1986) Exposure in vivo with panic management for agoraphobia: treatment rationale and longterm outcome. In: Hand I, Wittchen HU (eds) Panic and phobias. Empirical evidence of theoretical models and longterm effects of behavioral treatments. Springer, Berlin Heidelberg New York
Klepsch R (1987) Das Hamburger Zwangsinventar: Entwicklung zweier computer-dialogfähiger Kurzformen: HZI-K, HZI-UK. Dissertation, University of Hamburg
Lambert MJ, Bergin AE (1978) The evaluation of therapeutic outcome. In: Garfield SC, Bergin AE (eds) Handbook of psychotherapy and behavior change: an empirical analysis. Wiley, New York
Manecke C (1986) Agoraphobie: Verläufe und Tendenzen 6–9 Jahre nach der Kurzzeit-Verhaltenstherapie. Psychology thesis, University of Hamburg
Marks IM (1969) Fears and phobias. Academic Press, New York
Marks IM (1971) Phobic disorders four years after treatment: a prospective follow-up. Br J Psychiatry 118:683–688
Marks IM (1987a) Fears, phobias and rituals. Panic, anxiety, and their disorders. Oxford University Press, New York
Marks IM (1987b) Behavioral aspects of panic disorder. Am J Psychiatry 144:1160–1165
Mathews AM, Johnston DW, Shaw PM, Gelder MG (1974) Process variables and the prediction of outcome in behaviour therapy. Br J Psychiatry 129:256–264
Mathews AM, Teasdale J, Munby M, Johnston D, Shaw P (1977) A home-based treatment program for agoraphobia. Behav Ther 8:915–924
Mathews AM, Gelder M, Johnston D (1981) Agoraphobia. Nature and treatment. Guilford, New York
McPherson FM, Brougham L, McLaren S (1980) Maintenance of improvement in agoraphobic patients treated by behavioral methods – a four-year follow-up. Behav Res Ther 18:150–152
Munby M, Johnston DW (1980) Agoraphobia: the long-term follow-up of behavioural treatment. Br J Psychiatry 137:418–427
Smail P, Stockwell T, Canter S, Hodgson R (1984) Alcohol dependence and phobic anxiety states: a prevalence study. Br J Psychiatry 144:53–57
Stern RS, Marks IM (1973) Brief and prolonged flooding: a comparison in agoraphobic patients. Arch Gen Psychiatry 28:270–276
Strian F (1983) Angst. Grundlagen und Klinik. Springer, Berlin Heidelberg New York
Tearnan BH, Telch MJ (1984) Phobic disorders. In: Adams HE, Sutker PB (eds) Comprehensive handbook of psychopathology. Plenum, New York
Thorpe GL, Burns LE (1983) The agoraphobic syndrome. Behavioral approaches to evaluation and treatment. Wiley, New York
Watson JP, Marks IM (1971) Relevant and irrelevant fear in flooding – a crossover study of phobic patients. Behav Ther 2:275–293
Wittchen HU, von Zerssen DV (1987) Verläufe behandelter und unbehandelter Depressionen und Angststörungen – Eine klinisch-psychiatrische und epidemiologische Verlaufsuntersuchung. Springer, Berlin Heidelberg New York
Zaworka W, Hand I, Jauernig G, Lünenschloss K (1983) Das Hamburger Zwangsinventar, HZI. Manual und Fragebogen. Beltz, Weinheim
Zerssen von DV, Koeller D-M (1976) Klinische Selbstbeurteilungsskalen (KSb-S) aus dem Münchener psychiatrischen Informationssystem. Beltz, Weinheim

20. Prediction of Outcome Following In Vivo Exposure Treatment of Agoraphobia

D. L. CHAMBLESS and E. J. GRACELY

Introduction

The development of in vivo exposure treatment for agoraphobia has led to a significant increase in our ability to successfully treat these previously refractory clients. Jansson and Ost (1982), in their review of the literature on exposure, concluded that approximately 60%–70% of clients who complete a trial of exposure are clinically improved at both posttest and follow-up. However, these authors also pointed to the dearth of research on prognostic variables which might help us understand the variability of outcome. That 30%–40% of clients fail to improve poses an important problem clinically and theoretically.

A review of the literature since 1982 indicates that behaviorists have become more concerned with understanding treatment failures (see, for example, Foa and Emmelkamp 1983). Nevertheless, there are a number of consistent problems with studies in this area that limit their contribution:

1. There are frequently too few subjects in a treatment trial to provide sufficient power for statistical tests of predictors. Variables showing substantial correlations with outcome, for example, $r = 0.40$, are rejected as nonsignificant because there were only 12–15 clients in the study. Studies conducted with small numbers of subjects are likely to lead to unstable findings, adding to the confusion in the field.
2. When conflicting results are obtained by various investigators, comparisons are made even more difficult by the many different instruments used to measure similar variables.
3. Different criteria are used across centers for the measurement of treatment success or failure. Often the definition of success is arbitrary and idiosyncratic. Cut-off points on one or more questionnaires are employed in the absence of a solid empirical basis for their selection.
4. Frequently statistical approaches to the data are inadequate. Raw change scores or raw outcome scores are used as the criteria against which the success of predictors is tested. Raw outcome scores are influenced by pretreatment variability in subjects' responses and the frequent correlation of pretest and posttest scores on the criterion. Raw change scores are sometimes problematic because the same degree of change may have different meaning depending on the subject's pretest score. Consequently, such data are generally confounded making interpretation difficult (Mintz et al. 1979).
5. When significant effects are found for a predictor variable, these are often not reported in correlational form, making it difficult to interpret the clinical significance of a predictor by evaluating the strength of its association with the criterion.

In this paper we will report the results of a series of studies with two samples of agoraphobic clients who received in vivo exposure, taking into account the points we have raised above. We examined a number of predictor variables that have been identified by other researchers, as well as variables predicted to be of importance on theoretical grounds.

Sample I: Temple University Agoraphobia Program Sample

Method

Subjects

Subjects were 134 outpatients (113 women, 21 men) who entered and completed the 2-week intensive treatment program at the *Agoraphobia and Anxiety Program of Temple University Medical School.* All met DSM-III criteria for agoraphobia with panic attacks, based on diagnosis from an interview with a psychologist specializing in agoraphobia. Clients averaged 33.5 years in age (SD = 9.2) and reported having been agoraphobic for a mean of 9.7 years (SD = 8.6). On the average clients were middle-class as indicated by a mean score of 33.1 (SD = 17.1) on the Hollingshead two-factor index of social status, but they spanned the entire range of social class. Clients who participate in this intensive 2-week program have been shown to be somewhat more disabled than those who select a less intensive treatment format (Chambless and Mason 1986).

Sixty-five of these clients have reached the 1-year follow-up point and participated in follow-up data collection. These clients do not differ from those who did not participate in follow-up when compared at pretest or posttest (Chambless et al. 1986). Drop-out is unusual in this program; over the 9 years it has been offered, three clients have left before the end of the 2-week program. Hence the data presented may be considered representative of the results of the treatment program.

Measures

In addition to demographic information, self-report measures collected before and after treatment with this sample included: Agoraphobic Cognitions Questionnaire, Body Sensations Questionnaire, Gambrill–Richey Assertion Inventory, Beck Depression Inventory, Fear of Negative Evaluation Questionnaire, Social Avoidance and Distress Scale, Marks and Mathews' Fear Questionnaire, Mobility Inventory for Agoraphobia, and State-Trait Anxiety Inventory - Trait Form. The Marital Satisfaction Questionnaire was administered only at pretest. Reliability and validity data for these measures have been summarized elsewhere (Chambless et al. 1986).

Procedure

The treatment program for these subjects has been described extensively by Chambless et al. (1986). Clients are tested before and 1 week after participation in the program, and subsequently mailed follow-up questionnaires at 6 months and 1 year posttreatment. Clients are treated 6–8 h daily for 10 days during the 2-week period. The composition of the program has varied somewhat over the data collection period, but has consistently included approximately 27 h of in vivo exposure conducted in 3-h groups. Additional treatment includes anxiety and panic management training (e.g., respiratory control, relaxation, cognitive techniques), as well as eclectic individual and group psychotherapy. Clients beginning the program on psychotropic medication are typically withdrawn over the course of the 2 weeks. Spouses and family members are routinely included in educational sessions and a brief series of therapeutic sessions. With rare exception they agree to participate. Clients have been shown to improve from pre- to posttest on all measures administered except the fear of negative evaluation scale (Chambless et al. 1986). Most continue in ad lib treatment once the 2-week program has been completed. Fifty-two percent had additional exposure in the follow-up period for a median of 20.5 sessions (range, 1–62); 78% had additional individual therapy for associated problems for a median of 24 sessions (range, 1–52).

Results

Statistical Procedures

One criterion for improvement with treatment, whether at posttest or follow-up, was the corresponding score on avoidance alone from the Mobility Inventory. The score reflects the average of 1- to 5-point ratings of avoidance of 26 typical phobic situations for agoraphobics when they are not accompanied by a trusted companion. This measure yields a broader assessment of agoraphobia than does the typical main phobia rating, and is somewhat less sensitive to changes with treatment (Chambless et al. 1985).

The second criterion was a dichotomous measure of change, the Reliable Change (RC) Index (Jacobson et al. 1984; as amended by Christensen and Mendoza 1986), based on avoidance alone scores. The RC Index provides a stringent criterion for assessing improvement with treatment. According to the RC Index standard, the posttest score minus the pretest score divided by the standard error of the difference scores (corrected for reliability) must equal or exceed 1.96. At the 0.05 level of confidence, such change is unlikely to have occurred by chance, hence the name Reliable Change. This measure thus indicates the number of clients who may be considered to be reliabl improved or to be treatment failures, and provides a rational basis for this categorization, as opposed to the idiosyncratic and arbitrary definitions used by many investigators. While the regression using avoidance alone as a continuous measure allows us to examine degrees of improvement, the RC Index permits us to look at treatment failures per se. (That is, all clients might conceivably improve, and differ only in the degree to which they improve.) The RC Index was calculated for posttest and follow-up scores.

Since demographic variables were not found to be significantly correlated (all *P*s > 0.10) to the criteria, these variables were not considered further in data analyses. All other measures listed were considered for their utility as predictors of outcome. Sample sizes varied across variables and were considerably larger for posttest than for follow-up analyses. Measures on which less than 20 subjects were available were not analyzed. An estimate of power based on simple correlations reveals that, at the lower limit ($n = 20$), we would have slightly over 60% power to detect correlations of 0.50. Fortunately, sample sizes at posttest always exceeded 50, often substantially, providing 70%–80% power to detect a correlation as low as 0.30 for most variables. Even at follow-up, sample sizes were generally at least 23, which provides 70% power for a correlation of 0.50.

Degree of Improvement

The average improvement at posttest was 35.4%. Prediction of the posttest avoidance alone score was accomplished through a series of regression analyses. The pretest score on avoidance alone was always entered first to control for the effects of initial differences among clients. The second variable entered was the predictor in question. Due to sample size limitations, each predictor was analyzed in a separate regression. Alpha was set at 0.05, despite the number of analyses conducted, in order to reduce the probability of type II error.

The following variables were significant predictors of degree of improvement: Marital Dissatisfaction (standardized beta $= -0.17$, $n = 57$, $P < 0.04$), and the Body Sensations Questionnaire (standardized beta = 0.18, $n = 74$, $P < 0.03$). In addition there was a strong trend for the physical concerns factor on the Agoraphobic Cognitions Questionnaire to be associated with outcome (standardized beta = 0.17, $n = 75$, $P = 0.058$). Marital dissatisfaction was not itself related to either pre- or posttest scores on avoidance; rather it appears to operate as a suppressor variable, appearing as a significant predictor of posttest only once pretest score variance is removed. Depression, trait anxiety, panic frequency, severity of agoraphobia on the Fear Questionnaire and the social/behavioral factor of the Agoraphobic Cognitions Questionnaire, assertiveness, and social anxiety failed to predict outcome despite generous sample sizes of 73 to 119 on these measures.

Success/Failure on the RC Index

At posttest, 39.67% of the clients were reliably improved. Since pretest scores are already taken into account in the calcuation of the RC Index, the regression in this case was reduced to a point biserial correlation. There were trends (Ps < 0.10) for two of the same variables to predict success: Marital Dissatisfaction and the Body Sensations Questionnaire. In addition, the Fear Questionnaire - agoraphobia factor tended to predict outcome ($P < 0.10$).

Follow-up

Degree of improvement was analyzed in a similar fashion to posttest improvement. These analyses, however, required two additional control variables. Because clients continued as desired in exposure and/or other eclectic psychotherapy (individual or couples) after the end of the 2-week intensive program, they varied as to the amount of treatment they received in the follow-up period. Consequently, number of exposure sessions and number of psychotherapy sessions were included as control variables and forced into the regression equation after the pretest score and avoidance alone, and before the inclusion of the predictor of interest. Sample sizes ranged from 25–45. There were no trends for any of the pretest measures to predict outcome (all Ps $>$ 0.10), with the exception of one measure. Subjects with higher pretest panic frequency ($\geqq 2$ attacks per week) tendend to improve less (standardized beta = 0.22, $n = 42$, $P < 0.08$). Panic frequency was treated as a dichotomous variable in these analyses (0–2 or >2 per week) due to its extremely skewed distribution.

Posttest scores on the various predictors were also examined controlling for posttest avoidance alone scores and number of treatment sessions during follow-up. Sample sizes ranged from 22 to 38. A single trend emerged for assertion probability on the Assertion Inventory (standardized beta = 0.27, $n = 24$, $P < 0.09$). The average improvement at follow-up was 50.2%).

Success/Failure on the RC Index. At follow-up, 53.85% of clients were reliably improved. Regression analyses on the RC index were conducted using numbers of sessions of additional treatment as control variables. No significant predictors of treatment success were discerned.

Sample II: American University Phobia Program Sample

Study 1

Method

Subjects

Subjects were 30 outpatients (24 women, 6 men) at the *Phobia Program of the American University,* all of whom had received a diagnosis of agoraphobia with panic attacks based on a diagnostic interview with a clinical psychologist specializing in treatment of anxiety disorders. Their mean age was 36.5 years ($SD = 11.0$), and they reported having been agoraphobic for a mean of 10.5 years ($SD = 9.5$). They averaged 30.3 on the Hollingshead Two-Factor Index of Social Position ($SD = 16.9$), ranging from the lowest possible class to middle class, with no upper middle class clients. Exclusionary criteria were alcohol and substance abuse, suicidal intent, and depression or life crisis so severe as to preclude cooperation with treatment.

Measures

The Fear Questionnaire (global phobia and main phobia - avoidance) and performance on a three-item individualized behavioral avoidance test were used as outcome measures. On each item on the behavioral avoidance test, clients are scored 0 for total avoidance, 1 for partial avoidance or escape, or 2 for completion of item. The items are summed, yielding a score ranging from 0 to 6. Predictors were demographic variables as well as the measures listed in the previous measures section. Additional predictor variables were expectancy/credibility (adapted from Borkovec and Nau 1972) of treatment (as assessed after 1 treatment session) and intensity of panic attacks in the week preceding assessment, taken from the revised Mobility Inventory (Chambless, in press).

Procedure

Before and after ten sessions of treatment, all clients completed self-report and behavioral assessment, the latter conducted by an unfamiliar research assistant. Treatment consisted of ten sessions of individual, therapist-conducted, in vivo exposure with training in respiratory control. Each session contained 90 min of exposure and was conducted according to a research protocol proscribing interventions other than exposure and coping techniques. (For example, clients raising interpersonal problems were redirected to a focus on overcoming their phobias). The six clients who entered the program taking antidepressants, beta blockers, or tranquillizers were required to maintain stable dosages throughout the treatment and assessment, and were not allowed to begin treatment before a stable dosage had been achieved.

Results

Significant change with treatment was observed on all outcome measures. The criterion for improvement in the prediction analyses was a composite of global phobia (disability rating) and main phobia (avoidance rating) as reported on the Fear Questionnaire and performance on the behavioral avoidance test, constructed by normalizing scores on each component before summing them. Since demographic variables and drug use were not correlated significantly with outcome, these variables were not considered further in the data analyses which follow ($Ps > 0.17$). Analyses were conducted as for the Temple sample at posttest, using the composite measure as a continuous variable. The RC Index could not be calculated, as it requires reliability coefficients, which were not available for the behavioral avoidance test. One-tailed tests were used in analysis of variables that had been significant in the Temple sample.

Sample sizes ranged from 26 to 30 for these analyses. An estimate of power indicates that 28 subjects are needed for 80% power to detect a correlation of 0.50. None of the predictor variables significantly predicted posttest outcome, but there was a trend for higher scores on the

Agoraphobic Cognitions Questionnaire - physical concerns factor to be associated with less improvement (standardized beta = 0.25, $n = 28$, $P = 0.06$, one-tailed). Only 18 subjects were married or cohabiting upon entry to the study, 2 less than our minimum for data analysis. Nevertheless, in light of the anomalous findings on the Temple sample, marital dissatisfaction was analyzed in a confirmatory regression analysis. Although nonsignificant with this sample size, the standardized beta was comparable in size to that of the Temple sample (0.16 vs - 0.17, respectively), but in the opposite direction.

Study 2

Twenty-three of the clients in the American University sample who were not taking psychotropic medication also participated in a study of affect changes during their in vivo exposure treatment (DeMarco and Chambless 1987). Therapists asked clients to rate their subjective anxiety levels on the SUDS scale (0–100) every 10 min throughout the exposure sessions. In addition, clients completed the Stiles' Session Evaluation Questionnaire - Positive Affect Section immediately before and after each exposure session. Outcome criteria were residualized gain scores (controlling for pretest scores) on performance and anxiety on the behavioral avoidance test, and the main phobia rating on the Fear Questionnaire. Negative affect predictors were the average anxiety rating during each exposure session as well as the number of high anxiety ratings during each session (over 60 on a 0–100 scale). Positive affect predictors were the postsession good feelings score on the Stiles' Session Evaluation Questionnaire, and the change in good feelings score on the same questionnaire as assessed by residualized gain scores (controlling for the effects of presession levels of good feelings on postsession good feelings scores). Neither positive nor negative affect predicted outcome beyond chance levels. (Occassionally higher SUDS averages were correlated with poorer outcome.)

Study 3

Williams and Chambless (1987) examined characteristics of the therapist-client relationship, as perceived by the client, as predictors of outcome for 25 agoraphobic clients in the American University sample. Outcome was assessed by means of residualized gain scores on the behavioral avoidance test performance. Clients completed a confidential questionnaire concerning their perceptions of the therapist and their relationship after the fourth session of treatment. This 66-item questionnaire, taken in part from the Barrett-Lennard Relationship Inventory, yielded six factors which were relatively independent and demonstrated good internal consistency. Test-retest reliability (2–4 weeks) was modest, but was contaminated by additional treatment during the test-retest interval. These factors were: a large "nice therapist" cluster comprised of items reflecting tolerance, empathy, warmth, respect for the client, and congruence; modelling; unconditionality of regard; presenting challenges; therapist's willingness to be known; and explicitness.

The residualized gain scores were correlated with the therapist variables using Kendall nonparametric correlations, due to the skewed distributions of the latter. One-tailed P values were used where predictions had been made. Contrary to prediction, explicitness (tau = 0.18, $P > 0.12$) and unconditionality of regard (tau = 0.01, $P > 0.46$) were not related to positive outcome, nor was willingness to be known (tau = 0.14, $P > 0.17$), about which no prediction had been made. Predictions were confirmed in the case of the "nice therapist" cluster (tau = 0.27, $P < 0.04$), modelling (tau = 0.25, $P < 0.05$), and presenting challenges (tau = 0.32, $P < 0.02$).

Discussion

When failure in treatment was defined according to the RC Index, no predictors of outcome emerged from these investigations. Consequently, the remainder of this discussion will involve consideration of degrees of success in treatment, that is, prediction of change on phobia severity analyzed as a continuous variable.

Biographical Variables

Consistent with the results of prior investigations (e.g., Emmelkamp and van der Hout 1983), demographic characteristics of clients and duration of phobia were not associated with differential success in treatment. The one exception is a study by Mavissakalian (1985) in which ten men were found to have improved less than ten women on one measure of agoraphobia: global phobic disability at 1-month follow-up. Since Mavissakalian's results differ from the two samples in this study, one of which was considerably larger than his, as well as from data reported by Hafner (1983), it is likely that sex effects on phobia change are the exception rather than the norm. It should be noted, however, that both Hafner and Chambless and Mason (1986) found sex effects on panic frequency such that women improved less with treatment. Subjects in the latter study were a subset of those in the present Temple University sample.

Data from these analyses and those of prior studies permit us to assuage the concern of clients who frequently believe they cannot change because they are too old or have been phobic for too long. These findings call into question the use of these variables for matching subjects before assignment to treatment groups, as has been done in several investigations. Matching on irrelevant variables is of little benefit.

Phobic Severity and Dysphoria

The present results are in agreement with those of Emmelkamp and van der Hout (1983) in indicating that pretreatment severity of phobia does not predict treatment outcome. Severity of affective disturbance as measured by depression, chronic anxiety, and panic frequency and intensity did not affect treatment outcome. (In addition, affect during and immediately after exposure bore no relationship to treatment outcome.) These findings are congruent with those of Emmelkamp and van der Hout, but in disagreement with those of Watson et al. (1973). The latter study, however, involved correlations of these variables with raw outcome scores rather than with change with treatment. Thus, clients who are more depressed, anxious, and panicky at pretreatment may indeed be more phobic at outcome, but this is probably because they are highly likely to be more phobic before treatment as well (see Chambless 1985 for the relationship of avoidance behavior to these variables). It should be noted, however, that clients with major depressive disorder were excluded from the present investigations and from most other studies in the field. These findings should not be taken to mean that such clients are appropriate for exposure treatment.

Expectancy

The importance of expectation of improvement and credibility of treatment to the actual effectiveness of therapy has been emphasized by a number of authors (e.g., Kazdin and Wilcoxin 1976). The results of the present study are in keeping with those of Emmelkamp and Wessels (1975). In the latter study pretreatment expectancy ratings were not correlated with end-state functioning after 8–12 sessions of in vivo exposure; nor was expectancy/credibility related to change with ten sessions of treatment in the present study. In contrast Emmelkamp and Emmelkamp-Benner (1975) and Emmelkamp and Wessels found expectancy did predict end-state functioning after four sessions of exposure. These data suggest that expectancy may play a role in changes early in therapy, but that this effect washes out as treatment progresses. It is sometimes difficult to assess the real impact of expectancy on exposure treatment because the credibility of the treatment rationale appears to be so compelling that virtually all clients have high expectations. In the present study, however, there was a reasonable range on the measure (16–40 on a 4–40 point scale).

Social Anxiety and Assertiveness

The relationship of interpersonal anxiety and assertiveness has been investigated in several studies. Consistent with the present results, Emmelkamp (1980) and Emmelkamp and van der Hout (1983) failed to find any association of pretreatment assertion with change on avoidance. Similar findings were obtained for measures of social anxiety in the present study and in the follow-up study by Emmelkamp and Kuipers (1979). The current data indicate, however, that if subjects continue to be unassertive at posttest, there is a trend for them to fare less well in the follow-up period.

Unfortunately the number of subjects available for this analysis was rather small. In light of the study by Kleiner et al. (1987) demonstrating positive effects of adding interpersonal problem-solving to exposure for agoraphobics, these findings warrant further investigation.

Marital Relationship

Prior studies have yielded conflicting results on the utility of marital dissatisfaction as a predictor of poor treatment outcome. The present results add to this mixed picture, even though the same measure of marital dissatisfaction was used for both samples. There was no trend for dissatisfaction to be associated with outcome for the American University sample, whereas for the Temple University sample, a small but significant relationship was detected in which higher marital dissatisfaction was related to greater change with treatment at posttest although not at follow-up. The latter finding is a counterintuitive one which may simply reflect type I error, that is, a chance finding. One possible interpretation, however, may be derived from an examination of the nature of the Temple treatment program. Whereas the American University program involved straightforward exposure, the Temple program is heavily interpersonal in focus. Thus, the Temple program may be most successful for clients whose difficulties fit the underlying model of the program – those whose anxiety is in part caused or maintained by interpersonal conflict, particularly with the spouse.

The most commonly cited study in the literature supporting marital dissatisfaction as a contributor to treatment outcome at follow-up is that by Milton and Hafner (1979). These authors, however, compared more or less maritally satisfied clients on raw outcome without controlling for pretreatment differences. The maritally dissatisfied appear to have been a more disturbed group on a number of dimensions. Similar results at 2-year follow-up were reported by Monteiro et al.

(1985) who also examined raw outcome or raw change scores. Monteiro et al. explicitly note that the more maritally satisfied were better adjusted in general, and that good overall adjustment was related to better outcome. Similar findings at 3- and 6-month follow-up were obtained by Bland and Hallam (1981) who followed comparable statistical procedures. Thus, it seems that maritally dissatisfied agoraphobics generally fare worse at follow-up ranging from 3 months to 2 years. This relationship may well result from the overall poorer pretreatment adjustment of the maritally dissatisfied client. In the present study, the findings of which run counter to prior research, maritally dissatisfied clients were not more poorly adjusted overall. Indeed they scored as significantly less pathological on several measures than did the less dissatisfied.

In several other studies the effects of marital dissatisfaction on change in treatment have been examined with controls instituted for pretreatment differences among clients on initial severity of phobia (Arrindell et al. 1986; Emmelkamp 1980; Himadi et al. 1986). Findings of these studies do not support the hypothesis that the more maritally unhappy change less in treatment. Indeed, Arrindell et al. found trends in accord with our data from the Temple sample: the more dissatisfied changed more on their phobia. Thus, self-report measures of marital satisfaction (and confounded other variables) may predict end-state functioning, but they do not forecast how much clients will gain from treatment.

As a set, the results from these investigations suggest that investigators interested in the relationship of the interpersonal system to the agoraphobic's functioning need to look beyond self-report measures of marital satisfaction. Scales of various types have failed to yield meaningful findings, and the scales do not seem to tap what clinicians are responding to in their assessment of marital quality, as indicated by the poor relationship between these two methods of assessment (e.g., Monteiro et al. 1985). That Arnow et al. (1985) found marital communications training to add significantly to the effects of exposure in ameliorating agoraphobia suggests, although it certainly does not confirm, that the interpersonal climate affects the agoraphobic's progress in overcoming phobia. On the whole, investigators have yet to apply the more sophisticated methods which have been developed for assessment of interpersonal interaction to research on agoraphobia. Nevertheless, the results of two recent studies lend tentative support to the notion that a change in methodology might lead to more fruitful data. Emmelkamp and van den Hout (1983) found that clients who complained more about their spouses during treatment according to therapist's records were less likely to be treatment successes. Unfortunately, the nature of these complaints was not reported. Thomas-Peter et al. (1983) examined the relationship of the spouses' behavior to treatment outcome for agoraphobics, appropriately controlling for pretest severity. Therapists interviewed spouses and rated them on their ability to manage the agoraphobics' symptoms effectively. Agoraphobics whose spouses received more positive ratings on this measure were more likely to improve with treatment.

Therapist Factors

Additional support for the importance of the agoraphobics' interpersonal context for therapeutic outcome comes from this study's findings of the relationships between therapists' characteristics as perceived by the clients and change with treatment. Therapists who were described as warm, empathic, tolerant, and respectful, yet who were challenging and modelled assertion had clients who improved more. The size of the correlations would indicate these effects are but modest ones. However, the effects were difficult to measure, since almost all clients described their therapists in very positive terms. Emmelkamp and van den Hout (1983) found therapist characteristics to be highly predictive of end-state functioning. Interpretation of these findings is problematical because one-half of the clients refused to provide these ratings, saying the items were too personal. In addition the ratings of therapists were obtained at follow-up, making a halo effect on these ratings probable (Emmelkamp, personal communication), that is, clients who improved more might remember their therapists in a more positive fashion. The only other study of therapists' characteristics as perceived by the clients suffers from similar problems (Rabavilas et al. 1979). In addition, the utility of the Rabavilas et al. study to our discussion of outcome for agoraphobia is limited, since the sample was a mixture of obsessive-compulsives and phobics. In the only study to use objective ratings of therapist characteristics, Gustavson et al. (1985) did not find positive therapist behaviors to predict outcome. However, their statistical power was very limited (only 12 subjects), and the data analysis was somewhat problematical. At present, the conclusion that therapist effects, at least as perceived by clients, have some impact on outcome seems warranted, but replication is highly desirable.

Cognitive Factors

As predicted by cognitive theories of agoraphobia (Beck and Emery 1985; Clark 1986; Goldstein and Chambless 1978), there were consistent trends for measures of "fear of fear" to predict change with treatment. Thus, clients who were more fearful of their autonomic signs of anxiety (e.g., dizziness) and who reported higher frequency of physically focused maladaptive thinking about their anxiety (e.g., "I'll faint") improved less from pre- to post-treatment. Cognitions concerning social or behavioral consequences of anxiety (e.g., "I'll go crazy") were not associated with change during treatment. These findings reinforce our previous findings (Chambless and Gracely 1987) that fears of physical symptoms are of central importance to the agoraphobic syndrome. In our earlier study, the Body Sensations Questionnaire was found to distinguish those with agoraphobia from dients with all other anxiety disorders, including those with panic disorder. It is notable that in the present investigation, fear of the effects of panic was more consistently predictive of outcome than was reported frequency and intensity of actual panic. That is, panic seems to be less important than the client's reactions to panic. The fear of fear variables were no longer significant predictors at follow-up, at which time many subjects had had considerable additional treatment. These findings suggest that clients who are more fearful of their anxiety fare worse in the short run but, at least with continued cognitively oriented treatment, ultimately have equal chance of success in treatment.

Conclusions and Summary

In this series of investigations, as in previous studies, it proved difficult to discern factors which account for the variability of outcome in the treatment of agoraphobia. Although the size of our samples gave us far more power than is typical in such investigations, the power analyses we conducted indicated that only large correlations could be detected in most of our analyses, indeed larger correlations than it is reasonable to expect. These findings highlight the difficulty in conducting prediction research and suggest that multicenter studies may be necessary for meaningful progress. The richest area for future exploration suggested by these data is the impact of fear of fear on success with treatment. In addition, our findings indicate that behavior therapists should be more attentive to therapist effects on treatment response.

Acknowledgement: The authors wish to thank the following for their assistance in the preparation of this manuscript: Deborah Dowdall, Wendy Greve, Laura Hillman, Emily Hauck, and Philip Levin

References

Arnow BA, Taylor CB, Agras WS, Telch MJ (1985) Enhancing agoraphobia treatment outcome by changing couples communication patterns. Behav Ther 16:452–467

Arrindell WA, Emmelkamp PMG, Sanderman R (1986) Marital quality and general life adjustment in relation to treatment outcome for agoraphobia. Adv Behav Res Ther, pp 139–185

Beck AT, Emery G (1987) Anxiety disorders and phobias: a cognitive perspective. Basic, New York

Bland K, Hallam RS (1981) Relationship between response to graded exposure and marital satisfaction in agoraphobics. Behav Res Ther 19:335–338

Borkovec TD, Nau SD (1972) Credibility of analogue therapy rationales. J Behav Ther Exp Psychiatry 3:257–260

Chambless DL (in press) The mobility inventory for agoraphobia. In: Bellack AS, Hersen M (eds) A dictionary of behavioral assessment measures, Plenum, New York

Chambless DL (1985) The relationship of severity of agoraphobia to associated psychopathology. Behav Res Ther 23:305–310

Chambless DL, Caputo GC, Jasin SE, Gracely EJ, William C (1985) The mobility inventory for agoraphobia. Behav Res Ther 23:35–44

Chambless DL, Goldstein AG, Gallagher R, Bright P (1986) Integrating behavior therapy and psychotherapy in the treatment of agoraphobia. Psychotherapy 23:150–159

Chambless DL, Gracely EJ (1987) Fear of fear and the anxiety disorders. To be published

Chambless DL, Mason J (1986) Sex, sex-role stereotyping and agoraphobia. Behav Res Ther 24:231–235

Clark DM (1986) A cognitive approach to panic. Behav Res Ther 24:461–470

Christensen L, Mendoza J (1986) A method of assessing change in a single subject: an alteration of the RC index. Behav Ther 17:305–308

DeMarco D, Chambless DL (1987) An examination of the opponent process theory as applied to in vivo exposure treatment of agoraphobia. Unpublished manuscript, Department of Psychology, The American University, Washington, DC, USA

Emmelkamp PMG (1980) The role played by agoraphobics' interpersonal problems in the effects of exposure in vivo. Arch Gen Psychiatry 37:1303–1306

Emmelkamp PMG, Emmelkamp-Benner A (1975) Effects of historically portrayed modelling and group treatment on self-observation: A comparison with agoraphobics. Behav Res Ther 13:135–139

Emmelkamp PMG, Kuipers A (1979) Agoraphobia: a follow-up study for years after treatment. Br J Psychiatry 134:352–355

Emmelkamp PMG, van den Hout A (1983) Failure in treating agoraphobia. In: Foa EB, Emmelkamp PMG (eds) Failures in behavior therapy. Wiley, New York, pp 58–81

Emmelkamp PMG, Wessels H (1975) Flooding in imagination vs flooding in vivo: A comparison with agoraphobics. Behav Res Ther 13:7–15

Foa EB, Emmelkamp PMG (1983) Failures in behavior therapy. Wiley, New York

Goldstein AJ, Chambless DL (1978) A reanalysis of agoraphobia. Behav Ther 9:47–59

Gustavson B, Jansson L, Jerremalm A, Ost L-G (1985) Therapist behavior during exposure treatment of agoraphobia. Behav Modif 9:491–504

Hafner RJ (1983) Behavior therapy for agoraphobic men. Behav Res Ther 21:51–56

Himadi WG, Cerny JA, Barlow DH, Cohen S, O'Brien GT (1986) The relationship of marital adjustment to agoraphobia treatment outcome. Behav Res Ther 24:107–116

Jacobson NS, Follette WC, Revenstorf D (1984) Psychotherapy outcome research: methods for reporting variability and evaluating clinical significance. Behav Ther 15:336–352

Jansson L, Ost L-G (1982) Behavioral treatments for agoraphobia: An evaluative review. Clin Psychol Rev 2:311–336

Kazdin A, Wilcoxin L (1976) Systematic desensitization and nonspecific treatment effects: a methodological evaluation. Psychol Bull 83:729–758

Kleiner L, Marshall WL, Spevack M (1987) Training in problem solving and exposure treatment for agoraphobics with panic attacks. J Anxiety Disorders 1:219–238

Marks IM, Mathews AM (1979) Brief standard self-rating scale for phobic patients. Behav Res Ther 17:263-267

Mavissakalian M (1985) Male and female agoraphobia: Are they different? Behav Res Ther 23:469-471

Milton F, Hafner J (1981) The outcome of behaviour therapy for agoraphobia in relation to marital adjustment. Arch Gen Psychiatry 36:807-812

Mintz J, Luborsky L, Christoph P (1979) Measuring the outcomes of psychotherapy: Findings of the Penn psychotherapy project. J Consult Clin Psychol 47:319-334

Monteiro W, Marks IM, Ramm E (1985) Marital adjustment and treatment outcome in agoraphobia. Br J Psychiatry 146:383-390

Rabavilas AD, Boulougouris JD, Perissaki C (1979) Therapist qualities related to outcome with exposure in vivo in neurotic patiens. J Behav Ther Exp Psychiatry 10:293-294

Thomas-Peter BA, Jones RB, Sinnott A, Scott Fordham A (1983) Prediction of outcome in the treatment of agoraphobia. Behav Psychother 11:320-328

Watson JP, Mullet GE, Pillay H (1973) The effects of prolonged exposure to phobic situations upon agoraphobic patients treated in groups. Behav Res Ther 11:531-545

Williams Ke, Chambless DL (1987) The association of clint-perceived therapists' characteristics with outcome of in vivo exposure treatment of agoraphobia. Meeting of the Eastern Psychological Association, Arlington, VA

21. Intra- and Interpersonal Characteristics Predictive of Long-Term Outcome Following Behavioral Treatment of Obsessive-Compulsive Disorders

G. Steketee

Introduction

Although exposure to feared situations with the inclusion of response prevention has been shown to be a highly effective treatment for obsessive-compulsive disorder (OCD), reports of relapse rates from 25% to 30% are common (see Foa et al. 1985 for review). Still others refuse to participate (25%) or drop out of treatment (12%; Foa et al. 1983b). Such difficulties in treatment appear to be even greater when drugs are added to behavioral therapy (Foa et al. 1987). In view of the severe disability typically imposed by OCD symptoms, such failure is of considerable concern to the psychiatric and lay communities. Several studies have searched for variables that might explain the poor outcome of these patients in the hope that identification of such factors will lead to both better matching of patients with appropriate treatments and to improved treatment programs. The present study is focused on prediction of relapse following behavioral treatment for OCD. Previous research on this issue is reviewed below.

There is general agreement that most demographic variables, including age, sex, intelligence level, and marital status are at best minimally predictive of outcome (e.g., Basoglu et al. 1986; Foa et al. 1983a; Mavissakalian and Michelson 1983). Degree of religiosity but not type of religious affiliation has proven predictive: more devout patients had poorer outcome (Schwartz 1982; Steketee et al. 1985). Several studies have examined mood state as a predictor of outcome. Pretreatment depression and anxious mood have been found negatively related to immediate treatment gains in some studies (e.g., Marks et al. 1980; Foa et al. 1983a) but not others (e.g., Steketee et al. 1985); but little association with long-term benefits has been reported (Foa et al. 1983a; Mavissakalian and Michelson 1983; Steketee et al. 1985). Similar results have also been reported for agoraphobics (see Chambless and Gracely 1986). It is noteworthy, however, that Steketee et al. (1985) found that some measures of mood were predictive of long-term gains, but in an unexpected direction: Greater depression and anxiety led to better outcome. This finding appeared, on further study, to be due to the association of improvement in mood from pre- to posttreatment with better long-term maintenance of gains. Marks (1986) has reported similar findings in some drug studies.

In a preliminary study conducted in Philadelphia, we found that greater economic satisfaction was associated with immediate outcome: more financially comfortable patients improved more (Steketee et al. 1985). Several measures of social functioning showed a significant relationship with long-term benefits; again, *improvement* in social leisure, family, and total adjustment scores were predictive of better treatment gains 6 months later. These findings suggest that poor initial social functioning may not be problematic, but may be merely indicative of the degree to which obsessive-compulsive symptoms have disrupted an individual's lifestyle. When such functioning improves during exposure treatment, long-term prognosis appears to be good. An additional variable that has been found positively associated with long-term gains for OCD patients is their level of marital satisfaction (Hafner 1982; Schwartz 1982). The above findings suggest that social factors may have more bearing on relapse than internal ones and that further study of these variables and their interaction with intrapersonal ones is needed.

To this end, in the present study several internal and interactional characteristics of patients with OCD were examined for their relationship to follow-up outcome. In particular, since both anxious and depressive mood states have been identified as predictors of outcome in some studies of anxiety- disordered patients (although not in others), these variables were examined. Rarely have patients' social skill and anxiety or their social functioning in the environment in which they reside after treatment been studied with respect to relapse or maintenance of gains. Particularly for OCDs, whose symptoms have often interfered with their social development in adolescent years, such factors may impair their ability to access needed social reinforcers at home and in the larger community. The absence of such access may in turn reduce their capacity to engage in appropriate social activities, rather than succumbing to strong urges to ritualize, and thus may prevent them from soliciting or obtaining the aid of others to reinforce nonobsessive behaviors and appropriate coping strategies. Social skill and social anxiety were therefore investigated as possible outcome predictors in the present study. The present data are part of a larger study of the effect of social support on long-term outcome of obsessive-compulsives; results of these data are reported separately (Steketee 1987a) and are summarized here in relation to their association with mood state and social variables.

Procedure

Subjects

Forty-three obsessive-compulsives and their closest significant other participated. All patients had a primary diagnosis of OCD according to DSM-III (American Psychiatric Association 1980) and all were engaged in ongoing studies of exposure and response prevention treatment for this disorder. In the present study, 15 spouses (5 wives and 10 husbands) 18 parents (mothers), 3 siblings, and 7 friends participated as close informants. Thirteen patients were also participating in a concurrent trial of imipramine vs placebo given prior to and during behavioral treatments. Since preliminary analyses indicated that the outcome for drug-treated patients did not differ from that of nondrug patients, data from both samples are combined in the present study. Subjects ranged in age from 18 to 62 years (mean, 32.7 years) and had had their symptoms for an average of 13 years. Nineteen men and 24 women participated; one-half were employed outside the home or were students, one-quarter worked in the home, and the remainder were unemployed.

Measures

Two measures of *obsessive-compulsive symptoms* were collected:

1. Averaged ratings of obsessive fear and target rituals on 0 (no symptoms) to 8 (severe symptoms) scales, composited across three raters: patients, therapist, and independent assessors; and
2. the Compulsive Activity Checklist (CAC; Philpott 1975; Freund et al.

1987) of 38 daily activities rated by an independent assessor from 0 (no problem) to 3 (severe interference, unable to complete or attempt activity).

Correlations between these two measures ranged from $r = 0.33$ ($P < 0.05$) at pretreatment to $r = 0.72$ ($P < 0.001$) at follow-up. Both measures were employed since the use of target symptom ratings alone tends to overestimate the degree of improvement because treatment was directed specifically at these areas. The CAC provides a broader measure of obsessional difficulties commonly found in OCD patients.

Measures of *mood state* were the 21-item Beck Depression Inventory (BDI, Beck et al. 1961) and the Spielberger State-Trait Anxiety Inventory (STAI, Spielberger et al. 1970). Only the *state* anxiety score was used.

Social functioning was scored according to the Social Adjustment Scale-self report from (SAS-SR, Weissman and Bothwell 1976) from the following four areas: work (employment, student role, or houseperson role), social and leisure activities, extended family relationships, and total adjustment. High scores indicated worse functioning. Marital adjustment and current family unit functioning were omitted since the number of married subjects in the sample were too few to allow meaningful statistical analyses of these data. In addition, the therapist rated patients on Likert-like scales from 0 (no problem) to 8 (severe difficulty) on home management, work, family relationships, and social activities. Since the SAS subscales and the therapists ratings did not measure the same areas, they were not composited for the present study. When a total social functioning score was needed, the SAS total score was used.

Social skill was measured using the Social Performance Survey Schedule (SPSS) completed by the patient and a close informant (Lowe and Cautela 1978). The total score derived from both the positive and negative subscale scores was used. High scores indicate greater maladjustment. *Social anxiety* was measured according to the Social Anxiety Inventory (SAI, Curran et al. 1980) which assesses specific types of social anxiety, as well as total anxiety across social situations. In the present study, three subscales and the total score were considered to be of particular interest and were therefore studied: disapproval, anger, and conflict with parents.

In order to examine the possible relationship of the above variables to general *social suport* and to the specific responses of the closest significant other to the patient, additional measures were included. These are described in detail elsewhere (Steketee 1987a) and include: the Interview Schedule for Social Interaction (ISSI, Henderson et al. 1980), which assesses the availability and adequacy of social attachments and social integration; the Interpersonal Support Evaluation List (ISEL, Cohen et al. 1985), which measures total social support based on tangible aid, appraisal and esteem support, and belongingness; and the Perceived Social Support (PSS) scales for both family and friends (Procidano and Heller 1983). To study the impact of social support in general, the two adequacy of support scores from the ISSI, the total ISEL score and both PSS scores were converted to Z scores and composited across all five measures to yield and single social support score. Finally, the patient's closest available significant other was interviewed regarding his or her reactions to the patient when the latter evidenced obsessional symptoms and their general view of household interactions. Both patients and significant others rated the other's criticalness and angry reactions, and the degree of negative interactions in the household. Patient- and informant-rated negative responses were converted to Z scores and composited separately and to Z scores and composited separately and together for correlational and regression analyses.

Procedure

Subjects were assessed before treatment, after 4 weeks of intensive exposure and response prevention therapy, and again 6 to 14 months after treatment ended (mean = 9.3 months). In vivo- and imaginal exposure to feared obsessional situations and instructions not to ritualize were provided for 90 min daily for 15 sessions, followed by a visit to the home to continue exposure for 8 h over 2 additional days. Exposure and response prevention homework was also assigned. Patients in the drug trial received imipramine 6 weeks prior to behavioral procedures and continued it for a total of 22 weeks, after which drugs were withdrawn. During follow-up, the use of psychotropic medications was not restricted and therefore their impact on follow-up outcome is unknown. On average, subjects received 21 additional psychotherapy sessions; the impact of these sessions also cannot be determined. Measures of social skill, social anxiety, and social support were collected at pretreatment only and were available for only 27 of the 43 patients. Thus, findings regarding these data must be viewed with greater caution. It should be noted that missing data on some of the measures reduced the sample size slightly and variably across the analyses reported below.

Results

Outcome

Outcome results are given in Fig. 1. According to mean scores on both measures of obsessive-compulsive symptoms, behavioral treatment led to considerable overall improvement for this patient sample immediately after treatment. Seventy-five percent of patients were only mildly symptomatic and the remaining 25% were moderately so at posttest; a decline in severity of at least 2 points on the 9 point rating scale of target symptoms was evident in all subjects at posttreatment. However, at follow-up although mean scores showed little loss of gains, two patients had relapsed completely and the number who were moderately symptomatic had grown to 50% of the sample. Thirteen of the 43 patients were identified as relapsers (at least a 2-point loss on target symptoms and at least a 20% loss on the CAC) and 17 as maintainers (loss of 1 point or less on target ratings and less than 20% on the CAC).

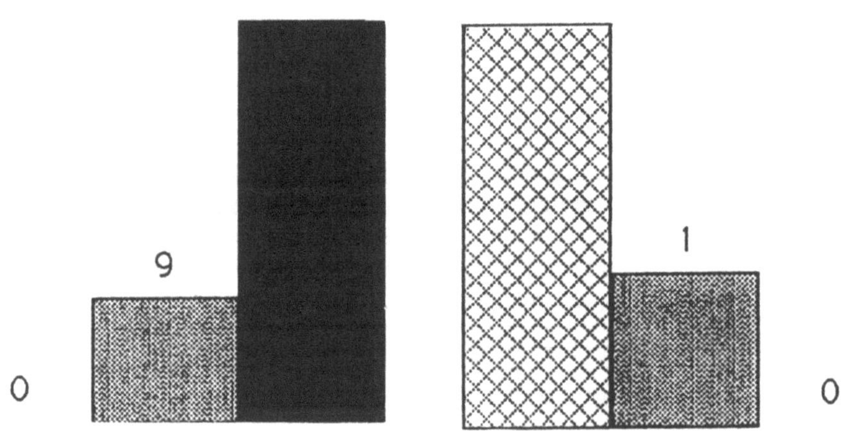

Fig. 1

Statistical Analyses

Residualized gain scores on target symptoms and on the CAC were selected as the dependent variables in order to study prediction of long-term outcome while controlling for initial level of symptoms. Since relapse was the issue of primary concern, scores from posttreatment and follow-up were used to compute residual gain in OCD symptoms, rather than scores at pretreatment and follow-up. Correlations used to examine the strength of the relationship of predictor variables to outcome were calculated according to a formula for part correlation provided in Manning and DuBois (1962) for use with residual gain scores. Two-tailed *t*-tests were also employed to compare scores of relapsers with those of maintainers. The predictors accounting for the largest proportion of variance were sought via regression analyses in which the pretreatment outcome score was forced into the analyses on the first step to control for differences in initial levels of severity. Other variables were then entered in a stepwise fashion and regressed into the follow-up outcome score. Where a single measure of obsessive-compulsive symptoms was needed (e.g., in comparisons of relapsers with maintainers or in regression analyses), the composite target symptom rating was employed.

Correlations and *t*-Tests

Correlations of dependent and independent variables are presented in Table 1. On average, patients scored in the severe range on depression (BDI: mean = 22.2; SD = 11.2) and on state of anxiety at pretreatment (STAI: mean = 55.7; SD = 14.5), but neither measure was associated with long-term gains. However, measures of both *mood states at posttreatment* were strongly predictive; state anxiety accounted for most of the relationship of negative mood and poor outcome (r's = 0.49 and 0.57; $P < 0.002$ for the two outcome measures); correlations of depression and outcome were lower (r's = 0.30 and 0.42; $P < 0.05$).

Correspondingly, improvement in anxiety during behavioral treatment was strongly related to better maintenance of gains, and again, state anxiety was the strongest predictor (r's = 0.49 and 0.46; $P < 0.01$ vs $r = -0.35$; $P < 0.04$ and $r = 0.24$ [NS] for BDI). Comparisons of relapsers and maintainers via *t*-tests supported the above findings: Relapsers were considerably more anxious after treatment than maintainers (means were 50.2 and 31.2 respectively, $t\,[20] = 3.27$, $P < 0.02$) but were not significantly more depressed. No differences were evident at pretreatment.

With respect to *social functioning* at pretreatment mean SAS scores ranged from 2.26 (SD = 0.73) for extended family functioning and to 2.84 (SD = 0.83) for social leisure adjustment, indicating marked difficulty for most patients. Similarly, average therapist-rated functioning with regard to home, work, family, and social activity ranged from 4.1 to 5.4 on 9-point scales (SDs were 2.1 to 2.6), suggesting moderate difficulty. Like mood state, pretreatment ratings of social functioning were not significantly associated with follow-up outcome, with the exception of therapist-rated home management and family functioning for the CAC only (see Table 1). However, when assessed after treatment, several of these variables were predictive: positive relationships with long-term outcome were found for SAS work, social leisure (with the CAC only), and overall adjustment (with the CAC), and therapist-rated home management (target ratings only) and family relations. Correlations were somewhat lower than those for mood state. In comparing relapsers and maintainers, *t*-tests supported these findings: no social adjustment measures taken at pretreatment distinguished groups; at posttest, therapist-rated family functioning was predictive ($t[24] = 2.34$, $P < 0.03$; means were 1.92 for relapsers and 0.64 for maintainers). However, scores on this measure indicated only mild difficulty, even for the former group.

To further study the contribution of social functioning to outcome, change scores from pre- to posttreatment were calculated for each measure. Improvement during treatment in two areas, work and social leisure, on the SAS was moderately positively related to maintenance of gains: $r = 0.49$, $P < 0.01$ for work and the CAC; r's = 0.29 and 0.34, $P < 0.10$ for social

Table 1. Correlaton of predictor variables with measures of relapse in obsessive-compulsive disorder, controlling for initial severity of symptoms (n = approximately 43 cases except where noted; correlations of $P < 0.10$ are in bold)

Predictor variables		Residual gain scores: Target ratings		Compulsive activity checklist	
		r	*P*	*r*	*P*
Beck depression inventory	Pre	−0.13	0.393	−0.03	0.838
	Post	**0.30**	0.044	**0.42**	0.007
Spielberger state anxiety	Pre	−0.04	0.790	0.02	0.911
	Post	**0.49**	0.002	**0.57**	0.001
Social adjustment					
Work	Pre	0.11	0.488	0.05	0.758
	Post	**−0.33**	0.034	**−0.47**	0.003
Social/leisure	Pre	−0.23	0.126	−0.07	0.693
	Post	0.06	0.705	**0.36**	0.040
extended family	Pre	−0.21	0.158	0.04	0.827
	Post	−0.02	0.886	0.24	0.200
Overall adjustment	Pre	−0.19	0.179	0.01	0.957
	Post	0.13	0.381	**0.41**	0.017
Therapist-rated functioning					
Home management	Pre	0.19	0.228	**0.36**	0.022
	Post	**0.32**	0.013	0.20	0.174
Work	Pre	0.11	0.488	0.02	0.906
	Post	0.10	0.524	0.11	0.553
Family relationships	Pre	0.09	0.589	**0.37**	0.028
	Post	**0.37**	0.018	**0.42**	**0.01**
Social activities	Pre	0.11	0.514	0.26	0.125
	Post	0.14	0.374	0.20	0.239
Social performance (n = 27)					
Patient		0.24	0.237	0.18	0.476
Informant		−0.14	0.531	0.25	0.292
Social anxiety inventory (n = 27)					
Dissaproval		0.05	0.796	0.08	0.720
Anger		0.07	0.714	0.04	0.853
Conflict with parents		0.08	0.666	−0.07	0.777
Total		−0.01	0.958	0.07	0.752
Social support composite (n = 27)		−0.05	0.801	0.03	0.891
Responses by significant other (n = 27)					
Negative composite (patient-rated)		**0.50**	0.017	**0.41**	0.097
Negative composite (other-rated)		0.23	0.277	**0.40**	0.060
Total negative composite		**0.56**	0.014	**0.42**	0.081

leisure with both outcome measures. That relatively few of these change scores on social functioning measures were predictive suggests that it is end-state functioning immediately after intensive treatment that has more impact on relapse. Comparisons of relapses with maintainers indicated that only on SAS social leisure did the latter improve significantly more during treatment than the former ($t\,[18] = -2.23$; $P < 0.04$). No other significant findings emerged.

To investigate the separate effects of posttreatment social adjustment and mood state independently of the effects of the other variable, partial correlations were calculated on raw scores on target ratings and the CAC at follow-up, controlling for initial severity of OCD symptoms. In general, when social adjustment was partialled out of mood state, correlations remained highly significant, particularly for state anxiety, across both outcome measures. The greatest reduction in the size of the relationship was obtained when therapist-rated family functioning was removed: anxiety remained significantly associated with follow-up OCD symptom levels (partial r's = 0.43 and 0.48 for target ratings and the CAC, $P < 0.01$), but correlations for depression were no longer significant (partial r's = 0.13 and 0.20, NS). When mood state was partialled out of the association of posttreatment social adjustment and outcome, a decline in the strength of the relationship was evident for several variables, with the exception of SAS work adjustment (partial rs = −0.36 and −0.41, $P < 0.04$, when STAI was removed and −0.37 and −0.51, $P < 0.03$, when BDI was removed) and therapist-rated family functioning (partial rs = 0.30, $P < 0.10$, and 0.46, $P < 0.01$ for STAI-removed and 0.38 and 0.48, $P < 0.04$ for BDI-removed). Removing BDI from other social functioning variables left several other significant relationships, but the pattern was inconsistent across the two measures of OCD symptoms.

With respect to *social skill,* according to both patient and informant reports, social behaviors were not significantly associated with relapse in either correlational analyses or a t-test. Similarly, neither the subscale scores nor the total score of the *social anxiety* scale were associated with maintenance of gains via correlations or t-tests. Thus, neither social skill nor social anxiety appeared to have a strong or consistent direct association with long-term outcome, although further research on a larger sample is needed to confirm these findings.

A possible indirect realtionship of these variables to outcome via an association with posttreatment mood state and social functioning was studied. The total score on social anxiety was significantly related only to posttreatment depression (r = 0.50, $P < 0.05$) but not to anxiety, and no association of social skill with mood state was found. Partialling social skill and anxiety out of the association of mood state with relapse did not significantly alter the size of the correlations. Both social skill and social anxiety were correlated positively with social functioning at posttreatment. A somewhat stronger relationship was evident for social anxiety: rs ranged from 0.69 to 0.75, $P < 0.002$ for SAS measures (except for work adjustment which was not significant) and rs = 0.35 to 0.44, $P < 0.05$ for therapist-rated functioning, with the exception of home functioning. Social skill was significantly related to family functioning on both the SAS and therapist ratings (rs = −0.47 and −0.41, $P < 0.04$) and to social adjustment on the SAS ($r = -0.53$, $P < 0.02$). Partialling social skill and anxiety out of the association of social functioning with outcome reduced all correlations to nonsignificant relationships, but sample size for these analyses were quite small. In summary, it does not appear that either social skill or social anxiety are directly associated with relapse in OCD patients. Some indirect association of social anxiety may be present, but further study on a larger sample would be needed to establish its relevance.

Detailed data on the relationship of *social support* variables to outcome on OCD patients are reported elsewhere (Steketee 1987a, b). For the present investigation, the composite score of social suport was correlated with follow-up residual gain scores. No relationship to outcome was detected (see Table 1), nor was a *t*-test comparing relapsers and maintainers significant. The possible relationship of general social support to other posttreatment variables which were predictive of outcome was studied using Pearson correlations. Social support was marginally negatively related to anxiety and depression ($rs = -0.27$, $P < 0.1$) and was significantly negatively related to several social adjustment variables, including SAS family ($R = 0.64$), social ($r = -0.59$) total score ($r = 0.44$, $Ps < 0.04$), and therapist-rated family ($r = -0.44$) and social functioning ($r = -0.55$, $Ps < 0.02$).

In studying the association of *reactions of the closest significant other* to maintenance of gains over time, correlations indicated that the total composite score of patient- and other-rated negative interactions (anger, criticalness, arguments, negative feelings in the household) were significantly associated with relapse on target ratings ($r = 0.56$, $P < 0.01$) and marginally so on CAC scores ($r = 0.42$, $P < 0.08$). This appeared to be more evident in patients' perceptions of other's behavior than in the latter's own ratings of communications. Comparing relapsers with maintainers, *t*-tests indicated that relapsers had experienced significantly more negative interactions according to both patient and informant reports ($t\,[11] = 2.34$, $P < 0.04$ and $t\,[15] = 2.34$, $P < 0.03$).

Regression Analyses

To further determine which variables explained the greatest variance in predicting long-term outcome, a series of stepwise regression analyses were conducted relating pretreatment, posttreatment, and change score measures of the above variables to follow-up outcome. The dependent measure employed in these analyses was status at follow-up, controlling for initial severity of OCD symptoms according to target symptom ratings. Independent variables were entered four at a time for analyses where $n = 43$ and three at a time for variables with smaller sample sizes.

At *pretreatment*, none of the mood state, social functioning, social skill, or social anxiety variables, nor the composite social support score were accepted into the regression equation. With respect to *posttreatment* variables, whenever state anxiety was entered with social adjustment scores, depression, social skill, social anxiety, or general social support, it alone was retained in the equation, accounting for about 30% of the variance (for variables with larger sample sizes, beta = 0.515, $P < 0.002$, multiple R = 0.571, adjusted $R^2 = 0.281$; for variables with smaller sample sizes, beta = 0.523, $P < 0.024$, multiple $R = 0.634$, adjusted $R^2 = 0.317$). (Since the sample size changed depending on the variables included in the analysis, some variation in the amount of explained variance for individual analyses was evident.) Measures of social skill, social anxiety, and general social support did not account for sufficient variance to be retained in any equation in which they were entered. Regression analyses on *change scores* from pre- to posttreatment yielded similar findings; change in state anxiety explained approximately 40% of the variance and no other social functioning or mood state change scores were retained in the equation (beta

= 0.662, $P < 0.001$, multiple $R = 0.686$, adjusted $R^2 = 0.436$).

Two exceptions to the dominance of state anxiety in explaining outcome exclusively were therapist-rated family functioning at posttreatment and negative interactions of significant other with the patient, particularly as rated by the patient. Family functioning after treatment when entered with all therapist-rated functioning variables yielded a beta of 0.449, $P < 0.017$, and a multiple $R = 0.488$, adjusted $R^2 =$ 0.178. However, when entered with state anxiety, it was no longer retained as an explanatory factor. By contrast, the patients' perception of the criticalness of the significant other explained 38% of the variance (beta = 0.649, $P < 0.012$, multiple $R = 0.676$, adjusted $R^2 = 0.37$), removing state anxiety from the equation. Although the patients' perception of angry reactions from the significant other and of general negative responses accounted for up to 25% of the variance when state anxiety was omitted from equations containing social adjustment variables, these two factors were not retained when state anxiety was added to the variable list. It appears, then, that both state anxiety and perceived criticism are approximately equally and strongly explanatory of relapse and share sufficient variance that their combined capacity is not significantly stronger than either alone.

When the above analyses were repeated using the CAC as the dependent variable, findings were essentially similar to those reported for target ratings: More variance was explained by state anxiety than any other variable (40% to 60% depending on sample size). Posttreatment work adjustment and change in social adjustment on the SAS, as well as family functioning rated by the therapist were consistent predictors, accounting together for 60% of the explained variance, but again, none of the factors was retained whenever state anxiety was introduced into the equation.

Discussion

The finding that posttreatment factors predicted long-term outcome has not been reported previously, perhaps because most efforts to identify predictive variables to date have examined the effect of only pretreatment and treatment process variables, mostly on short-term gains. Interestingly, one study has found that behavior 6 months after treatment was a much better predictor of follow-up outcome 5 to 9 years later than behavior prior to treatment (Munby and Johnston 1980). Similarly, Arrindell et al. (1986) found that social interaction factors (marital adjustment) attained greater explanatory powers at posttreatment and early in follow-up in explaining later agoraphobic symptoms. Attention to posttreatment status seems warranted, particularly in view of the substantial association of posttreatment OCD symptomatology with follow-up outcome (e.g., Foa et al. 1983a).

Mood state predicted outcome largely independently of functioning in a social context. In the present study, greater anxiety after treatment, more than depression, was associated with long-term loss of gains. This contrasts somewhat with prior literature in which the focus was on depression rather than anxious mood. It is noteworthy that in a previous study, we found anxious mood predictive of outcome, (e.g., Foa et al. 1983a), but anxiety was assessed *before* treatment and had its impact on *posttreatment* outcome. It may be that after intensive treatment is completed, depressed mood occurs in reaction to continued high anxiety and is therefore secondary to it. The latter response no doubt renders patients less able to engage in cognitive coping strategies (e.g., logical self-talk regarding the probability of danger or its importance) to reduce urges to ritualize which inevitably follow even a highly successful treatment.

The findings that several aspects of pretreatment general social support were significantly negatively associated with posttreatment anxiety and depression (Steketee 1987a), suggest that greater availability of support leads to better mood and perhaps thereby to better long-term outcome. In the present study, pretreatment social and familial functioning, as well as negative household interactions, were significantly correlated with posttreatment anxiety. The pathway by which posttreatment negative mood leads to which relapse requires further elucidation and may be related to prior levels of social functioning as well as social support. At present, a direct attack on negative mood state via psychotropic drugs (antidepressant or anxiolytic) during follow-up seems premature and potentially detrimental, in view of typical relapse rates on drug withdrawal and the failure of such drugs to improve short-term outcome (Foa et al. 1985). Rather, as their mechanism of action is identified, some attention to social support factors and social functioning may prove more beneficial.

As with mood state, although pretreatment *social adjustment* was generally not predictive, greater problems with home and familial functioning immediately *after* treatment did appear to lead to more return of obsessive-compulsive symptoms over time. Correspondingly, patients whose functioning in a variety of spheres (work, home, family, social leisure) did not improve with treatment fared less well at follow-up. Conversely, improvement in social functioning was related to better outcome, suggesting that increased social contacts and better familial relationships led to less relapse. It may be that reduced depression and anxiety and increased social functioning serve to facilitate various coping abilities, enabling patients to better resist obsessional thinking and the inevitable urges to ritualize which tend to reappear in the face of environmental stressors. If high levels of adverse mood state decrease resistance to such urges, social interaction may serve as a distractor, allowing urges to decline before the patient is able to act upon them. They may also provide positive reinforcement for not ritualizing, so long as social interactions are experienced as reinforcing events rather than unpleasant one (i.e., are not anxiety provoking or conflict ridden). Although many obsessive-compulsives do not appear to be socially fearful or deficient in their social skills, some (particularly those with early onset) do evidence considerable social difficulty. In view of the relationship found between social anxiety and depression and social functioning, for individuals who evidence considerable social anxiety, perhaps a therapeutic focus during follow-up on social anxiety and functioning may increase social contacts and secondarily forestall return of OCD symptoms.

The present research (see also, Steketee 1987a) points to an association of immediate family members' attitudes and behaviors with long-term outcome of OCD. Whereas measures of general social support were not associated with relapse, several of the informants' specific responses to the patients' obsessive-compulsive symptoms were related to long-term benefits. Greater criticism, anger, urging of confrontation with feared obsessional cues, negative interactions in the household, and the informant's belief that patients could control their symptoms if they wished were all predictive of poor outcome. Correspondingly, greater empathy and positive household feelings were indicative of a better prognosis. Consistent with previous findings regarding life events, more distress from life events during the follow-up period was associated with poorer long-term status. These findings suggest that among social environment factors, it is not the broader social network, but rather the specific reactions of close family members to patients after treatment, which influences maintenance or loss of treatment benefits. Such results are congruent with the literature on "expressed emotion" (criticism, emotional overinvolvement, and hostility) in family members as a predictor of long-term outcome for schizophrenic and depressed patients (cf. Hooley 1985).

Therapeutic efforts which improve the patient's capacity to access social reinforcement from significant others, more than from the general social environment, may be needed to enhance resistance to the return of problematic obsessions and rituals. Additional research corroborating the findings of this study is needed before we can confidently assert that a formal treatment program which includes such therapeutic efforts directed at familial relationships, as well as at other social capacities and interactions, is likely to be of benefit. Such research must at least be longitudinal, measuring specific aspects of social functioning and their association with social support and with mood state at several points in time.

References

American Psychiatric Association (1980) Diagnostic and statistical manual of mental disorders, 3rd edn. Washington DC

Arrindell WA, Basoglu M, Lax T, Emmelkamp PMG, Kasvikis Y, Sanderman R, Marks IM (1986) Patterns and predictors of improvement in obsessive-compulsive disorder. Unpublished manuscript.

Beck AT, Ward CM, Mendelson M, Mach J, Erbaugh J (1961) An inventory for measuring depression. Arch Gen Psychiatry 4:561–571

Chambless DL, Gracely E (1986) Follow-up research on agoraphobics. In: Steketee G Factors associated with success and failure in anxiety-disordered patients following behavioral treatment. Symposium at the meeting of the Society for Psychotherapy Research, Wellesley

Cohen S, Mermelstein R, Kamarck T, Hoberman H (1985) Measuring the functional components of social support. In: Saranson IG, Sarason BR (eds) Social support: theory, research and applications. Martinus Nijhoff, Dordrecht

Curran JP, Corriveau DP, Monte PM, Hagerman SB (1980) Social skill and social anxiety: self-report measurement in a psychiatric population. Behav Modif 4:493–512

Foa EB, Grayson JB, Steketee GS, Doppelt HG, Turner RM, Latimer PR (1983a) Success and failure in the behavioral treatment of obsessive-compulsives. J Consult Clin Psychol 51:287–297

Foa EB, Steketee GS, Grayson JB, Doppelt HG (1983b) Treatment of obsessive-compulsives: when do we fail? In: Foa EB, Emmelkamp PMG (eds) Failures in behavioral therapy. Wiley, New York

Foa EB, Steketee GS, Ozarow BJ (1985) Behavior therapy with obsessive-compulsives: from theory to treatment. In: Mavissakalian M (ed) obsessive-compulsive disorder: psychological and pharmacological treatment. Plenum, New York

Foa EB, Steketee GS, Kozak MJ, Dugger D (1987) Imipramine and placebo in the treatment of obsessive-compulsives: their effect on depression and on obsessional symptoms. Psychopharmacol Bull 23:8–11

Freund B, Steketee G, Foa EB (1987) The compulsive activity checklist (CAC)

Hafner RJ (1982) Marital interaction in persisting obsessive-compulsive disorders. Aust NZ J Psychiatry 16:171–178

Henderson S, Duncan-Jones P, Byrne DG, Scott R (1980) Measuring social relationships: the interview schedule for social interaction. Psychol Med 10:723–734

Hooley JM (1985) Expressed emotion: a review of the critical literature. Clin Psychol Rev 5:119–139

Lowe MR, Cautela JR (1978) A self-report measure of social skill. Behav Res Ther 9:535–544

Manning WH, Dubois PH (1962) Correlational methods in research on human learning. Percept Mot Skills 15:287–321

Marks IM (1986) Fears, phobias, and rituals. Oxford University Press, New York

Marks IM, Hodgson R, Rachman S (1975) treatment of chronic obsessive-compulsive neurosis by in vivo exposure. Br J Psychiatry 127:349–364

Mavissakalian M, Michelson L (1983) Tricyclic antidepressants in obsessive-compulsive disorder: antiobsessional or antidepressant agents? J Nerv Ment Dis 171:301–306

Munby M, Johnson DW (1980) Agoraphobia: the long-term follow-up of behavioral treatment. Br J Psychiatry 137:418–427

Philpott R (1975) Recent advances in the behavioral measurement of obsessional illness. Scot Med J 20:33–44

Procidano ME, Heller K (1983) Measures of perceived social support from friends and family: three validation studies. Am J Community Psychol 11:1-24

Schwarz VF (1982) Prognostische Kriterien bei der stationären Gruppenpsychotherapie neurotisch depressiver und zwangsneurotischer Patienten Z Psychosom Med 28:30-51

Spielberger ED, Gorsuch RL, Lushene RG (1970) The state-trait anxiety inventory. Consulting Psychologists Press, Palo Alto

Steketee G (1987a) Predicting relapse following behavioral treatment for obsessive-compulsive disorder: the impact of social support. Dissertation Abstracts International

Steketee G (1987b) Social support as a predictor of long-term outcome of obsessive-compulsives following a behavioral treatment program. Unpublished manuscript

Steketee G, Kozak MJ, Foa EB (1985) Predictors of outcome for obsessive-compulsives treated with exposure and response preventions. European Association for Behavior Therapy, Munich, West Germany, September 1985

Weissman M, Bothwell S (1976) Assessment of social adjustment by patient self-report. Arch Gen Psychiatry 33:1111-1115

22. Marital Quality and Treatment Outcome in Anxiety Disorders

P. M. G. EMMELKAMP

Introduction

A number of therapists have suggested that interpersonal, particularly marital, difficulites play an import part in the development and maintenance of patients' phobic symptoms (Emmelkamp 1982; Goldstein and Chambless 1978; Hafner 1982). The partners of phobics have been described as impeding or reversing the positive effects of treatment or even developing psychiatric symptoms themselves. Further, it has been suggested that treatment-produced change in phobic symptoms may have a negative impact upon the client's marriage (e.g., Hafner 1982). On the basis of such clinical observations, it has been claimed that a system-theoretic interactional approach is needed to understand the etiology and maintenance of agoraphobia (Hafner 1982).

Interest in relationship problems of agoraphobics is not only recent. Fry (1962) suggested that the marital functioning of agoraphobics was affected by the feelings of inferiority and inadequacy of their spouses. Hafner, in a number of publications (1976, 1977a, 1977b, 1979, 1982, 1983, 1984a, 1984b; Hafner and Ross 1983; Milton and Hafner 1979), has stressed the importance of relationship problems in agoraphobia, but his studies are among "the most methodologically deficient and consistently criticized studies on marital adjustment and the behavioural treatment of agoraphobics" (Wilson 1984).

The publications of Hafner stimulated a research project at the Clinical Psychology Department of the University of Groningen. In a series of studies the following issues were investigated:

1. Are partners of agoraphobics themselves psychologically disturbed?
2. Are the marriages of agoraphobics qualitatively different from those of control couples?
3. Does the quality of marriage have an impact on the outcome of behavior therapy?
4. Is spouse-aided therapy more effective than individual treatment?

Partners of Agoraphobics

One of the first issues that was investigated was whether psychological characteristics of the partner of the agoraphobic patient are important factors in the development and maintenance of the patient's symptoms. Previous studies in this area had provided inconclusive results. The partners of agoraphobics have been described as "unstable" (Webster 1953), "typically negativistic, anxious, compulsive with strong withdrawal tendencies" (Fry 1962), "neurotic" (Schaper 1973), and "abnormally jealous" (Fry 1962; Hafner 1979). Others, however, found no evidence that partners of agoraphobics were themselves disturbed (Agulnik 1970; Buglass et al. 1977).

In the study by Arrindell and Emmelkamp (1985) partners of 32 female agoraphobics were compared with the partners of nonphobic psychiatric subjects and nonpatient normal controls on a large number of variables. The findings of this study indicated that the partners of female agoraphobics cannot be characterized as more defensive than those of nonphobic psychiatric or normal controls. Further, no evidence was found that partners of agoraphobics are more neurotic, more socially anxious, or more obsessive than partners of controls. Although the partners of agoraphobics were found to be more intropunitive than the partners of nonpatient female subjects, further analyses revealed that their scores fell within normal ranges. Fry has suggested that the agoraphobic patient and the spouse resemble one another and that the partners of agoraphobics have symptoms very similar to those of the patient. Contrary to suggestions by Fry (1962), Arrindell and Emmelkamp (1985) found in agoraphobic couples the largest between-spouse differences on those variables dealing with the target symptoms, i.e., agoraphobia, anxiety, and somatization. The agoraphobics appeared to be less comparable to their partners in terms of personality and symptoms than were spouses from the control groups. Thus, there is no evidence that the partners of agoraphobics are psychologically disturbed themselves.

Marital Relationship of Agoraphobics

A second question that was addressed in our research program was whether the marital relationship of agoraphobics is qualitatively different from that of control couples, as suggested by a number of authors. Most of the studies emphasizing the importance of quality of marital relationships in the etiology of agoraphobia (e.g., Fry 1962; Goldstein 1973; Hafner 1981; Holmes 1982; Webster 1953) lack adequate control groups, are retrospective in nature, and are based on interviews of unknown reliability and validity.

The aim of the Arrindell and Emmelkamp (1986) study was to investigate whether the marriages of agoraphobics differ from those of controls. Thirty female agoraphobics and their partners filled out a number of questionnaires, including the Maudsley Marital Questionnaire and a communication questionnaire, measuring intimate communication, destructive communication, discongruent communication, and avoidance of communication. Three control groups also participated in this study:

a) nonphobic psychiatric controls and their partners,
b) maritally distressed couples and their partners, and
c) nondistressed females and their partners.

The results revealed that agoraphobics and their spouses tend to be more comparable to happily married subjects in terms of intimacy (e.g., marital and sexual adjustment and satisfaction, and quality of communication), while nonphobic psychiatric patients are more comparable to maritally distressed couples.

Marital Quality and Treatment Outcome

A third question that was addressed by our research group was the impact of the quality of the marital relationship on the outcome of behavior therapy. Previous studies in this area found a significant impact of relationship problems of agoraphobics on the outcome of behavioral treatment (e.g., Emmelkamp and Van der Hout 1983; Hudson 1974; Milton and Hafner 1979; Monteiro et al. 1985; Bland and Hallam 1981), while others found no relationship between initial marital ratings and improvement (Cobb et al. 1984; Emmelkamp 1980; Himadi et al. 1986). The studies that evaluated the impact of marital quality on the outcome of exposure in vivo are hampered by a number of methodological problems, the most important being the lack of norms for marital measures. In the previous studies in which the decision had to be made with respect to classifying couples as maritally satisfied or maritally dissatisfied, this was based on a median split (that is, in relation to other couples in the sample) or on some other arbitrary criterion rather than on an externally validated cut-off score. Unfortunately, this raises the possibility of classifying subjects or couples erroneously as satisfied or dissatisfied. Other methodological problems in previous studies involved a combination of exposure in vivo and drug treatment, lack of adequate follow-up, and lack of reliable clinical ratings of marital quality in addition to self-report.

In acknowledging the limitations of previous studies on a number of points, special attention was paid to the following aspects in a study by Arrindell et al. (1986):

1. The administration of an exposure-based therapy not combined with drugs
2. The use of a relatively long follow-up assessment period (1 year)
3. The utilization of a reliable and valid marital measure widely employed in the area for which norms exist; namely the Maudsley Marital Questionnaire (MMQ)
4. The use of a better alternative to trivial cut-off scores for distinguishing satisfied from dissatisfied marriages (MMQ > 20)
5. The focus on female patients only as subjects
6. The inclusion of an independent observer rating of marriage quality

Patients were treated by means of prolonged exposure in-vivo (ten 3-h sessions, three times a week). The details of this treatment are explained in detail in Emmelkamp (1982).

Results indicated that independent observers' marital rating and marital self-ratings on the Maudsley Marital Questionnaire predicted treatment failure neither at posttest nor at follow-up. A second question that was investigated was whether agoraphobic improvement is associated with a deterioration in marriage quality. Contrary to expectations from system-theorists, agoraphobics' marriage quality and sexual relationship did not deteriorate as a result of the improvement of the agoraphobic patient. Also the partner rated the marriage and the sexual relationship as unaffected by the improvement of his agoraphobic wife.

Finally, results of these agoraphobics on the marital relationship were compared with other groups. Agoraphobics scored in the range of normal community females, rather than in the range of either maritally distressed females or other psychiatric patients.

In sum: There is no evidence that agoraphobics are characterized by interpersonal problems in the relationship and it is thus not surprising to find that such problems do not predict failure or success of treatment by exposure in-vivo.

Spouse-Aided Therapy

The final question that was addressed was whether spouse-aided therapy is more effective than treatment of the patient alone. In a recent multicenter trial (Emmelkamp et al. 1988b), 58 severe agoraphobic patients with partners were randomly assigned to individual exposure treatment or to spouse-aided therapy. In the patient alone condition, the spouse was seen only for measurement. The patient alone was given a treatment manual (Mathews et al. 1981). Treatment started with one therapist-accompanied session of prolonged exposure in-vivo, and continued with homework tasks which the patient carried out between sessions. After the first two sessions (initial assessment and exposure session), the therapist used the treatment time to monitor progress, discuss difficulties, and decide on further exposure tasks. In the spouse-aided condition both patient and spouse were given manuals (Mathews et al. 1981), and both were present at all treatment sessions. Treatment focused on the phobia; discussion of relationship problems if necessary was postponed to after the experimental trial. The spouse was instructed to assist the patient with carrying out homework tasks. Treatment consisted of six sessions and was conducted within 1 month. There was a 1-month waiting period to control for the passage of time. Immediately after treatment another 1 month waiting period followed.

Agoraphobics were accepted for treatment if the partner was willing to cooperate and if they had a score of more than 17 on the agoraphobic scale of the fear questionnaire. One-half of the patients were treated in our department in Groningen, the other half in the psychiatric department of the University Hospital in Leiden.

Results revealed that treatment led to significant results on anxiety and avoidance scales, fear questionnaire, and behavioral measure. In addition to improvement of the main symptoms of agoraphobia, treatment was associated with significant changes of psychopathology as assessed by the SCL-90. Marital and sexual adjustment was neither found to improve nor to deteriorate as a result of treatment. As in our previous study (Arrindell et al. 1986), very few couples scored in the marital distressed range at the start of the treatment.

Was spouse-aided therapy more effective than treatment by the patient alone? The overall impression is that both treatments were equally effective not only on phobic symptoms but also on generalization measures. Thus, our results corroborate the results of Cobb et al. (1984) and Himadi et al. (1986) with a smaller number of patients, underscoring the conclusion of Cobb et al. (1984) that although there are no basic objections against including the spouse, there is no justification for trying to coerce a partner to be involved if lack of time or inclination makes it difficult.

In two studies we investigated the effects of partner-assisted exposure treatment with obsessive-compulsives. A study by Emmelkamp and Lange (1983) found exposure by the patient alone to be less effective than partner-assisted exposure, however, due to the small number of patients ($n = 12$) involved in that study, an additional study with a lager number of obsessive-compulsives is needed. In the Emmelkamp et al. (1988a) study, which was conducted at the Reijnier de Graaf Hospital in Delft, 50 obsessive-compulsives whose partners were willing to cooperate were randomly assigned to either partner-assisted exposure or patient-alone treatment. In both the Emmelkamp and Lange (1983) and Emmelkamp et al. (1988a) studies, exposure in vivo consisted of presenting patients with anxiety-evoking items or situations that trigger compulsive behavior in a gradual manner. Treatment consisted of homework assignments (for details see Emmelkamp 1982). In the patient-alone condition, the partner was only seen for assessment. In the couple condition the partner had to accompany the patient to each treatment session. The patient had to carry on his homework assignments with his partner present. The task of the partner was to encourage the patient and to have him confront the distressing stimuli until the patient got used to them. In addition, the partner was instructed to withhold reassurance, when the patient asked for it. As in the patient-alone condition, the patient was not allowed to perform his rituals, There was not any practising of the tasks during the treatment sessions at the hospital. In contrast to our pilot study, in the Emmelkamp et al. study, both conditions generally were found to be equally effective, thus corroborating results of studies with agoraphobics.

Discussion

The results of our studies into the marital relationship of agoraphobics can be summarized as follows:

1. Partners of agoraphobics are not psychologically disturbed themselves.
2. The marriages of agoraphobic couples are more comparable to normal community couples and nondistressed couples than to maritally distressed couples.
3. The impact of relationship dysfunction - if any - on treatment outcome is small and does not account for much variance.
4. Spouse-aided therapy is no more effective than treatment of the patient alone.

Taking together the data of our series of studies there is little empirical support for the propositions of Hafner (1982) that agoraphobics' spouses often initially resist the patient's symptomatic improvement, and that this is less likely to occur if the spouse is actively involved in the patient's therapy. Actually, Hafner's own data do not support his theory either. For example, Milton and Hafner (1979) reportet that: "... the marriages of nine (out of 15) patients appeared to be adversely influenced by their symptomatic improvement" (p. 807). However, inspection of their data (Milton and Hafner, Table 1, p. 808) reveals a totally different picture: Both patients and their partners show an improvement rather than a deterioration of marital and sexual adjustment. Thus, the idea of a worsening of the marriage was based on clinical anecdotal material rather than on the more objective measures used.

It should be noted that the large series of publications by Hafner (1976, 1977a, 1977b, 1979, 1982, 1983, 1984a, 1984b; Milton and Hafner 1979; Hafner and Ross 1983), purporting to demonstrate the interactional model of agoraphobia, are all based on only *two* independent sets of data. Ironically, their results have not always been interpreted uniformly, which is rather curious given the interdependency of the data sets and the relatedness of the hypotheses being tested (Arrindell et al. 1986). The interpretations of the data in studies by Hafner have also been heavily criticized by Stern (1977), Monteiro et al. (1985), Wilson (1984), and Kleiner and Marshall (1985). In commenting on the finding of the Hafner and Ross (1983) study that the more friendly the partners were, the less their agoraphobic wives improved, Wilson (1984) notes: "In a manner characteristic of Hafner's previous idiosyncratic analyses ..., Hafner and Ross are able to interpret the husbands' friendliness and vigor as reflections of their 'capacity to deny aspects of their negative feelings'. ... One wonders how these ill-fated husbands would have been viewed had they been unfriendly and passive" (Wilson 1984). In a similar vein, Kleiner and Marshall (1985) note that Hafner seems to interpret a denial of marital dissatisfaction as meaning that agoraphobics may be covering up real problems and state that disconformation of this hypothesis may be hard to come by.

How to explain the findings that in the Arnow et al. (1985) study couples communication training resulted in significant improvement of phobias as compared to relaxation control? First, it should be noted that relatively few of the marriages (25%) appeared distressed at pretest, which corroborates our findings. Further, marital adjustment scores remained largely unchanged throughout the study despite significant positive changes in communication among those couples who underwent communication training. Thus, it seems that communication training - rather than dealing with marital problems - dealt with discussing and changing interactional patterns that may have been impeding the agoraphobic's progress in overcoming the symptoms. One may wonder whether this communication approach is actually that much different from the spouse-aided therapy program of Mathews et al. (1981).

Another possibility suggested by Arrindell et al. (1986) is that the positive effects of communication training can be interpreted as resulting from the positive functions of a supportive social network which is provided by the partner. Research in the area of stressful life events and social support indicates that any change in a person's life, whether related to a positive or a negative event, constitues a state of risk in that it carries the need for readjustment (Murphy 1986). Actively involving the partner of phobics in the treatment may reduce this risk by increasing the quality of the social support system. Further research along this line seems promising.

References

Agulnik PL (1970) The spouse of the phobic patient. Br J Psychiatry 117:59-67

Arnow BA, Taylor CB, Agras WS, Telch MJ (1985) Enhancing agoraphobia treatment outcome by changing couple communication patterns. Behav Res Ther 16:452-467

Arrindell WA, Emmelkamp PMG (1985) Psychological profile of the spouse of the female agoraphobic patient: personality and symptoms. Br J Psychiatry 146:405-414

Arrindell WA, Emmelkamp PMG (1986) Marital adjustment, intimacy and needs in female agoraphobics and their partners: a controlled study. Br J Psychiatry 149:592-602

Arrindell WA, Emmelkamp PMG, Sanderman R (1986) marital quality and general life adjustment in relation to treatment outcome in agoraphobia. Adv Behav Res Ther 14:139-185

Bland K, Hallam RS (1981) Relationship between response to graded exposure and marital satisfaction in agoraphobics. Behav Res Ther 19:335-338

Buglass D, Clarke J, Henderson AS, Kreitman N, Presley AS (1977) A study of agoraphobic housewives. Psychol Med 7:73-86

Cobb JP, Mathews AM, Childs-Clarke A, Blowers CM (1984) The spouse as co-therapist in the treatment of agoraphobia. Br J Psychiatry 144:282-287

Emmelkamp PMG (1980) Agoraphobics' interpersonal problems. Arch Gen Psychiatry 37:1303-1306

Emmelkamp PMG (1982) Phobic and obsessive-compulsive disorders: theory, research and practice. Plenum, New York

Emmelkamp PMG, De Lange I (1983) Spouse involvement in the treatment of obsessive-compulsive patients. Behav Res Ther 21:341-346

Emmelkamp PMG, van der Hout A (1983) Failure in treating agoraphobia. In: Foa EB, Emmelkamp (eds) Failures in behavior therapy. Wiley, New York, pp 53-75

Emmelkamp PMG, De Haan E, Hoogduin CAL (1988a) Spouse-aided therapy with obsessive-compulsives. (In preparation)

Emmelkamp PMG, Van Dijck R, Bitter M, Heins R (1988b) Spouse-aided therapy with agoraphobics. (In preparation)

Fry WF (1962) The marital context of an anxiety syndrome. Fam Process 4:245-252

Goldstein A (1973) Learning theory insufficiency in understanding agoraphobia. In: Brengelmann JC, Turner W (eds) Behaviour therapy. Urban and Schwarzenberg, München

Goldstein A, Chambless DL (1978) A reanalysis of agoraphobia. Beh Res Ther 9:47-59

Hafner RJ (1976) Fresh symptom emergence after intensive behaviour therapy. Br J Psychiatry 129:378-383

Hafner RJ (1977a) The husbands of agoraphobic women: assortative mating or pathogenic interaction? Br J Psychiatry 130:233-239

Hafner RJ (1977b) The husband of agoraphobic women and their influence on treatment outcome. Br J Psychiatry 131:289-294

Hafner RJ (1979) Agoraphobic women married to abnormally jealous men. Br J Med Psychol 52:99-104

Hafner RJ (1981) Agoraphobia in men. Aust NZ J Psychiatry 15:243-249

Hafner RJ (1982) The marital context of the agoraphobic syndrome. In: chambless DL, Goldstein AJ (eds) Agoraphobia: multiple perspectives on theory and treatment. Wiley, New York

Hafner RJ (1983) Behaviour therapy for agoraphobic men. Behav Res Ther 21:51-56

Hafner RJ (1984a) The marital repercussions of behavior therapy for agoraphobia. Psychotherapy 21:530-542

Hafner RJ (1984b) Predicting the effects on husband of behaviour therapy for wives' agoraphobia. Behav Res Ther 22:217-226

Hafner RJ, Ross MW (1983) Predicting the outcome of behaviour therapy for agoraphobia. Behav Res Ther 21:375-382

Himadi WG, Cerny JA, Barlow DH, Cohen S, O'Brien GT (1986) The relationship of marital adjustment to agoraphobia treatment outcome. Behav Res Ther 24:107-115

Holmes J (1982) Phobia and counterhobia: family aspects of agoraphobia. J Fam Ther 4:133-152
Hudson B (1974) The families of agoraphobics treated by behaviour therapy. Br J Social Work 4:51-59
Kleiner L, Marshall WL (1985) Relationship difficulties and agoraphobia. Clin Psychol Rev 5:581-595
Mathews A, Gelder M, Johnston D (1981) Agoraphobia. Guilford, London
Milton F, Hafner J (1979) The outcome of behavior therapy for agoraphobia in relation to marital adjustment. Arch Gen Psychiatry 36:807-811
Monteiro W, Marks IM, Ramm E (1985) Marital adjustment and treatment outcome in agoraphobia. Br J Psychiatry 149:383-390
Murphy JM (1986) Trends in depression and anxiety: men and women. Acta Psychiatry Scand 73:113-127
Schaper W (1973) Some aspects of the interaction between phobics and their partners. In: Brengelman JC, Turner W (eds) Behaviour Therapy. Urban and Schwarzenberg, München
Stern R (1977) Letter. Br J Psychiatry 130:418
Webster AS (1953) The development of phobias in married women. Psychol Monogr Gen Appl 67 (367): 1-18
Wilson GT (1984) Fear reduction methods and the treatment of anxiety disorders. In: Wilson GT, Franks CM, Brownell KD, Kendall PC (eds) Annual review of behavior therapy. Theory and practice, vol 9. Guilford, New York

23. Patterns of Patient-Spouse Interaction in Agoraphobics: Assessment by Camberwell Family Interview (CFI) and Impact on Outcome of Self-Exposure Treatment

H. PETER and I. HAND

Introduction

The Concept of Expressed Emotion

The concept of Expressed Emotion (EE) was developed by George Brown and his colleagues from their work with schizophrenic patients.

They found the relatives' attitudes towards the patient to be the single most powerful predictor of the course of the patient's illness. This attitude is assessed by means of a semistructured interview, the Camberwell Family Interview (CFI). In a series of studies (Brown et al. 1966, 1972; Vaughn and Leff 1976, 1982; Vaughn et al. 1982, 1984), high expressed emotion appeared to be this predictor of relapse. Patients living with "high EE" relatives who were either very critical or emotionally overinvolved, relapsed four times more often within a 9-month follow-up period than patients with "low EE" relatives. Recently, similar results were reported for the course of manic disorder (Miklowitz 1985) and for depression (Vaughn and Leff 1976; Hooley et al. 1985).

For young first and second breakdown schizophrenics though, Dulz and Hand (1986) found EE ratings of relatives to fluctuate strongly over short periods of time and not to be reliable predictors of relapse. A similar result was reported from a study with a much larger sample of first breakdown schizophrenics in England (McMillan et al. 1986).

As EE is an "empirical", and not a theory-derived construct, the question arises whether EE reflects intrapersonal or interpersonal factors. Brown assumed that a relative's EE reflects a persistent attitude towards the patients' personality rather than towards his illnes behavior. Over the last few years, an association between dyadic interaction patterns and EE ratings has been shown for schizophrenics as well as for depressives and their relatives or spouses (Halweg et al. 1985; Hooley and Hahlweg 1986). Hooley found that the interaction style of couples with "high EE" spouses is characterized by more negative affects, more personal and specific criticism, more disagreement, and more negative mutual reinforcement than in couples with low EE spouses.

The CFI may therefore also be useful to assess the quality of marital relationship in patients with anxiety disorders, perhaps more so than marital self-rating questionnaires.

Agoraphobia and Marriage

Despite effective interventions for agoraphobia, like exposure in vivo, most outcome studies report failure rates of about 30% (Marks 1971; Emmelkamp and Kuipers 1979; McPherson et al. 1980; Barlow et al. 1984; Cohen et al. 1984; Hand et al. 1986). Another problem is the rate of treatment refusals after an intake interview and of treatment drop-outs, together accounting for about another 25% of agoraphobics (Barlow et al. 1980; Hand 1988b). Considering these results, one can assume that 50% of all agoraphobics looking for behavioral therapy have a poor or an unknown prognosis. Why is this so?

The importance of interpersonal problems in the development and maintenance of agoraphobia has been discussed for many years. Generally, interpersonal problems are described to be the most frequent stressor before the onset of symptoms (Last et al. 1984).

Like others (Lazarus 1966, 1972; Everaerd et al. 1972; review in Hafner 1986), we found that a high proportion (66%) of agoraphobics reported marital problems (Hand et al. 1974; Hand and Lamontagne 1976). But reported marital problems may not differ between agoraphobics and "normals" (Buglass et al. 1977; Emmelkamp 1980, this volume; Fisher and Wilson 1985). Studies examining the dependence of treatment outcome on marital interaction or marital satisfaction give contradictory results. Some authors found a poor outcome of exposure treatment for agoraphobics to be related to disturbed relationships (Milton and Hafner 1979; Bland and Hallam 1981), whereas other authors could not find such a correlation (Emmelkamp 1980; Cobb et al. 1984; Monteiro et al. 1985; Himady et al. 1986). In a study by Hand and Lamontagne (1976), marital problems did affect the immediate posttreatment development of several patients, but there was no consistent negative effect upon 6-month follow-up results. Comparison of these studies is difficult because of the different assessments of marital relationship. A particularly puzzling problem arises where symptoms have a "protective function" in covering marital dissatisfaction or conflicts (Haley 1963). In case of such a function, the couples' self-ratings of their marriages are bound to be "good," i.e., misleading (Hand et al. 1977). What then is the impact of interpersonal tension (marital distress) on the formation and maintenance of symptoms in agoraphobics? We will present the first results from a new attempt to tackle this apparently old problem.

Design

Subjects

Subjects were selected from agoraphobic patients of the Behavior Therapy Outpatient Unit of the Hamburg University Hospital. Diagnosis of agoraphobia was made after an extensive intake interview. All patients had to be married or had to be living in a marriage-like relationship for at least a year. Within a short period of time, 22 female and three male agoraphobics who met these criteria were found. The mean age was 34.2 years (range 22–51), the mean duration of symptoms was 5.7 years (range 0.5–20) the mean duration of the relationship was 12.8 years (range 1–30).

Treatment

All patients – except one, who participated in therapist-aided group exposure in vivo (Hand et al. 1974) – received manual-aided home-based-treatment (HBT, Mathews et al. 1977). While group exposure in vivo is based on the flooding paradigm, HBT much more resembles a desensitization approach, allowing avoidance when anxiety exceeds a certain level. During 4 weeks of daily self-exposure, patients with HBT received five in-office contacts with their therapist to discuss proper use of the manual program. One patient dropped out while on the waiting list, two patients dropped out from treatment.

It is important to emphasize that patients in this part of our large-scale project on anxiety disorders received HBT *without* spouses participating as cotherapist - while in the original program by Matthews et al. spouses were involved. Two of the three drop-outs participated in the follow-up testing. These data are included in the outcome study.

Assessments

Assessments were based on:
a) symptom self-rating scales,
b) marital self-rating questionnaires, and
c) the Camberwell Family Interview (CFI).

1. *Symptom self-ratings*

- Agoraphobia (Fear Survey Schedule, FSS; Hallam and Hafner 1978)
- Additional phobia meassurements: total phobia (from FSS), behavioral resistance to phobic advoidance, and hindrance in daily-life activities by phobic anxiety (details in Hand and Zaworka 1982; Fisher et al., this volume)
- Depression (v. Zerssen and Koeller 1976)
- Obsessive-compulsive symptoms (Hamburger Zwangs-Inventar, HZI; Zaworka et al. 1983)

2. *Marital self-rating questionnaires*

- Dyadic Adustment Scale (DAS; Spanier 1976)
- Marital Happiness Scale (MHS; Azrin 1973)

3. *The Camberwell Family Interview*

This is a semistructured interview lasting for about 1 h. The topics of the interview are the relative's (spouse's) behavior in everyday life (e.g., household tasks, financial arrangements, and family time management), the course of the illness, irritability, physical complaints, and the relationship. Questions refer to concrete events, mostly within the last 3 months. The audiotaped interview is then rated on five separate scales:

a) the number of critical comments,
b) hostility
c) emotional overinvolvement (EOI),
d) the number of positive remarks, and
e) warmth.

All CFI interviews and ratings were done by the first author (H. Peter), who was trained by Christine Vaughn and successfully completed post training rater reliability testing.

In our study, the CFI was done with spouses *and* patients separately and at pretreatment only. To our knowledge, this is the first and so far only study, that adds the CFI assessment of patients attitudes toward their spouses to the usual assessment of spouses' attitudes toward the patients. Most CFI were conducted before self-rating scales were applied.
All symptom and marital self-rating scales were rated by patients at the pretreatment, posttreatment, and follow-up stages (1-2 years after treatment). Spouses only rated the marital questionnaires and the criticism scale on all these occasions.

Results

Several ratings have not been analyzed in the context of this study. On the CFI scale "hostility" was omitted, as almost none of the patients or their spouses scored on this scale. Of the self-ratings on neurotic symptomatology we only used agoraphobic and additional phobic symptomatology.
For the evaluation of agoraphobic symptomatology we mainly relied on the FSS agoraphobia scale as a valid and reliable indicator for the severeness of agoraphobic anxiety as well as of multisymptomatology and other illness behaviors (see

Hand et al. 1986). The items "total phobia," "resistance to phobic anxiety," and "hindrance of daily-life activities by phobic anxiety" were added for additional information.
In the first step of the statistical analysis we used the Pearson correlation, to examine whether any correlations exist between marital factors (CFI, marital self-rating questionnaires) and agoraphobic symptomatology at the pretreatment and follow-up stages. In the second step we applied analysis of varianc (MANOVA) to reveal more specific results regarding the dependence of treatment outcome on marital variables.

Pretreatment Assessments

Correlations Between CFI Ratings and Agoraphobic Anxiety

There is a positive correlation between *patients* criticism toward their spouses and their degree of agoraphobic anxiety, and a negative correlation between *patients'* warmth toward their spouses and agoraphobia. *Patients'* EOI or positive remarks do not correlate with the severeness of agoraphobia. The *spouses'* CFI ratings do not correlate with agoraphobic anxiety on any scale (Table 1).

Correlations Between CFI Ratings and Additional Phobia Measurements

Patients' warmth is positively correlated with behavioral resistance to phobic advoidance and negatively correlated to the hindrance of daily life activities by phobic symptoms, whereas *patients'* criticism is positively correlated with the FSS total phobia score.
There is also a significant correlation between *patients'* EOI and hindrance, and *patients'* positive remarks and behavioral resistance.

Table 1. Pearson correlation (r) between pretreatment agoraphobic anxiety (FSS) and CFI ratings of patients ($n = 24$) and spouses ($n = 23$)

	CFI ratings	
FSS-agoraphobia	Patients	Spouses
Critical comments	0.53**	−0.14
Emotional over-involvement	0.21	0.15
Warmth	−0.56**	−0.06
Positive remarks	−0.31	0.02**

** $P \leqq 0.01$

While *spouses'* CFI ratings are not correlated with the level of agoraphobic anxiety, there is a positive correlation between *spouses'* criticism and patients' behavioral resistance and a negative correlation between *spouses'* positive remarks and patients' hindrance (Tables 2, 3).

Correlations Between Marital Self-Ratings and Agoraphobic Symptomathology

There is no significant correlation between the patients' and the spouses' self-ratings on DAS and MHS and the patients' degree of agoraphobic anxiety. But spouses' ratings on DAS and MHS are negatively correlated with patients' resistance (Table 4).

Follow-up Assessments

Correlations Between CFI Ratings and Agoraphobic Symptomatology

While at pretreatment phobic symptoms are clearly associated with *patients'* criticism, this correlation no longer applies at the follow-up stage. Even more surprising, the strong negative correlation ($r = -0.56$, $p \leqq 0.05$) between *patients'* warmth ratings and their agoraphobic anxiety at the pretreatment stage turned into the opposite at follow-up ($r = 0.37$, $p \leqq 0.05$).

Table 2. Pearson correlation (r) between additional phobia measurements at pretreatment and patients' CFI ratings

	Patients' CFI ratings			
Pretreatment phobia measurements	Critical comments	Emotional overinvolvement	Positive remarks	Warmth
Total phobia (FSS) ($n = 24$)	0.36*	0.28	−0.26	−0.24
Behavioral resistance to phobic symptoms ($n = 19$)	−0.28	−0.03	0.43*	0.47*
Hindrance by phobic symptoms ($n = 19$)	0.38	0.42*	−0.22	−0.39*

* $P \leqq 0.05$

Table 3. Pearson correlation (r) between additional phobia measurements at pretreatment and spouses' CFI ratings

	Spouses' CFI ratings			
Pretreatment phobia measurements	Critical comments	Emotional overinvolvements	Positive remarks	Warmth
Total phobia (FSS) ($n = 23$)	−0.17	0.03	0.03	−0.15
Behavioral resistance to phobic symptoms ($n = 18$)	0.44*	0.03	−0.36	−0.52*
Hindrance by phobic symptoms ($n = 18$)	0.17	−0.21	−0.43*	−0.16

* $P \leqq 0.05$

Table 4. Pearson correlation (r) between agoraphobic symptomatology at pretreatment and self-ratings on marital questionnaires (DAS, MHS)

	Patients' ratings		Spouses' ratings	
Agoraphobic symptomatology at pretreatment	DAS	MHS	DAS	MHS
Agoraphobia	−0.07	0.23	0.07	−0.24
Total phobia (FSS)	0.16	0.08	0.14	−0.36
Behavioral resistance against phobic symptoms	−0.08	0.08	−0.45*	−0.48*
Hindrance by phobic symptoms	−0.24	−0.29	−0.30	−0.15

* $P \leqq 0.05$

There is still no correlation at follow-up between *spouses'* CFI attitude and agoraphobic anxiety, and the significant correlation with additional phobic symptomatology at pretreatment has disappeared at follow-up.

Correlations Between Marital Self-Ratings and Agoraphobic Symptomatology

Like at pretreatment, there is no significant correlation between self-ratings on MHS and agoraphic symptomatology. However at follow-up there were positive correlations between *patients'* as well as *spouses'* ratings on DAS and patients' total phobia ($r = 0.39$, $P \leqq 0.05$; $r = 0.54$, $P \leqq 0.05$). Spouses' ratings on MHS are not included because of too many missing data.

CFI Ratings and Treatment Outcome for Agoraphobic Anxiety

In previous CFI studies, *relatives'* criticism toward the patients was the decisive single predictor for the course of schizophrenic and (neurotic) depressive disorders. Classification into high and low EE was made by a trial and error search for cut-off points of relatives' ratings on criticism, the population being best divided according to the predictive power for relapse in patients. For schizophrenia, the cut-off point was fixed at seven critical comments, for (neurotic) depression at two critical comments. The "high EE" relatives, defined this way, turned out to be a high-risk indicator for relapse in patients.
In this study, we chose a similar approach to identify the cut-off point best suited for prediction of relapse or nonresponse in agoraphobics, using ANOVA and MANOVA for each CFI scale.

Patients' Warmth and Outcome. Patients' warmth towards their spouses turned out to have a significant impact on the treatment outcome. The population was divided into two groups with a cut-off point of four, which at pretreatment stage showed a difference in agoraphobic anxiety. *Patients'* with low warmth ($\leqq 3$) had a higher score for agoraphobic anxiety. At posttreatment, this difference was equalized, and during the follow-up period patients with initial low warmth continued to reduce agoraphobic symptoms, while high warmth patients remained almost at the posttreatment level. Interaction between the groups over time is significant (Table 5).

Patients' Criticism and Outcome. Also, patients' criticism towards spouses turned out to have a significant impact on the treatment outcome. At a cutoff point of 8 the sample was divided into two groups with a significant difference of agorapho-

Table 5. Development of agoraphobic anxiety (FSS) over time: effects of patients' warmth (cut-off point 4)

	Agoraphobia								
Patients' warmth	At pretreatment			At posttreatment			At follow-up		
	$\bar{x}$	SD	n	$\bar{x}$	SD	n	$\bar{x}$	SD	n
0–3	26.2	8.07	18	16.1	5.08	16	10.8	7.45	15
4–5	20.8	4.79	6	15.4	4.39	5	16.8	7.20	6
Group 1 vs 2 (ANOVA)	NS ($P = 0.14$)			NS ($P = 0.80$)			NS ($P = 0.11$)		

Interaction between groups over time (MANOVA): F-test = 3.80; $P \leqq 0.05$; $n = 18$;

bic anxiety at the pretreatment stage. High critical patients scored higher on agoraphobic anxiety with a mean score of almost 30, while low critical patients only scored 22 in the FSS. At the posttreatment stage, high critical patients reached similar anxiety levels as low critical patients. During the follow-up period, high critical patients seemed to continue with symptom reduction. Interaction between groups over time is significant (Table 6).

Spouses' Criticism and Outcome. Although spouses' criticism is not correlated with pretreatment agoraphobic anxiety, it does seem to influence the long-term outcome. Dividing the population with a much lower cut-off point for criticism (2), the mean scores of agoraphobia in both groups are almost identical at pretreatment and posttreatment. But at follow-up, there is a highly significant difference between the two groups. Patients with critical spouses did fare better during the follow-up period in terms of reduction of agoraphobic symptoms. In spite of this result, interaction fails to be significant (Table 7).

Dyadic CFI Patterns and Treatment Outcome for Agoraphobic anxiety

With regard to dyadic CFI patterns, there are two different combinations of variables by which all couples can be classified.

1. Dyads with high criticism levels in patients, in spouses, or in both (high EE dyads). In these

Table 6. Development of agoraphobic anxiety (FSS) over time: effects of patients' criticism (cut-off point 8)

Patients' critical comments	Agoraphobia								
	At pretreatment			At posttreatment			At follow-up		
	$\bar{x}$	SD	*n*	$\bar{x}$	SD	*n*	$\bar{x}$	SD	*n*
0–7	22.0	6.27	15	15.6	4.54	14	13.7	7.52	13
≧ 8	29.7	7.68	9	16.6	5.68	7	10.6	8.16	8
Group 1 vs 2 (ANOVA)	S ($P = 0.01$)			NS ($P = 0.67$)			NS ($P = 0.39$)		

Interaction between groups over time (MANOVA): F-test= 3.77; $P \leqq 0.05$; $n = 18$;

Table 7. Development of agoraphobic anxiety (FSS) over time: effects of spouses' criticism (cut-off point 2)

Spouses' critical comments	Agoraphobia								
	At pretreatment			At posttreatment			At follow-up		
	$\bar{x}$	SD	*n*	$\bar{x}$	SD	*n*	$\bar{x}$	SD	*n*
0–1	24.5	7.93	11	16.2	5.10	10	16.4	6.50	10
≧ 2	25.0	8.09	12	15.0	4.55	10	7.8	6.37	10
Group 1 vs 2 (ANOVA)	NS ($P = 0.89$)			NS ($P = 0.59$)			ss ($P = 0.01$)		

Interaction between groups over time (MANOVA): F-test = 2.46; NS; $n = 18$

couples, there is considerable (open and covered) tension, disharmony, and dissatisfaction with the marital relationship, in some couples having reached a crisis point.
2. Dyads with remarkably high levels of harmony, understanding, and warmth toward each other, and with corresponding low critical and sometimes even no critical attitudes (low EE dyads).

We operationalized these two types of dyads by CFI criticism which showed the best predictive power for treatment non-response. Cut-off points of dyadic CFI are slightly different from those of single CFI, coming close to the mean scores of criticism ratings in patients (x = 6.40) and spouses (x = 3.04) respectively:

a) high EE dyads are defined as CFI critical comments in patients > 6 and/or in spouses > 2, and
b) low EE dyads are defined as CFI critical comments in patients < 7 and in spouses < 3.

Out of 24 couples, 11 ended up in the low EE and 13 in the high EE dyad group.

With regard to the assessment of outcome, we defined two criteria of success:

a) Total symptom reduction of at least 14 points on the FSS agoraphobia scale from the pretreatment to the follow-up stage.
   Following the criterion, we found 8 out of 12 (66%) patients from high EE couples to have a successful outcome whereas the same held true for only three out of nine (33%) patients from the low EE couples. This result failed to be significant (Chi-Square = 2.27).
b) Symptom reduction to or below an FSS agoraphobia score at follow-up, of 10 (within "normal" range).
   We chose this extreme criterion, as even after a reduction of 14 points on the FSS agoraphobia scale, patients may still show rather high levels of agoraphobic anxiety; taking this extreme criterion we got higher differences between groups. Out of 12 patients of the high EE couples eight (66%) could still be rated as having a successful outcome, but only one out of nine (11%) low EE couples (Chi-Quadrat = 8.18, $P \leqq 0.05$) had such a rating.

Analyses of Variance (ANOVA and MANOVA). Comparing both EE dyads by analyses of variance, there seemed to be a slight difference in agoraphobia pretreatment levels, similiar scores at the posttreatment stage, and a significant difference at follow-up. Both groups seemed to make similiar progress during the intervention period, while during the follow-up period only high EE dyads continued to enjoy a reduction in symptoms. Interaction between the groups over time is significant (Table 8).

Table 8. Development of agoraphobic anxiety (FSS) over time: effects of patients' and spouses' combined (dyadic CFI) criticism (patients' cut-off point 7; spouses' cut-off point 3)

Patients' and spouses' critical comments combined	Agoraphobia								
	At pretreatment			At posttreatment			At follow-up		
	$\bar{x}$	SD	*n*	$\bar{x}$	SD	*n*	$\bar{x}$	SD	*n*
Low EE couples	23.2	6.34	11	16.0	5.01	10	16.8	6.78	9
High EE couples	26.2	8.65	13	15.8	4.90	11	9.3	7.00	12
Group 1 vs 2 (ANOVA)	NS (*P* = 0.36)			NS (*P* = 0.93)			s (*P* = 0.02)		

Interaction between groups over time (MANOVA): F-test = 3.45; $P \leqq 0.05$; $n = 18$

Marital Questionnaires and Outcome

There is no significant correlation between patients' and spouses' marital self-ratings (DAS, MHS) and outcome.

Discussion

The CFI has so far mainly been applied for the prediction of relapse in schizophrenic and, more recently, in (neurotic) depressive patients. This study is the first attempt to apply the CFI for the prediction of relapse (or treatment nonresponse) in agoraphobic patients. It is also the first CFI study that gathered not only data about the family members' attitudes toward the patients, but additionally about the patients' attitudes toward the most significant family member - in our sample, the spouse ("dyadic" CFI).

With this extension of the CFI method, and with the additional application of two widely used marital self-rating scales - the DAS and the MHS - we have conducted the first comparative assessment of direct (DAS and MHS) and indirect ("dyadic" CFI) measures of the quality of marital relationships in agoraphobics. Thus, this study is not only an investigation into the applicability of CFI as a predictor of relapse in agoraphobics, but also a contribution to the ongoing research about the measurement and the impact of relationship problems on treatment outcome with exposure in vivo for agoraphobics. In the latter context, to our knowledge this is the first experimental investigation of a problem emphasized as early as a decade ago (Hand et al. 1977): If psychoanalytic and systemic theories about the protective function of agoraphobic symptoms in marriages at risk hold true for at least a certain proportion of agoraphobics, then direct marital self-ratings are bound to show good marriages despite a bad relationship.

In this case, all studies using only direct self-ratings of spouse relationships may have produced results that are difficult to interpret, as the proportion of such couples in the total sample investigated would be unknown.

Several aspects of our results are surprising.

1. On the *direct marital self-rating scales* (DAS, MHS) our results confirm those of most of the previous studies in this area:
   Marital happiness or dissatisfaction at the pretreatment stage does not seem to correlate with the severity of the *agoraphobic anxiety* before treatment (cf. Milton and Hafner 1979; Emmelkamp 1980; Chambless 1985) or at the follow-up stage (cf. Marks 1987; Emmelkamp, this volume). There are only correlations in a few scales of "additional phobia measurements," indicating a slight relationship betwen rather low "dyadic adjustment" and a low level of "marital happiness" (in patients and in spouses) on the one hand and higher phobic symptomatology (in patients) on the other.
2. *Indirect assessment of marital relationship* ("dyadic" CFI) reveals important contrasting results.
   Patients' attitudes toward spouses in particular, show several specific correlations with the patients' agoraphobic symptomatology both before and after treatment. *Patients'* high criticism and, correspondingly, low warmth correlate significantly with:
   - significantly higher agoraphobic symptomatology, at the pretreatment stage, than in patients with opposite ratings (low criticism, high warmth),
   - significantly higher reduction of agoraphobic anxiety during the treatment period.

   Spouses' high criticism correlates with a significant reduction in the patients' symptoms during the follow-up period.
3. CFI results allow the identification of two different types of dyadic relationships (*"dyadic" CFI patterns*):
   a) Couples with high criticism towards each other and with considerable open or hidden tension within their relationships (high EE dyads),
   b) couples with low or no criticism and remarkably high harmony in their relationships

   Patients in high EE dyads show a significantly better treatment outcome than patients in low EE dyads, especially during the follow-up period.

We would like to propose some tentative, preliminary hypotheses from our data. The assumption that "symptoms may cover marriages at risk" appears to be supported, but how could this have affected the outcome? High criticism/low warmth/severely agoraphobic patients may be particularly good candidates for exposure treatment for the following reasons:

1. Pretreatment high criticism of patients toward their spouses may reflect dissatisfaction with their perceived dependence on their spouses and with the lack of outside activities - due to hindrance by phobia in daily-life activities.
2. Expression of high criticism by patients during CFI may have been a first step towards more open communication with their spouses.
3. High criticism in patients who accept behavioral symptom treatment may thus indicate a high motivation for change.
4. Experience of learned anxiety-management skills during exposure training may increase awareness of self-efficacy and thus encourage patients to establish a more general "problem/conflict approach behavior" instead of the previously learned phobic and general avoidance behavior.
5. Increased self-efficacy may: (a) change patients' interactional style with spouses and, (b) increase their independent outside activities. In the first case, this may improve the relationship or it may lead to seperation. In the second case, increased outside activities may reduce suffering from an unsatisfactory marital relationship even when the relationship itself remains unchanged.
6. High criticism with high motivation for change in patients may be the reason for impressive progress especially during the treatment period, whereas changes in relationship may be the reason for progress especially during the follow-up period. Changes in relationship are more likely to occur in couples where spouses also express higher criticism which may be an important precondition for a lasting change in couples' interactional style.

These hypotheses are supported by our clinical impression: four out of 13 high EE couples separated after treatment, whereas one patient in a high EE couple got pregnant; in unchanged marriages, the patients definitely took part in more outside activies.

In contrast, patients from low criticism/high warmth dyads, with lower agoraphobic anxiety, may not have gained as much from exposure treatment for the following reasons:

1. Motivation for change is rather low, as the anxiety level is lower and at the same time the spouses' support of phobic avoidance is greater (i.e., they have adapted better to a housebound life-style).
2. Role compatibility may be higher in these dyads: patients want a very caring, supportive spouse, while husbands are happy with a wife who does not want to exhibit more dependent behavior. A moderate (follow-up anxiety level of FSS $\approx$ 15) agoraphobia is a safeguard for both partners in this kind of relationship.
3. Patient and spouse may both prefer a more housebound life-style, possibly because of general avoidance of stressful life situations (Hand 1988a).

High critical patients may be comparable to discontented agoraphobics (see Hafner 1986) who wish to work outside their home. In 1970, Marks and Herst found that discontented agoraphobics were significantly more phobic than contented (low critical/high warmth) agoraphobics. Contented agoraphobics were happy to remain full-time housewives, but rated their premorbid personality as less sociable, more anxious, and more dependent. Caution in the interpretation of these results is required for several reasons:

- Some methodological problems remain to be solved in CFI research (c.f., Dulz and Hand 1986).
- There was only one interviewer/rater for CFI.
- These results are from a study with HBT solo (without spouses); they might be different when spouses are involved and even more different in therapist-guided group exposure.
- With regard to initial high anxiety, results in this study contradict other studies from our own group (Hand et al. 1986; Fischer et al., Chapter 19).

In spite of all these restrictions, we hope that our results will stimulate further research in an area that seemed to have reached a "dead end," with controversial, inexplicable results. Replications of the comparative applications of direct and indirect measurements of dyadic relationship are particularly warranted.

References

Arzrin N, Naster B, Jones R (1973) Reciprocities counseling: a rapid learning based procedure for marital counceling. Behav Res The 11:365-382

Barlow DH, Mavissakalian M, Hay RH (1980) Couples treatment of agoraphobia: Changes in marital satisfaction. Behav Res Ther 19:245-255

Barlow DH, O'Brien GT, Last CG (1984) Couples treatment of agoraphobia. Behav Ther 15:41-58

Bland K, Hallam RS (1981) Relationship between response to graded exposure and marital satisfaction in agoraphobics. Behav Res Ther 19:335-338

Brown GW, Rutter M (1966) The measurement of family activites and relationships. Hum Relations 19:241-263

Brown GW, Birley JLT, Wing JK (1972) Influence of family life on the course of schizophrenic disorders: a replication. Br J Psychiatry 121:241-258

Buglass D, Clarke J, Henderson AS, Kreitman N (1977) A study of agoraphobic housewives. Psychol Med 7:73-86

Chambless DL (1985) The relationship of severity of agoraphobia to associated psychopathology. Behav Res Ther 23:305-310

Cobb JP, Mathews AM, Childs-Clarke A, Blowers CM (1984) the spouse as co-therapist in the treatment of agoraphobia. Br J Psychiatry 144:282-287

Cohen SD, Monteiro W, Marks IM (1984) Two-year follow-up of agoraphobics after exposure and imipramine. Br J Psychiatry 144:276-287

Dulz B, Hand I (1986) Short-term relapse in young schizophrenics: can it be predicted and affected by family (CFI), patient, and treatment variables? An experimental study. In: Goldstein MJ, Hand I, Hahlweg K (eds) Treatment of schizophrenia. Family assessment and intervention. Springer Verlag, Berlin Heidelberg New York

Emmelkamp PMG (1980) Agoraphobics' interpersonal problems. Their role in the effects of exposure in vivo therapy. Arch Gen Psychiatry 37:1303-1306

Emmelkamp PMG, Kuipers AC (1979) Agoraphobia: a follow-up study four years after treatment. Br J Psychiatry 134:352-355

Everaerd W, Rijken HM, Emmelkamp PMG (1972) A comparison of "flooding" and successive approximation in the treatment of agoraphobia. Behav Res Ther 11:105-117

Fisher LM, Wilson GT (1985) A study of the psychology of agoraphobia. Behav Res Ther 23:97-107

Hafner RJ (1986) Marriage and mental illness: A sex roles perspective. Guilford, New York

Hahlweg K, Nuechterlein KH, Goldstein MJ, Magana A, Doane JA, Snyder KS, Mintz J (1985) Parental expressed emotion attitudes and intrafamilial communication behavior. Conference on "The impact of family research on our understanding of psychopathology." Schloß Ringberg, West Germany, 2-6 Sept 1985

Haley J (1963) Strategies of psychotherapy. Grune and Stratton, New York

Hallam RS, Hafner RJ (1978) Fears of phobic patients: factor analyses of self-report data. Behav Res Ther 16:1-6

Hand I (1988) Verhaltenstherapie als Kurzzeit-Psychotherapie: In: Prax Psychother Psychosom (in press)

Hand I (1988b) Verhaltenstherapie und Psychopharmaka bei chronifizierten Angststörungen. In: Hand I, Wittchen HU (eds) Verhaltenstherapie und Medizin. Springer-Verlag, Berlin Heidelberg New York (in press)

Hand I, Lamontagne Y (1976) The exacerbation of interpersonal problems after rapid phobia-removal. Psychother: Theory Res Pract 13:405-411

Hand I, Zaworka W (1982) An operationalized mulitsymptomatic model of neuroses (OMMON): towards a reintegration of diagnosis and treatment in behavior therapy. Arch Psychol Neurol Scie 232:359-379

Hand I, Lamontagne Y, Marks IM (1974) Group exposure (flooding) in vivo for agoraphobics. Br J Psychiatry 124:588–602

Hand I, Spoehring B, Stanik E (1977) Treatment of obsessions, compulsions and phobias as hidden couple-councelling. In: Boulougouris JC, Rabavilas AD (eds) The treatment of phobic and obsessive-compulsive disorders. Perganon, Oxford

Hand I, Angenendt J, Fischer M, Wilke C (1986) Exposure in vivo with panic management for agoraphobia: treatment ratinale and long-term outcome. In: Hand I, Wittchen HU (eds) Panic and phobias. Empirical evidence of theoretical models and long-term effects of behavioral treatments. Springer Verlag, Berlin Heidelberg New York

Himady WG, Cerny JA, Barlow DH, Cohen S, O'Brien GT (1986) The relationship of marital adjustment to agoraphobia treatment outcome. Behav Res Ther 24:107–115

Hooley JM, Hahlweg K (1986) The marriages and interaction patterns of depressed patients and spouses: comparison of high and low EE dyads. In: Goldstein MJ, Hand I, Hahlweg K (eds) Treatment of schizophrenia. Family assessment and intervention. Springer Verlag, Berlin Heidelberg New York

Hooley JM, Orley J, Teasdale JD (1985) Levels of Expressed Emotion and relapse in depressed patients. Br J Psychiatry

Last CG, Barlow DH, O' Brien GT (1984) Precipitants of agoraphobia: role of stressful life events. Psychol Rep 54:567–570

Lazarus A (1966) Broad spectrum behavior therapy and the treatment of agoraphobia. Behav Res Ther 4:95

Lazarus A (1972) Phobias: broad-spectrum behavioral views. Semin Psychiatry 4:84–90

Marks IM (1971) Phobic disorders four years after treatment. Br J Psychiatry 118:683–688

Mathews AM, Teasdale J, Munby M, Johnston D, Shaw P (1977) A home-based treatment program for agoraphobia. Behav Ther 8:915–924 (A German version appears in Hand I, Wilcke [1988] Platzangst. Springer-Verlag, Berlin Heidelberg New York

McMillan JF, Gold A, Crow TJ, Johnson AC, Johnson EC (1986) Northwich Park Study of first episodes of schizophrenia. Part 4: Expressed Emotion and relapse. Br J Psychiatry 148:133–143

McPherson FM, Brougham L, McLaren S (1980) Maintenance of improvement in agoraphobic patients treated by behavioral methods - a four-year follow-up. Behav Res Ther 8:150–152

Miklowitz DJ (1985) The family and the course of recent onset mania. Conference on "The impact of family research on our understanding of psychopathology", Schloß Ringberg, Westgermany, 2–6 Sept 1985

Milton F, Hafner J (1979) The outcome of behavior therapy for agoraphobia in relation to marital adjustment. Arch Gen Psychiatry 36:807–811

Monteiro W, Marks IM, Ramm E (1985) Marital adjustment and Treatment outcome in agoraphobia. Br J Psychiatry 146:383–390

Munby M, Johnston DW (1980) Agoraphobia: the long-term follow-up of behavioral treatment. Br J Psychiatry 137:418–427

Spanier GB (1976) Measuring dyadic adjustment: new scales for assessing the quality of marriage and similar dyads. J Marr Fam 38:15–28

Vaughn CE, Leff JP (1976) The influence of family and social factors on the course of psychiatric illness. Br J Psychiatry 129:125–137

Vaughn CE, Snyder KS, Freeman W, Jones S, Falloon IRH, Liberman RP (1982) Family factors in schizophrenic relapse: a replication. Schizophr Bull 8:425–426

Vaughn CE, Snyder KS, Freeman W, Jones S, Falloon IRH (1984) Family factors in schizophrenic relapse. Replication in California of British research on Expressed Emotion. Arch Gen Psychiatry 41:1169–1177

Zaworka W, Hand I, Jauernig G, Lünenschloss K (1983) Das Hamburger Zwangsinventar, HZI. Manual und Fragebogen. Belz, Weinheim

Zerssen Dv, Koeller DM (1976) Klinische Selbstbeurteilungsskalen (KSb-S) aus dem Münchner psychiatrischen Informationssystem. Belz, Weinheim

Epilogue

Overview: Towards Integration in Panic and Phobia

I. M. Marks

The broad scope of new work in the field is well represented in this book. Although biological and psychological views seem to diverge, it may be possible to accommodate them within an integrated model. That we will try to build after reviewing salient points in the foregoing chapters.

The book opens with an epidemiological survey of a general population sample in Munich (Wittchen, Chap. 1). Of 1366 white 25- to 65-year-olds interviewed on the Diagnostic Interview Schedule (DIS), 657 were seen again 7 years later; 77 of these had an anxiety disorder. The diagnostic categories used were: agoraphobia, panic disorder, specific (simple) phobia and social phobia, obsessive-compulsive disorder (OCD).

Like the ECA studies in the USA, the Munich community sample had high prevalences (lifetime 14%, 6-month 8%) of anxiety disorders, the commonest being specific and/or social phobia (lifetime 8%, 6-month 4%) and agoraphobia (6%, 4%), panic disorder and OCD being less common (1%–2%). Agoraphobia without panic was common, as was found in the US (Weissman et al. 1985) and Basel (Angst and Dobler-Mikola 1986).

There was considerable overlap within DSM-III diagnostic categories, only one case each of panic and OCD having no other lifetime diagnosis of anxiety disorder. Forty percent of specific and agoraphobics had at least one severe panic. OCD and generalized anxiety disorder (GAD) overlapped 40% with other anxiety disorders. The 6-month comorbidity with anxiety disorders was lower but still high (42% vs. 66% for lifetime prevalence). Lifetime comorbidity with nonanxiety disorders was striking too, especially with depression. Of panic disorder cases, 71% also had affective disorder and 50% substance abuse; of agoraphobics, 65% had depression and 23% substance abuse; of specific phobics, 43% had depression. Depression and substance abuse in most cases began over 10 years after the phobias had appeared, and was far more common than in the general population.

Ages of onset of the disorders were much as in previous work. Specific phobias began often before age 10 and rarely after 30. Few cases of agoraphobia, panic disorder, and OCD began before age 10, most starting at ages 10–40. At the other end, few cases began after age 50, apart from panic disorder. Once begun, few cases were free of anxiety and avoidance for intervals of longer than 6 months, the most frequent course being very chronic and persistent (24 *years* for specific phobia, 19 years for agoraphobia, 10 years for agoraphobia with panic, 6 years for panic disorder, 13 years for OCD). The mean duration of agoraphobia was far longer than that of panic.

The striking role of depression agreed with many other studies (Marks 1987). Psychosocial impairment related highly to both present *and past* comorbid depression and not to duration of disorder. Past and present depression also related strongly to treatment, so much so that depression was practically a tracer for therapy. Of depressed cases, nearly all those of panic disorder and two-thirds of agoraphobics had treatment - usually small doses of medication over a short time.

Multiple diagnoses were associated with more impairment and less favorable outcome 7 years later, especially panic disorder plus depression, and substance abuse together complicated 52% of agoraphobia and panic disorder cases. Agoraphobics with or without panic disorder visited health carers more than did matched controls.

The epidemiological findings are daunting. They remind us how very common chronic anxiety disorders are, that overlap is frequent within the anxiety disorders and of them with depression and substance abuse, and that in the anxiety disorders much of the handicap and desire for treatment is associated with depression. The findings indicate the vast size of the problem these disorders pose for those planning to adequately deliver the effective treatments now available for them. This realization dawning in the late twentieth century parallels the way in which the huge scale of malnutrition and infectious diseases in the general population became apparent in the nineteenth century. It is a great challenge. And we know little about how to prevent anxiety disorders.

A different domain is entered in Chap. 2 (Uhde and Stein). They note that some drugs can reduce panic/anxiety but not how long this reduction is maintained as medication is continued. They hint at the paucity of data about long-term drug-free follow-up, a vital issue in disorders as chronic as agoraphobia with panic (Marks 1987).

Biochemical changes in panic disorder are surveyed. Dexamethasone suppresion test (DST) results are variable. In eight cases, basal adrenocorticotropic hormone (ACTH) was high and ACTH response to corticotropin releasing hormone was blunted as in depression, and basal cortisol was raised. Four out of ten cases had a low thyrotropic hormone response to thyrotropin-releasing hormone (without hyperthyroidism). This was as in depression, as was the blunted growth hormone response to clonidine in a few cases. Substances like lactate, caffeine, isoproterenol, and CO_2 can induce panic, but this is markedly modified by psychological manipulations (Margraf and Ehlers, Chap. 10; van den Hout, Chap. 11; Clark et al. Chap. 13; Hartl and Strian, Chap. 18). Uhde and Stein caution that biological perturbations can be epiphenomena, the product rather than the cause of chronic anxiety, though cognitive variables alone seem unlikely to explain why panics may arise during sleep and why sleep lactate infusions have wakened some patients. The authors point to the interaction of somatic, experiential, psychophysiological, and cognitive variables that may culminate in panic. In normals, an uncontrollable acoustic stress, compared to a controllable one, led to more subjective, neuroendocrine, and autonomic response. Patients who have somatic but not subjective symptoms of panic are less avoidant and seek treatment less.

The interaction of drugs and behavioral treatment is of growing interest. Mavissakalian (Chap. 3) reviewed six controlled studies of imipramine and exposure in agoraphobia. Most found a short-term imipramine effect, one (Mavissakalian and Perel 1985) finding this to be dose-dependent on several measures, though not on panic, where gains seemed due to exposure. There was slight worsening on withdrawal of imipramine, but overall gains were stable to 2-year followup, this being ascribed to self-exposure therapy, which also helped panic. In two studies the best outcome was with imipramine combined with self-exposure; antiexposure instructions virtually vitiated imipramine's benefit (Telch et al. 1985). One study (Marks et al. 1983) found no imipramine effect, improvement again being attributed to self-exposure, not therapist-aided exposure.

That baseline mood does not predict outcome with antidepressants is taken by Mavissakalian and by Uhde and Stein to mean that drug effects, when present, are unrelated to depression. This may be too simple a view, given that phobias, panic, and mood usually improve together (Marks 1987) and that the negative drug study had a sample with normal mood, while most positive drug studies had dysphoric agoraphobic samples. In anxiety disorders depression strongly relates to impairment and to seeking treatment (Wittchen, Chap. 1), which may affect outcome. The link between agoraphobia, panic, and mood is a complex puzzle.

Withdrawal effects on ceasing psychotropic medication are often neglected. This is remedied by Fyer (Chap. 4). Kramer in 1961 reported that on withdrawing from imipramine 56% of patients had nausea and vomiting, headache, giddiness, coryza, and chills. Discontinuation of alprazolam is commonly followed by a rise in panics – in 89% of the patients reported by Dupont. In Fyer's series only 25% were willing to come off alprazolam; 15 out of 17 had recurrence of panic and 9 out of 17 had malaise, insomnia, tachycardia, dizziness, lightheadedness, faitness, confusion, dysphoria, and irritability. (We find at the Maudsley Hospital that the number discontinuing alprazolam partly reflects the firmness of the clinician.)

Further caveats about alprazolam come from the randomized blind study by Klosko et al. (Chap. 5) of panic disorder (avoidance absent: 31% limited: 56%; extensive: 13%) with a problem duration of at least 6 months. Patients had, over 3 1/2 months, alprazolam (6 mg/day), or placebo, or cognitive behavior therapy (CBT), or waiting list placement. CBT included cognitive therapy (education, monitoring of automatic thoughts and self-statements, hypothesis testing, graded homework testing from low to high anxiety), relaxation, and exposure, both to actual external fear cues and to internal fear cues (hyperventilation training, running in place, spinning one's head, catastrophic interpreting), plus homework tasks between sessions. There were 57 completers (cell size 11–16); more patients dropped out of the placebo group than the other groups.

End of treatment outcome was sobering for alprazolam but fairly encouraging for CBT. Due to severity of withdrawal effects only one alprazolam subject was assessed drug-free pointing to dependence as an important drug drawback. Yet the number of patients who became panic-free was not significantly less with alprazolam (50%) than with placebo (36%) or waiting list (33%); in contrast, CBT yielded significantly more panic-free patients (87%) than did waiting list or placebo (though not alprazolam). Furthermore, alprazolam was similar (50%) to placebo (46%) on the number of patients becoming non-clinically severe, differing significantly only from waiting list (20%); on this measure 73% improved with CBT, significantly more than waiting list though not placebo or alprazolam. Not reported yet are the important issues of followup and of side effects other than dependence. That patients improved a bit more on placebo than on the waiting list suggests that a waiting list is a less desirable control for the "nonspecific" effects of therapy.

Consonant with the controlled results of Klosko et al. with CBT are those of Shear et al. (Chap. 6) with uncontrolled CBT in two series of patients with panic disorder. The first was a retrospective report of 11 patients, seven with limited and four with no avoidance. Mean problem duration was 3 years. CBT included education, panic management (slow breathing, relaxation, reframing of panic) with exposure to external cues and to internal cues evoked by exercise and hyperventilation. By the end of treatment 10 out of 11 patients had been free of panic for over 2 weeks and remained so over 3–12 months followup. Patients felt the most helpful aspects of therapy had been their education in the nature of panics and about abdominal breathing.

The second series was prospective in 21 patients (avoidance absent: 3; limited: 14; marked: 4) with a mean problem duration of 7 years. Three (12%) patients had dropped out. CBT was similar to that in the first series; exposure was mainly self-directed, and a weekly diary was kept. Therapy was individual and weekly to a maximum of 24 weeks or until there was no panic and avoidance. By the end of treatment patients had improved significantly on global severity, distress, number of symptoms, intensity of panics, freedom from spontaneous panic (17/21), total phobias, phobic avoidance, Hamilton and Trait Anxiety, and somatization, but not in depression. Follow-up was not reported.

Fyer reported to the Ringberg Conference that CBT abolished lactate-induced panic in five out of six panic disorder patients who had formerly panicked to lactate, even though their physiological changes continued. Similar abolition of lactate-induced panic by exposure therapy was found by Guttmacher and Nelles (1984). Such results indicate that lactate-induced and other panic can respond at least as well to psychological as to drug treatment.

Apart from exposure, the effective components of CBT including anxiety management (AM) await adequate dissection.

Mathews (Chap. 7) reviews three studies which compared AM with a nondirective counselling (NDC) control that gave warmth and empathy but no advice, merely reflecting back questions by rephrasing what clients said or asking them what would be best. The first (Blowers et al. 1988) studied 20 patients with generalized anxiety. It compared AM (relaxation + Beckian cognitive therapy + exposure instructions to test automatic thoughts or irrational beliefs in anxiety-evoking situations), NDC, and a waiting list, in eight individual sessions over 10 weeks. At post-treatment, AM was superior to waiting list but better than NCD only on peripheral measures of belief – a pattern persisting to 6 months follow-up. Overall change was small and less than that found by Butler et al. (1988) but like that of Barlow et al. (1984). The effect of AM was not attributable to relaxation or cognitive therapy.

The second study (Borkovec et al. 1988) used similar treatments in 30 student volunteers with GAD who all had relaxation, half continuing with cognitive therapy and half with NDC, over 12 individual sessions. Cognitive therapy + relaxation was superior to NDC + relaxation at post-treatment but not at follow-up on the 50% of clients who returned the followup questionnaire. Overall change was greater than in the first study.

The third study (Borkovec and Mathews 1988) was of 30 patients with GAD or nonphobic panic disorder. It contrasted cognitive therapy, NDC, and coping desensitization (imagine anxiety-evoking situations, evoke related somatic sensations, relax, practice in real life). All patients also had relaxation. At post-treatment and at 12 months followup, although gains were substantial and similar to those obtained by Butler et al. (1988), the three treatments did not differ, nor did outcome vary, either with the diagnosis of GAD or panic disorder (Mathews is unconvinced of the value of distinguishing between the two labels) or with the predominance of somatic or cognitive symptoms.

Mathews concludes that cognitive therapy is consistently superior to no treatment but not to NDC in clinic patients, and that it does not appear to act specifically on cognitive symptoms. He doubts whether cognitive therapy acts uniquely via verbalizable thought processes. His work raises questions about the value of the "cognitive" component in cognitive behavior therapy.

The long-term superiority of ungraded massed exposure vs. graded massed exposure is noted by Fiegenbaum (Chap. 8) in 127 patients who had DSM-III agoraphobia with panic. Mean problem duration was 11 years. Thirty-two percent of patients were housebound (their therapy began near their home) and 39% nearly so. After 4- to 8-h assessment and being told that avoidance maintained the problem, subjects had 4–8 h of pre-exposure preparation and then had a week or more to decide whether to have Therapy. Post-exposure "self-control" continued over 6–8 weeks (no details given). Therapy was refused by 14% of patients after assessment and 12% during preparation; none dropped out of exposure.

Mean clinician time per patient was 32 h. Of the first 48 subjects, 25 had ungraded and 25 graded massed exposure. The next 79 cases all had ungraded massed exposure. Follow-up ratings were blind regarding type of exposure. Graded exposure was intensive up a hierarchy; no more details are given.

Massed live exposure was like an assault course, over 6–10 days, with a therapist present at first. Subjects could not avoid the exposure targets, reduce exposure duration, or decide the sequence, and were asked to focus on and intensify their panic. Then, for example, on Day 1 patients were driven from home to the treatment center (Marburg) sitting in the rear of a 2-door car, confined in a narrow, dark room for 1–2 h, walked in a strange area for 1–2 h, flew in a sports plane for 3/4 h with 2–3 take-offs and landings, ate in crowded canteens, took a train to Frankfurt (1 h), travelled 3–4 h in the Frankfurt underground without the therapist, and took a 10-h train sleeper to Milan. Arrival in Milan was at 7 a.m. on Day 2. then for 11–12 h subjects had to go on the underground, bus, tram, paths through town, climb the cathedral, go into department stores and a cinema, eat in crowded restaurants, and fly to Munich. They spent the night in a Munich hotel. Day 3 morning exercises were the subway, the Olympic Tower, department stores. Afternoon tasks included a train, rack-railway (40 min in a tunnel), cablecar to the top of the Zugspitze (height 2962 m). Subjects then caught the night train home, followed by further exposure.

Ungraded patients showed *more* stress during training. At the end of treatment and 8-month follow-up ungraded and graded exposure subjects had done equally well. However, at 5-year followup (96% were found), ungraded was markedly superior to graded exposure, 76% vs. 35% being symptom free, 80% vs. 22% completing a stiff behavioral test. Five-year outcome of all massed patients combined was as good as in the first 25 cases. Seventy-five percent of the ungraded but only 13% of the graded subjects said they had learned to "Expose yourself to the situation until anxiety has gone" (a rule learned by most of the patients who completed the behavioral test but not by most who did not). In contrast, 2% of ungraded but 52% of graded subjects had learned "Cope with your anxiety step by step", which might leave room for partial avoidance.

Fiegenbaum's 5-year outcome after ungraded exposure is the greatest so far reported after exposure. Though gains can grow post-treatment, his is the first report of differential effects emerging so late – ungraded subjects improved similarly to graded ones up to 8-month followup but markedly more so by 5 years (no earlier ratings are available to judge when this superiority appeared). Intriguing questions arise. What proportion of all agoraphobics find such heroic ungraded exposure acceptable and feasible economically and practically? Was the mean of 32 h clinician time involved necessary, given recent good results with self-exposure. Were the homework instructions similar after the graded vs. ungraded exposure, including the last 6- to 8-week self-control phase? We have long known that massed is better than spaced exposure (Marks 1987), and Fiegenbaum's results suggest the need to study this further, with special attention to whether long-term outcome is best if sessions end with fear-abolition rather than just fear-reduction.

Another intensive exposure regime, plus more cognitive interventions, was given in the uncontrolled study by Andrews and Moran (Chap. 9) of 50 agoraphobics with panic. Mean problem duration was 8 years. Patients had 80 h of inpatient treatment in groups of six over 2 weeks. This included 40 h of exposure (half therapist-aided and half on their own) and 40 h learning about their illness, how to enter feared places, to breathe slowly during panic (6 h), relax, replace negative anticipations by positive ones, and to restructure irrational thoughts and be assertive (10 h).

After treatment the agoraphobics were markedly improved on phobias, panic, general anxiety, and the behavioral avoidance test, had become less neurotic and less externalized on locus of control, and had stopped medication. Most gains persisted 6 and 12 months later (92% follow-up rate); no patient was retreated during the year of follow-up. Without controls we cannot judge the therapeutic contribution of the various components in the therapy package. Andrews and Moran also review other studies of behavior therapies, finding that they reduced panic in the short and longterm, and little sign of antidepressants alone being lastingly effective.

More fear of fear and of internal bodily (interoceptive) cues is seen in agoraphobia and panic disorder than in GAD or specific phobia, and these fears disappear in agoraphobics after successful treatment (Foa, Chap. 14; Margraf and Ehlers, Chap. 10; van den Hout, Chap. 11; Clark et al., Chap. 13; Hartl and Strian, Chap. 18). We cannot conclude merely from their presence that fear of fear and internal cues cause agoraphobia. Compared with specific phobics, agoraphobics with panic also have more hypochondriacal and blood-injury fears and obsessive-compulsive symptoms (Fava et al. 1988a, b), loss of control, tonic anxiety, and depression (Marks 1969, 1987). We have no good reason to regard any of these as primary. If a particular facet of a protean syndrome were causal it should predate other symptoms[1]; this has not been shown for fear of fear in agoraphobia, nor for misinterpretations of body sensations. Already in 1871 Westphal called agoraphobia the "impossibility of walking through certain streets or squares, or possibility of so doing only with *resultant* dread of anxiety" (italics ours); his idea that fear of streets or squares *results* in fear of fear may be the right one. It accords with the way that fear of fear subsides as agoraphobia remits with prolonged exposure to public places.

Related to the focus on fear of fear is that on panic in DSM-IIIR and DSM-III, a topic reviewed by Margraf and Ehlers (Chap. 10). Clinical samples do not give the whole perspective. In the general population, only a minority of agoraphobics have panics, yet panics are frequent among students. Questionnaires in US students (Norton et al. 1985, 1986) found that 35% had had one or more panics in the past year and 2%–3% at least three in the past 3 weeks; panics were associated with other psychopathology (phobic and state anxiety, depression, fatigue, somatization, and anger/hostility) and with life stress and relatives who had panics. Infrequent panickers had similar panic and other symptoms to those in panic disorder, and responded to imagery and tasks

[1] Even fear of fear appearing first would not be conclusive – a rapid erection on seeing someone attractive is a sign of attraction, not its cause; Zajonc documented hedonic reactions occurring rapidly before cognitive ones.

with similar thoughts, symptoms, and physiology (heart rate, blood pressure, skin conductance, electromyograph).

In two German student samples, Margraf and Ehlers again found frequent panic with similar other symptoms. Information was reliable about panic number and intensity, stress at onset, avoidance, and family history, but was unreliable about unexpected (spontaneous) and social panics and about abruptness of onset. Compared to Norton's students, the questionnaires yielded even more who had had panics in the previous year (52%), and again 2% had had at least three panics over the last 3 weeks. However, only half the students noting panic on a questionnaire met panic criteria in a structured interview (Structured Clinical Interview for DSM-IIIR, SCID); the rest had milder forms of the same phenomenon short of the SCID's more conservative cut-off between panic and nonpanic. Compared to nonpanickers, panickers had more fear of fear, agoraphobic and injury fear, anxiety, depression, and somatization, but not more avoidance, social fear, separation anxiety, aggression, or hostility, and had similar heart rate and blood pressure at baseline and during hyperventilation.

Thus both US and German students often have panic, tonic anxiety, agoraphobic and other fears, depression, and other discomfort like that reported almost 40 years ago (Wheeler et al. 1950). There is no reason to single out panic as *the* feature in the spectrum of symptoms found. Not noted are the *sites* where discomfort begins. Lelliott et al. (1988) found that in panic with or without agoraphobia the first panic had begun outside home in the great majority of cases, mostly in public places. If confirmed, this might suggest that such places are prepotent cues for discomfort.

In panic, body sensations are often the first thing noticed and then continue. While this is often taken to mean that panic is a response to body sensations (van den Hout, Chap. 11; Ehlers et al., Chap. 12), those sensations could equally well be early signs of panic onset, just as an erection can be an early sign of sexual arousal. The sensations during panic are often misinterpreted; such misinterpretations could be the product rather than the cause of panic, though if present they may aggravate panic in a vicious spiral. The same is true for hyperventilation. Still to be controlled for is the level of baseline anxiety, which is higher in agora- than specific phobics. It has yet to be shown that, compared with specific or social phobics (not merely nonphobics), agoraphobics with panic show more body sensations, misinterpretations, and fear of fear during the severe panic induced by live exposure to their feared cues, or that their anticipatory anxiety is greater just before such exposure.

Instructions can reduce responses to lactate and CO_2 challenge in panic disorder. On inhaling CO_2 after either being informed that "normal" symptoms were expected to ensue, or without preparation, social phobics had little anxiety in either condition; compared to their uniformed counterparts, however, informed panic patients had less anxiety, dire thoughts, and similarity of the experience to natural panic. Responses by panic patients to CO_2 inhalations can also habituate on repetition.

Fear of fear and body sensations are returned to by Ehlers et al. (Chap. 12) and Clark et al (chap. 13). Problems with the idea that misinterpretations of body sensations are the cause rather than product of panic were discussed earlier. Some suggest that agoraphobics fear a large variety of situations mainly because of the panic induced by them, given the social or physical consequences of panic in such situations. This seems a bit implausible. Are the consequences of panic in a supermarket or a train really worse than of panic at a dinner party or being heard urinating or on seeing a tiny bird in the street? Such an idea seems imbued with the same "illusory correlation" with harmful consequences that students show to cues of spiders (Mineka and Tomarken 1988). Perhaps prepotency is common to both. This could be tested.

Ehlers et al. point out that positive feedback loops may aggravate panic, e.g., false feedback of tachycardia, and that interrupting such loops can reduce panic - this might be achieved by drug or psychological treatment. Neither biochemical nor cognitive abnormalities specific to a given disorder need be postulated to account for such effects, which might be seen with high anxiety from any cause - threat of examinations, or of attack, loss of job, spouse, or home. The authors point to the wealth of evidence that panic can be reduced by exposure without medication. They also cite cognitive therapy doing the same, cautioning that the mechanism of change remains unclear.

Clinicians have long known that phobics keenly scan their surroundings for phobia-relevant cues, which scanning disappears as they improve with treatment (Marks 1969). Such cognitive distortion is again not special to panic disorder but a wider feature of anxiety in general, as shown by the attentional bias towards threat cues related to their respective disorders found in obsessive-compulsives and in spider phobics. The bias disappeared once subjects lost their fears after exposure therapy, suggesting that the bias was a sign, not the cause, of the fear. Generalized anxiety patients had an attentional bias to social or physical threat; memory bias was not found.

Three papers examine predictors of outcome after exposure, two in agoraphobia and one in OCD (Chaps. 19–21). In German agoraphobics 1–9 years after exposure (Fischer et al., Chap. 19), outcome was worse in patients who had begun with many phobic and nonphobic symptoms. Not predictive were social anxiety, symptom duration, onset age, previous personality, or sociodemographic variables. In US agoraphobics 1 year after exposure (Chambless, Chap. 20), demographic variables were again not predictive of outcome, nor were initial severity of phobia, depression, anxiety and panic, or initial expectancy.

In US - obsessive-compulsive (OCs), outcome 6–14 months after exposure was not predicted by initial depression (which was marked), anxiety, work, social and family impairment, or social skill, social anxiety or social support (Steketee, Chap. 21). Outcome was worse in cases who had *post*-treatment anxiety (the best predictor) or work, social, or family impairment (pre–post change scores were less predictive), including family criticism and rows, which raised anxiety, or distress from life events during follow-up. That family criticism predicted relapse in OCs concurs with similar findings on expressed emotion in schizophrenics and depressives. In an OC whose relatives are hostile, relapse may be less likely if they are trained to become exposure cotherapists without being critical - in the author's experience this training need not take much time.

Marital adjustment and treatment outcome in anxiety disorders is reviewed by Emmelkamp (Chap. 22), whose conclusion largely agree with those of Marks (1987). In comparisons with controls, neither the partners nor the marriages of agoraphobics are disturbed (see also Peter and Hand, Chap. 23). Marital adjustment does not consistently predict outcome of live exposure. Exposure therapy for agoraphobia or OCD is usually effective whether spouse-aided or not. There is no harm in involving the spouse, but pressure to do this is unjustified if time or inclination are lacking, with one caveat; family criticism post-therapy predicts poorer outcome in OCD (Steketee, Chap. 21), so it may be helpful to train critical families how to promote exposure without hostility.

Towards a Synthesis

Some of the competing ideas about the etiology and treatment of panic and fear can be reconciled in an interactive framework including biological and psychosocial factors (Uhde, Chap. 2; Strian and Hartl, Chap. 18; Buller et al., Chap. 15). Adding an ethological dimension too might answer an important question – why is fear of public places associated with many more baseline anxiety symptoms (Marks 1969, 1987; Albus et al. Chap. 16), including fear of fear, misinterpretation of body sensations, and depression, than are specific phobias? Could it be because public places are harder to avoid in daily life than are spiders, heights, flying, thunderstorms, or public speaking, so that agoraphobics trying to continue their daily round more often become frightened? If so, "successful avoiders" like housebound agoraphobics who have given up going out should have less fear of fear and tonic anxiety, a point worth testing. If they do, it would be analogous to what is seen in animals having acquisition and extinction training in conditioned avoidance. During acquisition, fear appears early and subsides as animals become such slick avoiders that they never receive the unconditioned stimulus. During extinction, the conditioned stimulus is presented without the unconditioned stimulus while blocking avoidance; the fear then reappears with abortive avoidance attempts and dies down as the animal habituates to the conditioned stimulus. In contrast, repeated inescapable shock leads to persistent anxiety and helplessness in animals, analogous to the tonic anxiety and moderate depression of agoraphobics who are repeatedly frightended by, escape from, and then avoid, public places without allowing sufficiently long exposure to habituate well to them.

If this analysis is correct, we should also find in spider or snake phobics that presenting their phobic cue often while allowing lengthy escape should raise tonic anxiety and fear of fear that would remit if avoidance either became total or was blocked long enough for habituation to occur (but this test might be unethical). This explanation, that of all phobias agoraphobia is most associated with tonic anxiety, spontaneous panic, and other symptoms because the relevant cues are the hardest to avoid without disrupting daily life, still leaves a central point unexplained – why public places come to be feared in the first place. The same question applies to the origin of most other phobias and obsessive-compulsive worries. Perhaps evolutionary prepotency and preparedness partly explains our tendency to link certain discomforts more to some cues than to others. Agoraphobia could be a morbid form of the extraterritorial fear that many species show when outside their home range. This idea predicts that when in familiar public places, compared to being at home, normal people, especially young women, would

a) be more likely to become anxious when stressed by adverse life events or depression, or by discomforting procedures like hyperventilation or CO_2 inhalation, and
b) more likely to incubate fear and avoidance of those places.

In research of panic/fear a fuller perspective is obtained if we test whether any given feature is:

a) peculiar to a particular anxiety disorder, or found in a whole range of anxiety disorders during intense panic evoked by phobic but not normal threat, or found in such disorders and in intense normal anxiety too;
b) an antecedent or a later complication;
c) the first aspect of a disorder to improve before any other does so.

Such a broad perspective has yet to be achieved for biological features some think are relevant and for features like fear of fear and body sensations and catastrophizing. Until that perspective has been gained it will be hard to judge the contribution of the various etiological mechanisms postulated.

However fear/panic originates, once it has begun positive feedback loops like fear of fear, hyperventilation, and misinterpretations of sensations can develop to worsen the problem. These appear to be modifiable by exposing patients not only to external cues but also to internal ones like body sensations and cognitions associated with fear, along the lines noted by many authors in this book (Klosko et al., Chap. 5; Shear et al., Chap. 6; Andrews and Moran, Chap. 9; van den Hout, Chap. 11; Clark et al., Chap. 13). A matching hypothesis, that fear-reduction is greatest once all the cues habituated to during exposure match all the cues that were feared (centrally represented) when treatment began, could explain why outcome might be better if exposure involves internal as well as external cues, though claims that outcome is enhanced by adding internal to external cues during exposure need further testing. Claims for the value of cognitive manipulations per se (which not only expose to such internal cues but also try to cognitively transform them) require further contrasts with groups in which such cognitive manipulations are omitted while still including internal exposure to autonomic and catastrophizing cues.

One important development that has passed the test of controlled studies is only indirectly represented in this book (see Peter and Hand). That is the advent of self-exposure technology to the point where many phobics, including agoraphobics with panic, and obsessive-compulsives, can successfully treat themselves with the aid of a manual like *Living With Fear* (Marks 1978), without any therapist-aided exposure (Ghosh and Marks 1987; Ghosh et al. 1988; Marks et al. 1988). Another seminal area the book omits is the way some patients have "miracle cures" where very brief exposure induces rapid remission within hours or a couple of days, in contrast to the several days, weeks or couple of months usually required. We could help many patients far more quickly if we knew how to reliably help them attain the states of mind that allow such rapid change. Nevertheless, this book shows well how the field is advancing both in our understanding and in our ability to help sufferers.

References

Angst, Dobler-Mikola (1986) Assoziation und Depression auf syndromaler und diagnostischer Ebene. In: Helmchen H, Linden M, die Differenzierung von Angst und Depression. Springer, Berlin Heidelberg New York

Barlow DH, O'Brien GT, Last CG (1984) Couples treatment of agoraphobia. Behav Ther 15:41–58

Blowers C, Cobb J, Mathews A (1988) Generalised anxiety: a controlled treatment study (in press)

Borkovec T, Mathews A (1988) Treatment of nonphobic anxiety disorders: a comparison of nondirective, cognitive, and coping desensitization therapy (in press)

Borkovec T, Mathews A, Chambers A et al. (1988) Relaxation training with cognitive therapy or nondirective therapy and the role of relaxation-induced anxiety in the treatment of generalized anxiety (in press)

Butler G, Cullington A, Hibbert G et al. (1988) Anxiety management for persistent generalised anxiety (in press)

Fava GA, Kellner R, Zielezny MA (1988a) Hypochondriacal fears and beliefs in agoraphobia. J Affective Disord (in press)

Fava GA, Grandi S, Canestrari R (1988b) Blood-injury phobia and panic disorder: a neglected relationship (in press)

Fava GA, Zielezny M, Luria E, Canestrari R (1988c) Obsessive-compulsive symptoms in agoraphobia: changes with treatment. Psychiatry Res (in Press)

Ghosh A, Marks IM (1987) Self-treatment of agoraphobia by exposure. Behav Ther 18:3–16

Ghosh A, Marks IM, Carr AC (1988) Therapist-patient interaction and outcome to self-exposure: a controlled study. Br J Psychiatry 152:234–248

Guttmacher LB, Nelles C (1984) In vivo desensitization alteration of lactate-induced panic: a case study. Behav Ther 15:369–372
Lelliott P, Marks IM, McNamee G (1988) The onset of panic disorder with agoraphobia (in press)
Marks IM, Lelliott P, Basogulu M et al. (1988) Clomipramine, self-exposure and therapist-aided exposure in obsessive-compulsive ritualisers. Br J Psychiatry (in press)
Marks IM (1969) Fears and phobias. Academic, New York
Marks IM (1978) Living with fear. McGraw-Hill, New York
Marks IM (1987) Fears, phobias and rituals. Oxford University Press, New York
Marks IM, Gray S, Cohen D, Hill R, Mawson D, Ramm E, Stern R (1983) Imipramine and brief therapist-aided exposure in agoraphobics having self-exposure homework. Arch Gen Psychiatry 40:153–162
Mavissakalian M, Perel JM (1985) Imipramine in the treatment of agoraphobia: dose response relationships. Am J Psychiatry 142:1032–1036
Mineka S, Tomarken AJ (1988) The role of cognitive biases in the origins and maintenance of fear and anxiety disorders
Norton GR, Harrison B, Hauch J, Rhodes L (1985) Characteristics of people with infrequent panic attacks. J Abnorm Psychol 94:216–221
Norton GR, Dorward J, Cox B J (1986) Factors associated with panic attacks in nonclinical subjects. Beh Res Ther 17:239–252
Telch M, Agras WS, Taylor CB et al. (1985) Imipramine and behavioral treatment for agoraphobia. Beh Res Ther 23:325–335
Weissman MM, Leaf PS, Blazer DG, Boyd SH, Florio L (1986) The relationship between panic disorder and agoraphobia: an epidemological perspective. Psychopharmacol Bull 26:543–545
Wheeler EO et al. (1950) Neurocirculatory asthenia. 20 year followup study of 173 patients. J Am Med Assoc 142:878–889

Subject Index

MIX
Papier aus verantwortungsvollen Quellen
Paper from responsible sources
FSC® C105338

If you have any concerns about our products,
you can contact us on
ProductSafety@springernature.com

In case Publisher is established outside the EU,
the EU authorized representative is:
Springer Nature Customer Service Center GmbH
Europaplatz 3, 69115 Heidelberg, Germany

Printed by Libri Plureos GmbH
in Hamburg, Germany